Cochlear Implants in Young Deaf Children

COCHLEAR IMPLANTS IN YOUNG DEAF CHILDREN

EDITED BY

ELMER OWENS

AND

DORCAS K. KESSLER

UNIVERSITY OF
CALIFORNIA
SAN FRANCISCO

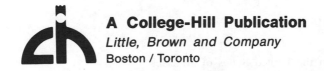

A College-Hill Publication
Little, Brown and Company
Boston / Toronto

College-Hill Press
A Division of
Little, Brown and Company (Inc.)
34 Beacon Street
Boston, Massachusetts 02108

Library of Congress Cataloging in Publication Data
Main entry under title:

Cochlear implants in young deaf children.

    "A College-Hill publication."
    Includes bibliographies and indexes.
    1. Cochlear implants. 2. Children, Deaf —
Rehabilitation.   I. Owens, Elmer. II. Kessler,
Dorcas K., 1942–   .   [DNLM: 1. Cochlear Implant —
in infancy & childhood. 2. Deafness — in infancy &
childhood. 3. Deafness — rehabilitation.
WV 271 C662]
RF305.C6293 1989   617.8'82059   88-13459

ISBN 0-316-67725-6

Printed in the United States of America

C O N T E N T S

P R E F A C E

T his volume evolved from a seminar at the annual convention of the American Speech-Language-Hearing Association (ASHA) in November 1984. Entitled "Cochlear Implants in Young Children: Issues and Alternatives," the question of cochlear implants in children was discussed and debated, and papers concerned with specific aspects of implantation in children were presented. Since that time, the number of children with implants has significantly increased and an alternative multichannel device, unavailable to children in 1984, is now being applied. Accordingly, although many of the original participants at that meeting have been retained, the choice of chapters and authors for inclusion in this volume has altered, and earlier papers have been revised to include state-of-the-art information. However, both the relevance and timeliness of the issues remain unchanged; it was agreed by the editors and contributors that a current work examining these issues would be an important and valuable resource for those involved in the welfare of children who are deaf.

The inspiration for the ASHA seminar was the ever-increasing media coverage of cochlear implantation in young children. For many of those engaged in implant work with adults and aware of the unresolved problems and areas of contention in all facets of cochlear implant research, the coverage seemed exaggerated. The popular press frequently portrayed implants in children as the panacea for childhood deafness — the single technological development that would immediately provide normal hearing and intelligible speech to the small deaf child, eliminating the need for rehabilitation and special services. Recently, with the advent of a multichannel children's implant program, the media has again focused on cochlear implantation in young children.

As popular coverage increases, so does the number of inquiries that must be answered by clinicians. This volume was conceived as a mechanism for bringing information about the implant to a wide range of professionals — mental health clinicians, speech pathologists, audiologists, teachers of the deaf, pediatricians, and otologists — who might increasingly come in contact with implant recipients and the parents of young deaf children seeking information about implants. The primary objective of the book is to provide a forum for the presentation and discussion of the many elements that must be considered in determining whether a particular child should receive an implant: the state of the art in both adults and children; the audiological assessment of very young children; issues relevant to language acquisition, speech perception, and speech production; medical and surgical considerations; and so forth. As the disciplines of the contributing authors each form one of the major areas of consideration in dealing with children who are deaf, it is hoped that the clinician or teacher might acquire a broader under-standing of the complexity of the issues at hand and a greater ability to counsel inquiring parents. At the same time, investigators in various fields associated with deafness and implant work should find this book rewarding, because the authors base their contributions on current research and indicate some directions for continuing studies.

Because of space constraints and the decision to address the broader clinical issues, several areas of implant work have been omitted, including the technical and engineering aspects of implant design, animal studies on the histopathology of electrical stimulation and the biocompatibility of materials, and the physiology of auditory mechanisms.

The issue of cochlear implantation in young children remains both controversial and complex, thus calling for the combined efforts of numerous disciplines to seek solutions to the problems. These efforts constitute a part of the continuing challenge in alleviating one of mankind's oldest, most agonizing, and most stubborn problems — that of childhood deafness. The aims of the editors are the dissemination of information concerning cochlear implants and the consideration of issues that surround their use in young deaf children.

E. O. and D. K. K.

CONTRIBUTORS

GRANT J. BATES, FRCS
  Radcliffe Infirmary,
  Oxford, England

ARTHUR BOOTHROYD, PH.D.
  City University of New York,
  Graduate School,
  New York, New York

SUSAN CURTISS, PH.D.
  University of California,
  Department of Linguistics,
  Los Angeles, California

J. WILLIAM EVANS, M.D.
  University of California,
  Center on Deafness,
  San Francisco, California

THOMAS J. FRIA, PH.D.
  Bricktown, New Jersey

ANN E. GEERS, PH.D.
  Central Institute of the Deaf,
  St. Louis, Missouri

ROBERT K. JACKLER, M.D.
  University of California,
  Department of Otolaryngology,
  San Francisco, California

DORCAS K. KESSLER, M.A.
  University of California,
  Department of Otolaryngology,
  San Francisco, California

GERALD E. LOEB, M.D.
  Queens University,
  Biomedical Engineering Unit,
  Kingston, Ontario, Canada

JEAN S. MOOG, M.S.
  Central Institute of the Deaf
  St. Louis, Missouri

MARY JOE OSBERGER, PH.D.
  Indiana University School of Medicine
  Department of Otolaryngology,
  Riley Hospital for Children,
  Indianapolis, Indiana

ELMER OWENS, PH.D.
  University of California,
  Department of Otolaryngology,
  San Francisco, California

ROSS J. ROESER, PH.D.
  Callier Center for Communication
  Disorders,
  University of Texas at Dallas,
  Dallas, Texas

JON K. SHALLOP, PH.D.
  Denver Ear Institute,
  Denver, Colorado

ROBERT V. SHANNON, PH.D.
  Boys Town National Institute for
  Communication Disorders in Children,
  Omaha, Nebraska

PAULA TALLAL, PH.D.
  University of California at San Diego
  Department of Psychiatry,
  La Jolla, California

WESLEY R. WILSON, PH.D.
  University of Washington,
  Seattle, Washington

ACKNOWLEDGMENTS

The editors would like to thank each of the contributors for their patience, cooperation, and participation in this project. Special thanks are owed to Jennifer L. Yanda for her invaluable assistance in the preparation of the manuscript.

E L M E R O W E N S
D O R C A S K. K E S S L E R

COCHLEAR IMPLANT SYSTEMS, AUTHOR CONTRIBUTIONS, AND TERMINOLOGY: AN OVERVIEW

The number of cochlear implant recipients around the world has increased from probably fewer than 100 in 1977, to a number that, according to some counts (D.J. Mecklenburg, personal communication, 1987), now exceeds 3000. The concept that the auditory system could be stimulated directly by an electric current is an old one, however, having been first demonstrated nearly 200 years ago by Alessandro Volta (1800). This early history has been extensively surveyed by Simmons (1966) and more recently summarized by Luxford and Brackmann (1985). The growing interest in cochlear implants has resulted in the development of a wide variety of implant devices and a proliferation of terms used to describe these systems.

Despite this variation, all cochlear implants operate on the same principle: in sensorineural deafness, although the hair cells are damaged or depleted, some cochlear neurons may remain intact, and these surviving neurons can be stimulated directly — that is, without hair cell involvement — by application of an externally produced electric current. The resultant nerve impulses travel along the auditory pathways to the cortical level and the brain interprets these impulses as sound.

Just as all cochlear implant systems operate on the same principle, they also share the same basic components (Figure 1-1). The sound is received by an external microphone that sends an electrical input to the signal processor. The processor transforms the electrical input into the desired pattern and shape of electrical stimuli. This information is then

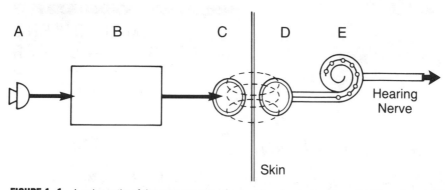

FIGURE 1–1. A schematic of the components of a cochlear implant system: (A) Microphone, (B) Processor, (C) Transmitter, (D) Receiver, and (E) Electrodes. Adapted from Pfingst, B. E. (1986). Stimulation and encoding strategies for cochlear prostheses. *Otolaryngologic Clinics of North America, 19,* 220.

transferred from the processor to the implanted system to excite the cochlear neurons of the auditory nerve. The transfer of information can happen either directly by wires through the skin or, more typically, across the skin by some form of inductive coupling.

For the most part, the use of cochlear implants has been restricted to adults who are post-lingually deafened, a small segment of the deaf population. Since 1980, however, implants have been increasingly applied to children who are deaf. Considering the present status of cochlear implants and implant research, it is probably an understatement to say that opinions differ on the advisability of implants in children. Even among those convinced that implants have already proven themselves, concern remains about how to select the candidates, how to choose the optimum time and the best device, and how to assure that the most efficacious postoperative training procedures will be followed. This volume is offered in the hope that, with the benefit of the work described and the opinions expressed, the reader will feel better informed about the complexity of decisions regarding whether, how, and when to consider a cochlear implant for a given child.

An effort has been made to include information on the major topics most pertinent to these decisions. In focusing on the issues surrounding the cochlear implantation of young children, however, justice could not be given to all of the various areas of implant research. For example, there is no section on the design and fabrication of cochlear implant systems, which have involved the collaboration of many disciplines, including anatomy, audiology, auditory neuroscience, electrophysiology, engineering, histopathology, manufacturing technologies, neuro-otology, psychoacoustics, and speech and hearing sciences. Neither is the contribution of animal studies to cochlear implant knowledge treated in a separate section. The reader is referred to Leake, Kessler, and Merzenich (in press) for a review specifically directed to animal research and to Miller and Pfingst (1984) who included a substantial account of animal studies in their broad overview of cochlear implants.

The contributed chapters are at once independent entities and interwoven pieces constituting the whole. As an independent entity, each chapter provides its own context for the terminology that is used. Not unexpectedly, however, some terms recur throughout the book with slightly different meanings. A threefold approach is taken in the present chapter: (1) a schematic of a cochlear implant is presented with notes on its functioning and the terminology of its component parts; (2) contributions of the authors are briefly introduced; and (3) short discussions are offered on some of the terms and issues that recur from chapter to chapter.

TRANSMISSION OF A SPEECH SIGNAL VIA A COCHLEAR IMPLANT SYSTEM

The notes accompanying the schematic shown in Figure 1–1 are based primarily on detailed descriptions by Fravel (1986) and Pfingst (1986). The *microphone* (*A*), worn externally, receives and transduces the acoustic speech signal into an electrical equivalent (analog). The wearable *processor* (B), also called the stimulator or the encoder, amplifies, compresses, filters, and shapes the electrical signal into the desired pattern of electrical stimuli. Compression is required in order that information in the signal be represented as fully as possible within the narrow dynamic range of hearing for electrical stimulation; filtering and shaping of the signal serve to control the range and weighting of frequencies to be transmitted. A variety of processing or speech coding schemes can be found among available cochlear implants. In some systems, the analog signal, a continuously changing waveform, is processed and transmitted to the electrode(s). In others, the analog waveform is converted into digitized information and stimulation occurs in pulses. A common strategy in multichannel analog systems is a vocoder approach in which a bank of filters splits the incoming signal into a number of frequency bands. The output from each filter determines the electrical signal that will be delivered to each electrode or electrode pair, positioned in different locations of the cochlea. Following the tonotopic arrangement of the cochlea, for example, low frequencies may be directed through one channel to the apical portion of the cochlea, and high frequencies through another channel to the basal portion. A vocoder approach can also be employed with multichannel, pulsatile systems, although generally these systems have used a variety of different schemes to deliver information to specific electrodes or electrode pairs.

In most implant systems, a *transmitter* (C), also called the antenna or outer coil, is used. It is placed on the mastoid for transmission of the processor signal across the skin to an inner coil, typically by some form of magnetic induction. Two modes of transmission from the processor to the implant are in use: percutaneous and transcutaneous. In *percutaneous* systems, transmission is accomplished by a direct connection through the skin via an external plug mounted on the skull. In such instances, of course, the outer coil or transmitter is not needed. The more common method of transmission is a *transcutaneous* system in which a receiver, placed under the skin, is inductively coupled with a wearable transmitter placed outside the skin.

In transcutaneous systems, the *receiver* (D), or internal coil, is surgically placed under the skin on the mastoid to ensure alignment with the removable outer coil. Many presently available systems incorporate magnets in both the internal and outer coils to facilitate their alignment and to hold the external transmitter in place. In percutaneous systems, direct hard-wired connection with the processor precludes the need for an internal receiver. Generally, the internal receiver or electronics package is housed in a hermetically sealed capsule, or *can,* most commonly made of titanium. It is mandatory that all internal wire leads from the receiver be protectively sealed from bodily fluids for the prevention of infection, a particularly challenging task with multichannel systems (see Merzenich, 1985, and Rebscher, 1985, for one solution).

Finally, the stimulus is delivered to the cochlear neurons via the *electrode(s)* (E). Cochlear implants may use either a single electrode or multiple electrodes. It must be clear that the terms *multichannel* and *multielectrode* are not synonomous and, therefore, cannot be used interchangeably. In a *multichannel* system, differently processed information is delivered to different electrodes through separate pathways (channels). By definition, a multichannel implant requires the insertion of multiple active electrodes. Conversely, if the same information is delivered to each electrode of a multielectrode array or if only one electrode is selected for stimulation, that system then functions as a single-channel implant. A *single-channel* system generally implies the insertion of a single electrode to which the signal is delivered through one pathway.

Electrodes may be placed exterior to the cochlea, in which case the implants are referred to as *extracochlear* systems. Usually, extracochlear devices are single-channel with the electrode placed at the round window niche or on the promontory. However, one extracochlear multi-channel device is presently in use (Banfai et al., 1986) and another is under development (Miller et al., 1987). *Intracochlear* stimulation refers to those systems, either single- or multichannel, in which an electrode or electrodes are inserted within the cochlea, usually through the round window into the scala tympani. The greatest variation in implant design occurs within the class of intracochlear, multichannel systems.

Two electrodes, an active and a ground (referent), are required to complete the electrical circuit. In most cochlear implants, either of two configurations of electrodes have generally been used. In *bipolar* stimulation, the active and ground electrodes are close together. In *monopolar* stimulation, the active electrode is distant from the referent; in multi-channel monopolar systems, the active electrodes generally share one common referent. Advantages and disadvantages of the two configurations relate to power requirements, interelectrode interference, and pitch specificity. For example, in monopolar stimulation a relatively broad sector of nerves is excited, whereas bipolar stimulation permits the stimulation of discrete segments of nerve fibers (van den Honert & Stypulkowski, 1987). Regardless of the configuration, nerve stimulation depends upon the relation of the voltage and resistance between electrodes. With multiple electrodes, careful design and attention to the arrangement and spacing between electrode contacts and their relationship to the target neurons is required to prevent interelectrode interactions. The electric field from current supplied by the active and referent electrodes induces a flow of current in the cochlear neurons, initiating a series of action potentials. The action potentials travel along the auditory (VIIIth) nerve to the central auditory system for decoding (central processing) of the signal and, hopefully, the interpretation of meaning inherent in the acoustic speech signal that had initially been received by the microphone.

AUTHOR CONTRIBUTIONS

The wide diversification of the 15 chapters that follow attests to the breadth of the questions surrounding cochlear implantations in young children and the varied professional skills that must be coordinated in addressing these questions. Shannon opens with a review of the psychophysical bases of electrically stimulated hearing in comparison with normal hearing parameters and stresses the importance of central processing by cochlear implant recipients. Owens presents an account of adults who have received cochlear implants, paying special attention to recently published results of multichannel stimulation as they compare with single-channel systems. In describing the behavioral auditory testing protocols for very young children, Wilson demonstrates that reliable, valid estimates of hearing thresholds can be obtained at very early ages. For children with hearing loss and no other disabilities, the earliest age for obtaining these estimates ranges from 6- to 12-months, well before surgery for an implant has typically been contemplated. Fria and Shallop review some of the known aspects of auditory evoked potentials and how they may apply to the diagnosis of children being considered for cochlear implants. They also discuss the application of electrically evoked potentials.

After a careful defining of terms, Boothroyd, establishes ranges of profound hearing loss for consideration of either a hearing aid or a cochlear implant in a child and predicts what the results might be. In either case, he urges a strong program of training that emphasizes the development of auditory/verbal skills. Roeser indicates the desirability of exploring a child's responses to tactile stimulation before cochlear implantation, especially in view of recent encouraging reports regarding the use of tactile stimulation in children and the introduction of easily wearable systems.

Loeb moves directly into the subject of cochlear implants in children, presenting a broad coverage of physiological developmental factors and engineering issues that must be considered in assessing the appropriate age for implantation and the type of implant to be used. He offers strong suggestions for present implant systems and for continuing implant research. Jackler and Bates follow with a comprehensive review of childhood deafness, including etiology, diagnosis, medical management, evaluative procedures with children who are cochlear implant candidates, and a discussion of surgical techniques for implantation as they relate to these young patients.

Approaching the question of the actual performance of children in response to electrical stimulation from an implant, Kessler surveys the status of children who have received either the 3M/House or Nucleus device. Included are observations on rationale, candidate selection, pre- and postoperative evaluations, and results. Geers and Moog are concerned with methods of evaluating speech reception in young children who are deaf and who have limited language and verbal skills. They define and offer validation for four speech perception categories, outline a series of tests in assigning young children who are profoundly deaf to these categories, describe tests for the evaluation of lipreading ability, and apply their test protocol to 12 of the most successful children using the 3M/House implant. Osberger summarizes present knowledge on the speech production abilities of profoundly hearing impaired children with hearing aids and, using a test battery suitable for children with minimal verbal skills, recounts some preliminary findings on these abilities in young children who have received implants.

The importance of central auditory processing skills is emphasized by Tallal, who offers a model for testing the ability to process the temporal aspects of the speech signal; this model might be applicable to young cochlear implant candidates. Curtiss surveys the acquisition of language in young children and, based on research in both spoken and signed language, the concept of a critical period for such acquisition. She extends her discussion to questions on the acquisiton of spoken language with respect to early audition that might be provided by a cochlear implant. In the penultimate chapter, Evans discusses some psychiatric and psychologic issues of cochlear implantation in both young children and teen agers that are crucial to their well being, and, as such, must be carefully considered with each child. In the final chapter, Kessler and Owens summarize the findings and conclusions of the various contributors, identifying the major questions surrounding cochlear implantation in young children that remain unresolved and require further research. Based on these conclusions, they contemplate the future direction of cochlear implantation in young children.

RECURRING TERMINOLOGY AND ISSUES

COCHLEAR NERVE TISSUE

One of the most pervasive comments throughout this book relates to the difficulty of identifying the amount and location of cochlear nerve tissue available for electrical stimulation. It is important to recall that the basic principle governing all cochlear implants is the direct electrical stimulation of the auditory nerve fibers. According to Pfingst and colleagues (1985), a high correlation exists between the presence of nerve tissue and the information that can be transmitted by an electrical signal. Presumably, implants can only be effective to the degree that there is a significant population of surviving cochlear neurons. Generally, radiographic techniques have not been helpful, although Magnetic Resonance Imaging (MRI) has been found useful in grossly determining whether the acoustic nerve is present and, if so, whether degeneration has occurred; improved techniques are anticipated (Balkany, et al., 1987). Histopathological studies have examined the number of surviving ganglion cells resulting from particular pathologies, but results have been contradictory. On the one hand, Otte, Schuknecht, and Kerr (1978) reported some general trends in the numbers of surviving spiral ganglion cells (cochlear neurons) with respect to differences in etiology. On the other hand, in more recent studies little or no relationship between etiology of hearing loss and the presence of neurons has been found (Hinojosa, Blough, & Mhoon, 1987; Hinojosa & Marion, 1983). Clinically, positive correlations between poor performance (presumably from minimal neuron survival) and specific pathologies have not been observed (Berliner, 1985; Schindler et al., 1986).

The primary method used in attempting to estimate the survival of auditory neurons and predict postoperative performance has been the preoperative electrical stimulation of the cochlea via the promontory or the round window. These investigations have taken two directions: electrophysiological and psychophysical. In the electrophysiological approach, electrically evoked auditory brainstem response (EABR) has been attempted, but has shown no consistent promise in verifying the presence and location of nerve tissue. Wave morphology of the EABR is highly similar to that of the conventional ABR, as demonstrated by Stypulkowski, van der Honert, and Kvistad (1986) in their EABR recordings of 44 implant subjects, except that Wave I, which is generated by auditory nerve activity and therefore would be helpful in assessing the status of cochlear neurons, is typically absent as the result of stimulus artifact (see Chapter 5 for further discussion on EABR). Concerning the psychophysical approach, preimplant promontory testing is no longer used at the House Ear Institute because of its unpredictability (House & Berliner, 1986). On the other hand, Shannon (Chapter 2) suggests some hope for eventual preoperative psychophysical measures using complex nonverbal stimuli, the responses to which can be compared with postimplant speech recognition measures, and the Nucleus and Vienna groups, among others, have continued to require promontory testing as part of the patient selection protocol. Most recently, Skinner and colleagues (in preparation) reviewed the difficulties thus far encountered in this approach and provided a strong rationale for the necessity of a reliable predictive estimate of neuron survival. These investigators compared preoperative electrical measurements using the Nucleus Promontory Stimulator with postimplant speech perception and lipreading scores in 5 postlingually deaf patients. Preoperative measurements included pitch discrimination, detection of a silent interval (gap) between two stimuli, and the ability to hear a stimulus over time with no appreciable decrement in loudness. Performance results in pitch discrimination, gap detection, and loudness adaptation were associated with improved postimplant ability in word recognition by sound alone and in lipreading. Of especial interest, in light of an earlier report of Hochmair–Desoyer, Hochmair, and Stiglbrunner (1985) and the comments of Shannon (Chapter 2), was the finding that mean gap detection threshold, particularly at a soft presentation level, seemed a good indicator of postimplant speech perception; that is, the shorter the gap detection threshold, the better the postoperative speech perception.

Miller and Pfingst (1984) suggested that appropriate tests for directly estimating the numbers and locations of surviving neural elements may evolve from studies of animals in which neural elements along the cochlea are systematically damaged to various degrees. Response to stimuli at various sites where the percentage of neural survival (or depletion) is known would then be compared with responses to middle ear stimulation at various sites.

PRELINGUAL VERSUS POSTLINGUAL HEARING LOSS

The terms *prelingual* and *postlingual* with respect to deafness seem to elude definition. The importance of definition hinges on the assumption that children who have learned speech and language with an intact auditory system before experiencing deafness have a better prognosis with an implant than those who lost their hearing before the acquisition of speech and language or those whose deafness was present at birth. As noted in several recent reports (Eisenberg et al.,1986; Mecklenburg, 1987; Northern et al., 1986), the problem of definition seems more prominent regarding *prelingual.* While it seems safe to say that a normally developed child who suffers a loss of hearing at 7 or 8 years of age has a postlingual loss, much uncertainty is involved when a child is labelled prelingual. For example, an 18-month-old with a vocabulary of 20 or 30 words, a 2-year-old using 2-word sentences, or a 4-year-old who uses most phonemes correctly in speech that is understandable, but who has not yet mastered complex syntax, may all be prelingual or postlingual depending on one's viewpoint.

The status of a child skilled in the language of sign raises another question. It is not known whether a child with an intact language base in sign, say at age 3 or 4 years, would be advantaged by an implant compared with a child much delayed in language acquisition, other things being equal whether by sign or otherwise.

In some texts, the terms *congenital* and *acquired* hearing loss are preferred (Northern et al., 1986). Congenital is used to define hearing loss present at birth, and acquired to define hearing impairment due to any postnatal etiology. Thus the term acquired is used broadly in referring to any loss that is not congenital; that is, it does not address the issue of a child's receiving an implant at a certain age to accommodate a presumed critical period for learning language. Although the term *adventitious* is seldom seen in association with implant subjects, it also refers broadly to hearing impairment acquired after birth and similarly fails to address the prelingual definitional problem. It remains to be seen whether the newer term *perilingual* — between prelingual and postlingual — will be helpful. In the meantime, emphasis must be placed on clear descriptions of language and speech levels in young implant candidates.

PROSODY

The term *prosody* is frequently used in discussing cochlear implant patient performance, although it is seldom defined. In speech acoustics, it is subject to various descriptions. It seems generally agreed that the prosodic features of speech extend over more than one phoneme segment and refer to the rhythmic and intonational patterns of speech (Moore, 1985; Pickett, 1980). Because the prosodic features extend over more than one phonetic segment, they are also called the suprasegmental features. The terms *rate, melody,* and *inflection* are commonly used in association with descriptions of speech prosody. The terms *pitch* and *intensity* might be subsumed under *intonation,* whereas *duration, stress, timing,* and *temporal cues* are aspects of *rhythm.* At the same time, *duration* and *intensity* are components of *stress.* Confusion arises because many of the terms are used interchangeably and because ability in the identification of prosodic elements is often measured not with running speech but with individual words.

In short, a multitude of terms, frequently interchangeable, can be used in referring to prosody. For ongoing speech, perhaps one satisfactory combination of terms would include intonation, stress, and pausal junctures (see Levitt, McGarr, & Geffner, 1987): intonation would be in the sense of rising-falling pitch; stress in the sense of intensity and duration differences among syllable strings; and pausal junctures in the sense that location and duration of pauses would relate to rhythm.

OPEN-SET AND CLOSED-SET TEST FORMATS

In discussing patient performance and the evaluation materials used with implant subjects, test items are frequently identified as either *open-set* or *closed-set.* Open-set is generally taken to mean that the test (target) stimulus is one of a large number of stimuli unknown to the patient, so that guessing becomes negligible; closed-set means that the target is one of a fairly small number of choices, usually four or five, which are clearly specified and shown to the patient, thus permitting guessing. Open-set materials are generally considered more difficult than closed-set items. The objective of most implant projects is to provide a device that affords open-set speech recognition; that is, the ability of the patient to achieve auditory speech understanding with hearing alone is considered the ultimate measure of implant success.

Although this distinction between terms is useful, the dichotomy is not perfect. For example, familiar spondee words presented randomly without a list of specific alternative choices for the patient to see may nevertheless function as a closed-set, because there are a relatively small number of such words in the language, thereby permitting a guessing effect. In addition, the same words may have been repeatedly administered to the patient in any number of audiologic evaluations, perhaps with inadvertent feedback as to the correct responses. Thus, familiarity with the items interacts with the distinction between closed- and open-set. On the other hand, if a monosyllabic word target is one of 15 or 20 choices shown to the patient in a closed-set, the guessing factor would be so low that the item might function more in the manner of an open-set.

TRACKING

The term *tracking* presents relatively few problems, but its occurrence in several chapters indicates the desirability of describing the procedure in this section. The clinician presents segments (phrases, clauses, sentences) of material from a prepared text and the task of the patient is to repeat the segment verbatim. If the patient fails to repeat a segment correctly, the clinician repeats the segment or works in other ways with the patient toward a correct repetition. Only after a verbatim response can the clinician proceed to the next segment. A tracking score is given in terms of the number of words per minute (wpm) repeated correctly.

Tracking serves as either an evaluative or rehabilitative measure, primarily for lipreading but also for audition. Using live-voice presentation, the clinician and patient (talker and receiver) typically sit face to face at a distance permitting easy visibility of the talker's lips and a comfortable loudness of the talker's voice as the receiver watches and listens. In cochlear implant evaluations, attention is focused on the enhancement of lipreading with auditory stimulation. Thus, tracking is administered in at least two conditions: vision alone (device off) and vision plus auditory (device on). In some instances, the patient's ability to do auditory-only tracking (without assistance from lipreading) is also tested. The difficulty of tracking can be affected by variables such as the textual materials (Hochberg, Rosen, & Ball, 1987), the "lipreadability" of the talker (some individuals seem naturally easier to lipread than others), and the motivation of the receiver. Two approaches to tracking have been described in DeFilippo and Scott (1978) and in Owens and Raggio (1987).

TERMINOLOGY FOR PROFOUND HEARING LOSS

Although the application of implants is generally restricted to those with profound or total hearing loss, the terminology is not correspondingly restricted. The terms *deaf, deafened, profound deafness, profound impairment, profound hearing loss, profoundly impaired, profoundly deaf, profoundly deafened,* and *totally deaf,* are used interchangeably in the literature and in this book.

Boothroyd (Chapter 6) specifically differentiates between *impairment* as any disorder of hearing and *loss* as a subnormal ability in detecting sound, defined in specified units. He further defines *profound* as referring to a hearing loss greater than 90 dB HL and *total* as referring to losses in which there is no residual hearing within the limits of 110 dB HL. Fairly good agreement among writers is found for the latter two definitions. Adherence to Boothroyd's few suggestions might help reduce the number of terms used interchangeably. Perhaps the use of *deaf* with congenital or prelingual loss, and the use of *deafened* with postlingual loss might add further clarity.

The recurring issues and terms in this section are only a few that appear throughout the following chapters. Unfortunately, definitions that have been agreed upon by all implant investigators and to which all of the contributors can adhere are not available. Therefore, each chapter defines its own terms and must be read with that particular author's usage in mind.

Terminology is perhaps among the least controversial of the issues calling for clarification in cochlear implant work. The various chapters in this book also attest to the great diversity in implant design, patient selection criteria, pre- and postoperative evaluation procedures and materials, rehabilitation methods, and reporting format. The concept of a conference or meeting at which implant workers from around the globe would gather for the purpose of defining terms and establishing uniform and standardized testing procedures is an appealing one. Realistically, however, the terminology and the pre- and postimplant evaluation protocols relating to cochlear implants will probably have to work themselves out gradually over time.

REFERENCES

Balkany, T., Dreisbach, J., Cohen, N., Martinez, S., & Valvassori, G. (1987). Workshop: Surgical anatomy and radiographic imaging of cochlear implant surgery. *American Journal of Otology, 8,* 195–200.

Banfai, P., Karczag, A., Kubik, S., Luers, P., & Surth, W. (1986). Extracochlear sixteen-channel electrode system. *Otolaryngologic Clinics of North America, 19,* 371–408.

Berliner, K. I. (1985). Selection of cochlear implant patients. In R. A. Schindler & M. M. Merzenich (Eds.), *Cochlear implants* (pp. 395–402). New York: Raven Press.

DeFilippo, C. L., & Scott, B. L. (1978). A method for training and evaluating the reception of ongoing speech. *Journal of the Acoustical Society of America, 63,* 1186–1192.

Eisenberg, L. S., Kirk, K. I., Thielemeir, M. A., Luxford, W. M., & Cunningham, J. K. (1986). Cochlear implants in children: Speech production and auditory discrimination. *Otolaryngologic Clinics of North America, 19,* 409–421.

Fravel, R. P. (1986). Cochlear implant electronics made simple. *Otolaryngologic Clinics of North America, 19,* xi–xxii.

Hinojosa, R., Blough, R. R., & Mhoon, E. E. (1987). Profound sensorineural deafness: A histopathologic study. *Annals of Otology, Rhinology and Laryngology, 96* (Suppl. 128), 43–46.

Hinojosa, R., & Marion, M. (1983). Histopathology of profound sensorineural deafness. In C. W. Parkins & S. W. Anderson (Eds.), Cochlear prostheses: An international symposium. *Annals of the New York Academy of Sciences, 405,* 459–483.

Hochberg, I., Rosen, S., & Ball, V. (1987). Effect of text complexity upon connected discourse tracking. *Annals of Otology, Rhinology and Laryngology, 96* (Suppl. 128), 82–83.

Hochmair-Desoyer, I. J., Hochmair, E. S., & Stiglbrunner, H. K. (1985). Psychoacoustic temporal processing and speech understanding in cochlear implant patients. In R. A. Schindler & M. M. Merzenich (Eds.), *Cochlear implants* (pp. 291–304). New York: Raven Press.

House, W. F., & Berliner, K. I. (1986). Safety and efficacy of the House/3M cochlear implant in profoundly deaf adults. *Otolaryngologic Clinics of North America, 19,* 275–286.

Leake, P. A., Kessler, D. K., & Merzenich, M. M. (in press). Application and safety of auditory prostheses. In W. F. Agnew & D. B. McCreery (Eds.), *Neural prostheses: Fundamental studies.* New Jersey: Prentice-Hall.

Levitt, H., McGarr, N., & Geffner, D. (Eds.) (1987). Development of language and communication skills in hearing impaired children. *ASHA Monographs, 26,* 5.

Luxford, W. M., & Brackmann, D. E. (1985). The history of cochlear implants. In R. F. Gray (Ed.), *Cochlear implants* (pp. 1–26). San Diego, CA: College-Hill Press.

Mecklenburg, D. J. (1987). The Nucleus children's program. *American Journal of Otology, 8,* 436–442.

Merzenich, M. M. (1985). UCSF cochlear implant device. In R. A. Schindler & M. M. Merzenich (Eds.), *Cochlear implants* (pp. 121–129). New York: Raven Press.

Miller, J. M., & Pfingst, B. E. (1984). Cochlear implants. In C. I. Berlin (Ed.), *Hearing science: Recent advances* (pp. 309–399). San Diego, CA: College-Hill Press.

Miller, J. M., Pfingst, B. E., Tjellstrom, A., Albrektsson, T., Thompson, P., & Kemink, J. L. (1987). Titanium implants in the otic capsule: Development of a new multichannel extracochlear implant. *American Journal of Otology, 8,* 230–233.

Moore, B. C. J. (1985). Speech coding for cochlear implants. In R. F. Gray (Ed.), *Cochlear implants* (pp. 163–179). San Diego, CA: College-Hill Press.

Northern, J. L., Black, F. O., Brimacombe, J. A., Cohen, N. L., Eisenberg, L. S., Kuprenas, S. V., Martinez, S. A., & Mischke, R. E. (1986). Selection of children for cochlear implantation. *Seminars in Hearing, 7,* 341–347.

Otte, J., Schuknecht, H. F., & Kerr, A. G. (1978). Ganglion cell populations in normal and pathological human cochlae. Implications for cochlear implantation. *Laryngoscope, 88,* 1231–1246.

Owens, E., & Raggio, M. (1987). The UCSF tracking procedure for evaluation and training of speech reception by hearing-impaired adults. *Journal of Speech and Hearing Disorders, 52,* 120–128.

Pfingst, B. E. (1986). Stimulation and encoding strategies for cochlear prostheses. *Otolaryngologic Clinics of North America, 19,* 219–236.

Pfingst, B. E., Glass, I., Spelman, F. A., & Sutton, D. (1985). Psychophysical studies of cochlear implants in monkeys: Clinical observations. In R. A. Schindler & M. M. Merzenich (Eds.), *Cochlear implants* (pp. 305–321). New York: Raven Press.

Pickett, J. M. (1980). *The sounds of speech communication: A primer of acoustic phonetics and speech perception.* Baltimore, MD: University Park Press.

Rebscher, S. J. (1985). Cochlear implant design and construction. In R. F. Gray (Ed.), *Cochlear implants* (pp. 74–123). San Diego, CA: College-Hill Press.

Schindler, R. A., Kessler, D. K., Rebscher, S. J., Yanda, J. L., & Jackler, R. K. (1986). The UCSF/Storz multichannel cochlear implant: Patient results. *Laryngoscope, 96,* 597–603.

Simmons, F. B. (1966). Electrical stimulation of the auditory nerve in man. *Archives of Otolaryngology, 84,* 24–76.

Skinner, M. W., Smith, P. G., Holden, T. A., Binzer, S. M., Leonetti, J. P., & Poler, S. M. (in preparation). Preoperative electrical stimulation of the cochlea with the Nucleus Promontory Stimulator.

Stypulkowski, P. H., van den Honert, C., & Kvistad, S. D. (1986). Electrophysiologic evaluation of the cochlear implant patient. *Otolaryngologic Clinics of North America, 19,* 249–257.

van den Honert, C., & Stypulkowski, P. H. (1987). Single fiber mapping of spatial excitation patterns in the electrically stimulated auditory nerve. *Hearing Research, 29,* 195–206.

Volta, A. (1800). On the electricity excited by mere contact of conducting substances of different kinds. *Transactions of the Royal Society of Philosophy, 90,* 403–431.

R O B E R T   V.   S H A N N O N

THE PSYCHOPHYSICS OF COCHLEAR IMPLANT STIMULATION

Psychophysical testing establishes a quantitative relationship between a physical sensory stimulus and an experienced sensation. Some psychophysical results can be interpreted in terms of underlying physiological mechanisms. For example, classical acoustic masking patterns are probably closely related to the traveling wave pattern on the basilar membrane (Wegel & Lane, 1924). Some simple auditory perceptions, such as threshold and loudness, depend primarily on the pattern of activity produced in the peripheral auditory nerve. Others, such as pitch perception and speech recognition, depend on complex processing of the peripheral information by the more central stages of the auditory nervous system.

When a cochlear implant activates the peripheral auditory nerve directly by electrical currents, the resultant pattern of nerve activity is quite distinct from the normal pattern of activity produced by acoustic stimulation. The perceptual importance of the differences between electrical and acoustical stimulation must be assessed. In order to accomplish this, those aspects of auditory perception that are dependent on peripheral activity patterns and those that are due to central transformations of the peripheral patterns must be determined. In postlingually deafened adults, it appears that the central processing stages of their auditory systems are relatively intact (Born & Rubel, 1985; Hinojosa & Marion, 1983), although their cochleas do not function. Therefore, it can be assumed that many of the differences in auditory perception demonstrated by postlingually deafened implant subjects are due to differences in peripheral neural patterns resulting from electrical stimulation.

In this chapter, the known psychophysical capabilities of adults with cochlear prostheses are summarized. Percepts that are quantitatively and qualitatively similar for both electrical and acoustical stimulation are distinguished from those that are not. From these results, inferences can be drawn regarding auditory percepts that are determined by the peripheral neural pattern and auditory percepts that require additional central processing. The implications of these findings for speech recognition and for implanting children are discussed.

COCHLEAR IMPLANT PSYCHOPHYSICS

The physical and physiological differences between acoustic and electrical activation of the auditory nerve cause differing perceptions. The following discussion compares the basic psychophysical measurements of dynamic range, intensity resolution, frequency resolution, pitch perception, and temporal resolution between normal hearing subjects and cochlear implant patients.

DYNAMIC RANGE

The dynamic range is defined as the usable range of sounds between absolute threshold and uncomfortable loudness. The dynamic range is much smaller with direct electrical stimulation of the auditory nerve than with acoustic stimulation. Electrically, the dynamic range is only 5 to 20 dB, whereas acoustically it is greater than 120 dB (Eddington et al., 1978; Hochmair-Desoyer & Hochmair, 1980; Pfingst & Sutton, 1983; Shannon, 1983a; Simmons, 1966). Furthermore, the electrical dynamic range, unlike the acoustical, varies as a function of the stimulating waveform. For brief (100 μsec) pulses, the electrical dynamic range is less than 5 dB; for low frequency sinusoidal stimuli or long (4 msec) pulses, it can be as large as 40 dB (Shannon 1983a; 1985a). Speech processing for cochlear implants requires compression of the auditory intensity range to accommodate the narrowed dynamic range of electrical stimulation. For maximum effectiveness and efficiency, this compression must be dependent upon the stimulating waveform.

INTENSITY RESOLUTION

Within the dynamic range, one psychophysical measure of the intensity resolution of the auditory system is the ability to discriminate small changes in intensity. Cochlear implant patients can detect a change in stimulus intensity of less than 1 dB (Muller, 1981; Shannon, 1983a), which corresponds closely to the performance of normal hearing subjects with acoustic stimulation. Nevertheless, because the electrical dynamic range is so small, implant patients can only discriminate 15 to 30 different levels of intensity, compared with over 100 levels discriminated by normal hearing listeners.

Frequency Resolution

One of the hallmarks of the normal auditory system is its exquisite frequency selectivity. The cochlea performs a type of spectral analysis with different frequencies producing maximum excitation at different locations along the basilar membrane. This frequency resolving mechanism is not present in the nonfunctioning cochleas of implanted patients. With implant stimulation, the electrical field from the electrodes spreads widely to activate a broad region of neurons (van den Honert & Stypulkowski, 1987). The extent of this electrical field is determined by the amplitude of the electrical stimulus, not by its frequency. Masking experiments with implanted patients have shown that there is no frequency selectivity for electrical stimulation in that a masker produces the same effect regardless of the frequency of the signal (Shannon, 1983a). It is important to emphasize that the electric analog of acoustic frequency is electrode position not electrical frequency.

Pitch Perception

In normal hearing listeners, pitch is closely related to the frequency of a sinusoidal stimulus and relatively independent of intensity. In implanted patients, changes in pitch with electrical frequency occur only up to about 300 Hz (Eddington et al., 1978; Muller, 1981; Shannon, 1983a; Simmons, 1966). All frequencies above 300 Hz, when balanced for loudness, have the same pitch. That pitch, however, may be much higher than what a normal hearing observer would hear at 300 Hz. The perceived pitch of an electrical stimulus is also influenced by the position of the electrode in the cochlea (Eddington et al., 1978; Tong et al., 1982). Stimulation of an electrode in the base of the cochlea results in a higher pitch sensation than stimulation of a more apical electrode. Thus, the multielectrode arrays of multichannel implants attempt to use varied electrode locations to achieve differing pitch sensations.

A complicating factor in electrical stimulation is that pitch can change dramatically with intensity (Shannon, 1983a; Townsend et al.,

1987). In some implanted patients, the pitch sensation of a single-frequency stimulus can change over several octaves as the intensity is increased.

TEMPORAL RESOLUTION

Temporal resolution is measured by several methods: gap detection, temporal integration, forward masking, and modulation detection.

GAP DETECTION. Gap detection measures the ability of listeners to detect a short gap in the middle of an ongoing stimulus. In normal hearing listeners, gap detection performance depends strongly on the intensity of the sounds surrounding the gap, decreasing from 30 msec or more near threshold to 2 to 3 msec for loud sounds. Some implant patients are able to detect gaps of 1 msec or less in a loud stimulus. Generally, implant patients can detect the same or smaller gaps than normal hearing listeners, when compared at equivalent loudness levels (Shannon, 1986).

TEMPORAL INTEGRATION. Temporal integration measures the time interval over which listeners integrate (or sum) stimulus energy. Thresholds are measured as a function of stimulus duration. For short durations, there is a trade-off between stimulus duration and intensity: the shorter the stimulus, the higher its intensity must be to maintain it at threshold. Normal hearing listeners need a constant amount of energy to detect a signal, with trade-offs between burst duration and signal power occurring for durations under 200 msec. In contrast, almost no temporal integration is observed with implanted patients — threshold changes little over a range of stimulus durations of 1 msec to 1000 msec (Shannon, 1986).

This difference is understandable in terms of a model of temporal integration developed by Zwislocki (1969). He proposed that the slope of the integration function should depend on the loudness growth function of the listener. Indeed, flatter integration functions are observed in impaired ears that have steep loudness growth functions (loudness recruitment). Because implant patients have dynamic ranges of only a few dB and steep loudness growth functions, a very flat temporal integration function is expected. According to the predictions of this model, temporal integration can also be described as appearing normal for both impaired ears and implant patients when the data are plotted in terms of loudness units.

FORWARD MASKING. Forward masking measures the recovery of sensitivity to a signal following the offset of a preceding sound (masker). In normal hearing listeners, the signal threshold recovers monotonically and completely by 300 msec after the offset of the masker. When plotted in the same coordinates, forward masking in implanted patients appears very different. Signal thresholds show little or no recovery for 20 to 50 msec after the masker offset and then recover slowly; measurable forward masking continues 500 msec after masker offset (Muller, 1981; Shannon, 1983a, 1986). However, when the implant forward masking data are plotted with an intensity scale that is more closely related to loudness, the curves look very similar to those of normal hearing subjects (Shannon, 1986). As with gap detection and temporal integration, then, temporal recovery appears to be relatively normal if plotted in loudness units.

MODULATION DETECTION. Modulation detection measures the ability to detect sinusoidal amplitude fluctuations in a stimulus. Normal hearers are quite sensitive in detecting slow fluctuations, but their performance deteriorates when the fluctuations are increased above 50 to 60 Hz (Viemeister, 1979). Implant patients can detect as small or smaller amplitude fluctuations than normal listeners at low fluctuation rates, and their performance does not decrease until the fluctuation rate exceeds 100 Hz.

SINGLE VERSUS MULTICHANNEL IMPLANTS

Some implants use multiple electrodes to take advantage of the tonotopic organization of the cochlea and to provide differently processed information to electrodes at different cochlear locations. Psychophysical experiments have shown little or no difference between measures from a single-electrode device or the individual electrodes of multielectrode devices. Most of the psychophysical results discussed here are not affected by the cochlear position of the stimulating electrodes (apical or basal), or by the distribution of the current in the cochlea (monopolar, bipolar, or distributed ground electrode configurations). The only psychophysical differences observed between single- and multichannel stimulation are the following: thresholds are higher for bipolar stimulation (localized current field) than for monopolar stimulation (broad current field), and perceived pitch changes as a function of the cochlear position of the electrodes with multiple electrode arrays.

IMPLICATIONS FOR SPEECH PERFORMANCE

Unfortunately, little or no correlation exists between the results of most psychophysical tests and speech recognition in the same patients (Tyler et al., 1982). Implant patients with identical psychophysical performance can have vastly different levels of speech recognition ability (Shannon, 1983a). Measures of the spread of current between electrodes or electrode pairs, that is, channel interaction (Shannon, 1983b, 1985b) may correlate with patients' speech recognition abilities, although data are insufficient for conclusive statements. Most psychophysical results are similar across devices and unaffected by electrode position, electrode configuration (monopolar or bipolar), or patient etiology. That is, psychophysical performance is apparently determined by basic mechanisms of electrical stimulation that are not sensitive to these specific parameters. It has been suggested (Clopton et al., 1983; Shannon, 1985a) that the factor limiting psychophysical implant performance is the biophysics of the electrode–neural interface. Physiological results with electrical stimulation (van den Honert & Stypulkowski, 1984) are compatible with this interpretation.

If psychophysical results are dependent on biophysical properties at the electrode neuron interface and do not correlate with speech recognition performance, then one implication is that the details of the peripheral neural activity pattern are not necessary for speech recognition. Speech recognition must therefore depend on central processing mechanisms.

If speech recognition performance depends on complex central processing of peripheral information, rather than psychophysical capabilities, then the differences observed between implant patients in speech reception abilities may be due to differences in the integrity of the patients' central processing systems. Tests of these central mechanisms probably require more complex stimuli and more complex tasks than are typically used in psychophysical experiments. Recent evidence obtained by the Vienna implant research group (Hochmair-Desoyer, Hochmair, & Stiglbrunner, 1985) showed a correlation between speech performance and the ability of the patient to detect a gap in noise. Detecting a gap in a temporally uncertain stimulus, such as noise, may require different central processing abilities than those used to detect a gap in a steady stimulus, such as a tone. It is possible that this simple psychophysical task might tap central processes that are also important for speech perception. Future psychophysical research with implant patients should concentrate on more complicated stimuli, attempting to evaluate the integrity of central speech processing mechanisms. Hopefully, tasks can be found that correlate with speech recognition. If measures of this type were found, they could be used as a screening procedure with electrical stimulation applied to a round window electrode prior to implantation.

IMPLICATIONS FOR THE IMPLANTATION OF CHILDREN

If the integrity of central mechanisms is essential for speech recognition, difficulties in the implantation of children are immediately apparent. Depending on factors such as age of onset, etiology, and progression of hearing loss, children may not possess the central processing mechanisms that are critical for speech recognition. Are these central mechanisms present in congenitally deaf children who have never received auditory stimulation? Can these mechanisms, even when stimulated within the presumed critical period, develop adequately when presented with the atypical patterns of activity generated by electrical stimulation? Can implanted children adapt to these new patterns by developing unique processing networks? If such development is possible, is it bound by an upper age limit? In order to provide usable auditory stimulation, at what age must implantation in children occur?

It is of great interest, not only in helping children who are deaf, but also for developmental neuroscience, to understand the role of sensory stimulation in the development of the brain's structure. Anatomical and physiological experiments in deafened chicks (Born & Rubel, 1985), kittens (Brugge, Kitzes, & Javel, 1981), and gerbils (Kitzes, 1984) have demonstrated that peripheral damage at an early age can delay or impair the development of more central neural structures (see Moore, 1985, for a general review). Based on these data, it can be inferred that the central auditory neural mechanisms of children who are congenitally deaf may be incompletely developed. In such cases, the electrical stimulation of the remaining auditory nerve may not result in interpretable sensations. Indeed, implants in a few congenitally deaf adults reveal that the sensations induced by the implant were not even perceived auditorally, but were experienced as sensations of dizziness or vibrations on the forehead (Eisenberg, 1982). Although speech processors that are capable of partially recreating "normal" peripheral neural patterns may be designed, if the central mechanisms are undeveloped because of a lack of early input, the child's brain may not be able to make use of the electrically induced information.

Knudson and colleagues (1984a, 1984b) demonstrated that barn owls with one ear plugged were unable to localize their prey. However, if the ear was plugged before they reached adulthood, young owls could modify their behavior to accommodate the impaired hearing and localize correctly. It was also demonstrated that when sensory function was restored by removing the earplug, normal functionality was recovered, provided that sensation was restored before the owl reached puberty. The conclusion was that there are different "critical" periods for adapting to damaged input and for adapting to restored input.

Deprivation experiments on the primate visual system (Harwerth et al., 1986) demonstrated that there are multiple sensitive periods in the development of visual function, depending on the complexity of the task. In general, the more centrally determined the visual function, the longer the critical period.

From these animal models, we might speculate that children could learn to use the implant stimulation in order to understand speech. The difference in this case, however, is that the implant provides an impoverished signal when compared to the richness of the normal acoustic environment employed in animal experimentation. It is not known whether the limited and "distorted" information provided by a cochlear implant is sufficient to allow children to learn to recognize speech, even if applied within the "critical" period.

Some adults who are postlingually deafened can recognize speech using only their implants (see Chapter 3), presumably because their central auditory systems have developed normally and they have a well-established reference system of auditory speech sounds within which to place the sounds heard with their implants. It is unclear whether children or adults with congenital or prelingual deafness can develop an auditory reference system for speech sounds with the limited information provided by a cochlear implant.

New psychophysical tests must be developed to evaluate the integrity and capability of the central auditory mechanisms that are important for speech recognition. These perceptual tests could then be used to evaluate implanted childrens' central auditory mechanisms and to document any changes in those measures as a function of implant use. Children who are implanted now should be closely monitored and their capabilities regularly tested so that some of these questions can be answered and the appropriate diagnostic tools developed for future application.

REFERENCES

Born, D. E. & Rubel, E. W. (1985). Afferent influences on brainstem auditory nuclei of the chicken: Neuron number and size following cochlear removal. *Journal of Comparative Neurology, 231,* 435–445.

Brugge, J. F., Kitzes, L. M., & Javel, E. (1981). Postnatal development of frequency and intensity sensitivity of neurons in the anteroventral cochlear nucleus of kittens. *Hearing Research, 5,* 217–229.

Clopton, B. M., Spelman, F. A., Glass, I., Pfingst, B. E., Miller, J. M., Lawrence, P. D., & Dean, D. P. (1983). Neural encoding of electrical signals. In C. W. Parkins & S. W. Anderson (Eds.), Cochlear prostheses: An international symposium. *Annals of the New York Academy of Sciences, 405,* 146–158.

Eddington, D. K., Dobelle, W. H., Brackmann, D. E., Mladevosky, M. G., & Parkin, J. L. (1978). Auditory prosthesis research with multiple channel intracochlear stimulation in man. *Annals of Otology, Rhinology, and Laryngology, 87* (Suppl. 53).

Eisenberg, L. S. (1982). Use of the cochlear implant by the prelingually deaf. *Annals of Otology, Rhinology, and Laryngology, 91* (Suppl. 91), 62–66.

Harwerth, R. S., Smith, E. L., Duncan, G. C., Crawford, M. L. J., & van Noorden, G. K. (1986). Multiple sensitive periods in the development of the primate visual system. *Science, 232,* 235–238.

Hinojosa, R., & Marion, M. (1983). Histopathology of profound sensorineural deafness. In C. W. Parkins & S.W. Anderson (Eds.), Cochlear prostheses: An international symposium. *Annals of the New York Academy of Sciences, 405,* 459–484.

Hochmair-Desoyer, I. J., & Hochmair, E. S. (1980). An eight channel scala tympani electrode for auditory prostheses. *IEEE Transactions on Biomedical Engineering, 27,* 44.

Hochmair-Desoyer, I. J., Hochmair, E. S., & Stiglbrunner, H. K. (1985). Psychoacoustic temporal processing and speech understanding in cochlear implant patients. In R. A. Schindler & M. M. Merzenich (Eds.), *Cochlear implants* (pp. 291–304). New York: Raven Press.

Kitzes, L. M. (1984). Some physiological consequences of neonatal cochlear destruction in the inferior colliculus of the gerbil, *Meriones,* unguiculatus. *Brain Research, 306,* 171–178.

Knudsen, E. I., Knudsen, P. F., & Esterly, S. D. (1984a). A critical period for the recovery of sound localization accuracy following monaural occlusion in the barn owl. *Journal of Neuroscience, 4,* 1012–1020.

Knudsen, E. I., Esterly, S. D., & Knudsen, P. F. (1984b). Monaural occlusion alters sound localization during a sensitive period in the barn owl. *Journal of Neuroscience, 4,* 1001–1011.

Moore, D. R. (1985). Postnatal development of the mammalian central auditory system and the neural consequences of auditory deprivation. *Acta Otolaryngologica* (Stockholm), *Suppl. 421,* 19–30.

Muller, C. G. (1981). Summary of cochlear implant work. *Journal of the Acoustical Society of America, 70,* S52.

Pfingst, B. E., & Sutton, D. (1983). Relation of cochlear implant function to histopathology in monkeys. In C. W. Parkins & S. W. Anderson (Eds.), Cochlear prostheses: An international symposium. *Annals of the New York Academy of Sciences, 405,* 490–501.

Shannon, R. V. (1983a). Multichannel electrical stimulation of the auditory nerve in man: I. Basic psychophysics. *Hearing Research, 11,* 157–189.

Shannon, R. V. (1983b). Multichannel electrical stimulation of the auditory nerve in man: II. Channel interaction. *Hearing Research, 12,* 1–16.

Shannon, R. V. (1985a). Threshold and loudness functions for pulsatile electrical stimulation of cochlear implants. *Hearing Research, 18,* 135–143.

Shannon, R. V. (1985b). Loudness summation as a measure of channel interaction in a cochlear prosthesis. In R. A. Schindler & M. M. Merzenich (Eds.), *Cochlear implants* (pp. 323–334). New York: Raven Press.

Shannon, R. V. (1986). Temporal processing in cochlear implants. In M. J. Collins, T. J. Glattke, & L. Harker (Eds.), *Sensorineural hearing loss: Mechanisms, diagnosis, treatment.* Iowa City: University of Iowa Press.

Simmons, F. B. (1966). Electrical stimulation of the auditory nerve in man. *Archives of Otolaryngology, 84,* 24–76.

Tong, Y. C., Clark, G. M., Blamey, P. J., Busby, P. A., & Dowell, R. C. (1982). Psychophysical studies for two multiple-channel cochlear implant patients. *Journal of the Acoustical Society of America, 71,* 153–160.

Townsend, B., Cotter, N., van Compernolle, D., & White, R. (1987). Pitch perception by cochlear implant subjects. *Journal of the Acoustical Society of America, 82,* 106–115.

Tyler, R. S., Summerfield, Q., Wood, E. J., & Fernandes, M. A. (1982). Psychoacoustic and phonetic temporal processing in normal and hearing-impaired listeners. *Journal of the Acoustical Society of America, 72,* 740–752.

van den Honert, C., & Stypulkowski, P. H. (1984). Physiological properties of the electrically stimulated auditory nerve: II. Single fiber recordings. *Hearing Research, 14,* 225–243.

van den Honert, C., & Stypulkowski, P. H. (1987). Single fiber mapping of spatial excitation patterns in the electrically stimulated auditory nerve. *Hearing Research, 29,* 195–206.

Viemeister, N. F. (1979). Temporal modulation transfer functions based upon modulation thresholds. *Journal of the Acoustical Society of America, 66,* 1364–1380.

Wegel, R. L., & Lane, C. E. (1924). The auditory masking of one pure tone by another and its probable relation to the dynamics of the inner ear. *Physics Review, 23,* 266–276.

Zwislocki, J. J. (1969). Temporal summation of loudness: An analysis. *Journal of the Acoustical Society of America, 46,* 431–441.

CHAPTER 3

ELMER OWENS

PRESENT STATUS OF ADULTS WITH COCHLEAR IMPLANTS

Experimental and clinical studies of hearing impaired adults with cochlear implants have a direct bearing on the issue of implants in young children. The present chapter, which focuses on adults with postlingual hearing loss who have had cochlear implants, includes the following subtopics: single-channel and multichannel implants; interpretation of implant reports; effects of implants on speech and voice; aural rehabilitation; prelingual loss; and implications for the implantation of children. Because of the plethora of recent publications on cochlear implants, many of which are duplicative, emphasis will be placed on those that are most recent and most encompassing.

SINGLE-CHANNEL IMPLANTS

3M/HOUSE

The 3M/House implant, a single-channel, single-electrode system described by Fretz and Fravel (1985) and widely used since 1982, functions basically in the same manner as the earlier House-Urban device. In the Report of the Ad Hoc Committee on Cochlear Implants (Hopkinson et al., 1986), it was concluded that several studies of the 3M/House device and its predecessor were in agreement on their findings (Edgerton, Prietto, & Danhauer, 1983; Englemann, Waterfall, & Hough, 1981; Gantz

et al., 1985; House et al., 1981; Owens, Kessler, & Raggio, 1983; Thielemeir, Brimacombe, & Eisenberg, 1982; and Thielemeir, 1985). The following summary statement therefore seems appropriate:

> cochlear implants for patients with postlingual hearing loss, with
> primary reference to the 3M/House device, can provide the follow-
> ing to various degrees: a general awareness of sound and the recog-
> nition of a few specific everyday sounds; enhancement of lipreading
> ability; temporal, durational, and intensity-difference (accent) cues;
> and pitch cues within a range below 300 Hz. Also, vocal self-moni-
> toring ability is usually improved. Speech understanding, as meas-
> ured by recognition of words or sentences in an open-set form, has
> not been attained to a consistent degree without visual or other spe-
> cial cues. General inability in vowel recognition is consistent with
> lack of spectral information. (Hopkinson et al., 1986, p. 33)

Of course, as with any cochlear implant system, there are no guaran-
tees for the individual patient who receives a 3M/House device. Although most patients will hear sound that is useful to a varying extent,
others will hear only noise, and a relatively small proportion will fail to
hear any sound. At present, no accurate prediction can be given to a prospective implant patient on the benefit he will receive. Preimplant testing, usually involving electrical stimulation of the promontory, can give
some indication whether neuronal tissue is present, but few clues regarding its extent and location along the cochlea (see Chapter 1 for further
discussion of preimplant testing).

According to Thielemeir, Brimacombe, and Eisenberg (1982), the
quality of sound provided by the House-Urban system, which eventuated
in the 3M/House, is initially described by patients as "static-like",
"scratchy", "tinny", and "crackling". The quality changes over time to
"more natural", but still not "normal", as increasing differentiation of
sounds occurs. Speech is described as "muffled"; sounds perceived as
natural include running water, footsteps, and clapping (p. 31).

It seems that the large majority of 3M/House patients have derived
some advantage from the implant. As supportive evidence of general sat-
isfaction, a followup on 269 consecutive patients was presented by
Thielemeir (1985). An interpretation of Thielemeir's tabled information
by Hopkinson and colleagues (1986) omits 21 patients *in process* and 7
deceased, for a derived total of 241, and includes 7 *biologic failures* (no response to stimulation) and 7 *device failures* (with no replacement) among
the *nonusers.* From the derived total of 241, then, users numbered 195 and
nonusers, 46, indicating that 81 percent of the patients have continued
using the implant.

3M/Vienna

The Vienna group has conducted studies on implant systems in which single-channel stimulation is directed to one of four intracochlear electrodes or to a single extracochlear electrode placed in the round window niche. The extracochlear system was used mainly for patients with some residual hearing to be preserved (Hochmair & Hochmair-Desoyer, 1985). Although the intracochlear device includes 4 electrodes, only one of the 4 — the one providing the best responses to various stimuli — was selected for permanent use in the studies reviewed here.

Hochmair-Desoyer, Hochmair, and Stiglbrunner (1985) presented results for a group of 12 patients (10 intracochlear and 2 extracochlear) who had been using their implant devices for 3 months. Vowel and consonant recognition was reportedly achieved by all 10 patients who took these two tests. Of the 12 patients in the study, 9 (including the 2 extracochlear patients) understood some open-set sentence materials, and 7 (including one of the two extracochlear patients) understood some open-set one-syllable words.

In a report by Burian, Hochmair-Desoyer, and Eisenwort (1986) on 56 postlingual and prelingual patients who received implants between 1978 and 1985 (31 intracochlear and 25 extracochlear), postimplant results were classified according to three groups: group 1 patients were capable of speech comprehension without the help of lipreading; group 2 patients were unable to understand speech without lipreading, but the auditory input improved their lipreading ability; and group 3 patients, although unlikely to achieve speech comprehension either with or without lipreading, were much improved in their orientation to everyday life. Most of the patients in group 1 were postlingually deafened and had received intracochlear implants. In an accompanying table of data on 42 of the patients (presumably the 42 who spoke German), 12 of 23 patients with intracochlear devices were in group 1, compared with only 5 of 19 patients with extracochlear devices, indicating a clear superiority for the intracochlear system. In an overall statement it was estimated that 60 percent of the postlingually deafened were able to understand open-set sentences and words without lipreading, provided that they were given at least 3 months implant use and appropriate rehabilitation. Fifty-one of the 56 patients were still using their implants in 1986.

In another report from the Vienna group (Hochmair-Desoyer, Hochmair, & von Wallenberg, 1987) the authors stated that "open list sentence and word understanding without lipreading can be achieved by 75% of the postlingually deafened implant patients." Specific data were not supplied.

Results by the Vienna investigators have not yet been supported in other centers outside Austria. The Vienna extracochlear system, now produced by the 3M company, was tested in the United States by Rose, Facer, King, and Fabry (1987) on a group of 5 patients. Test materials consisted of some selected closed-set tests of the Minimal Auditory Capabilities (MAC) battery (Owens et al., 1985). The MAC comprises a series of closed- and open-set materials, tape recorded by a male speaker, with stimuli graduated in difficulty from identification of accent, pitch change, noise versus voice, consonants, and vowels, to recognition of words and sentences. The high scores of one patient, particularly on the vowel test, suggested the possibility of some open-set speech understanding, but no open-set tests were administered. Compared to this patient's responses, those of the 4 remaining patients were clearly inferior. Similarly, the results for the first 2 of a planned series of 10 patients in Sweden using the 3M/Vienna extracochlear implant (Risberg et al., 1987) showed one patient scoring 57 percent on a list of food and vegetables presented in an open set and the other showing poor ability on this task. Details of the test materials and procedures were not given. At the University of Iowa, Tyler and colleagues (1985) studied 6 single-channel patients, 3 with the 3M/House device and 3 with the Vienna *intracochlear* device produced in Austria. These patients were tested on various subtests of the MAC and the Iowa Cochlear Implant Tests (Tyler, Preece, & Lowder, 1983). The Iowa tests, in addition to adaptations of selected MAC tests, include tests of everyday sounds, warning sounds, number of syllables, speaker discrimination, and lipreading. All patients in this series scored zero percent on open-set tests of speech understanding except for sporadic responses on the MAC Spondee Recognition test.

The conflicting results on the Vienna single-channel devices constitute an enigma. Although the results achieved in Austria can in no way be discounted, they must eventually be replicated in other centers before appropriate confidence can be placed in the Vienna group devices as systems that can afford speech understanding with some measure of consistency. Replication attempts must, of course, duplicate the implant system, the speech processing scheme, and the surgical approach. In addition, control must be exercised over both the selection of patients and the test materials and procedures. Regarding the former, one of the selection criteria (Burian et al., 1986) for Vienna candidates receiving an extracochlear device, is that thresholds must be higher than 85 dB (frequencies not specified). This criterion seems fairly lenient when it is realized that levels of 90 or 95 dB HL, assuming the inclusion of frequencies of 1000 Hz and higher, represent useful preimplant residual hearing (see Boothroyd, Chapter 6).

With respect to the testing procedure, Hochmair-Desoyer and colleagues (1985) offered a description of the test protocol that had been used for all Vienna postlingual implant patients. Lists of German one-syllable words, everyday sentences, and vowels were prerecorded on tape by a female speaker and, in the testing procedure, directed through a cable from the tape recorder to the patient's speech processor; that is, the stimuli were not presented auditorally through a speaker system. Each item was presented twice with approximately 3 seconds between presentations. For the vowel test, several practice runs on all the items, with feedback on the accuracy of the responses, were given before the actual test trial. On the consonant identification test, performed live voice, the full list was presented several times for practice, again with feedback of the correct response whenever an error was made. All tests were open-set with a write-down response.

Problems with live-voice aspects of the testing, limited to consonant identification, need no discussion, and the difficulty level of the Vienna materials in terms of vocabulary and familiarity is not known. However, the repetition of each test word and the practice given on the actual test items would no doubt serve to facilitate correct responses during the test ing session. In contrast, the usual protocol in American audiological clinics requires one presentation of each test word over a speaker system, no previous practice on test items (to say nothing of feedback), and no previous knowledge by a patient that a given item will be on a test list. Practice items are often employed to ensure that the patient understands and can accomplish the task, but the test items are typically not among them. In short, the Vienna test protocol may offer advantages to patients in Vienna that would not be provided in the United States when the usual audiologic procedures are followed.

A timely study by Tyler (in press), however, tended to discount suppositions that differences in test protocol can explain the surprising abilities of Vienna single-channel patients in open-set speech recognition. Tyler tested the word and sentence recognition of 9 users of the Vienna devices, all of whom had been bona fide implant candidates with little or no residual hearing and all of whom were considered to be among the "better" implant users. The testing was done in Austria with materials recorded in German by two Austrian speakers essentially unfamiliar to the patients. The patients were unaware of what the test materials would be, and other aspects of the test protocol were carefully controlled. Test words of 1 or 2 syllables and sentences of 3 to 6 words were presented open-set, and a write-down response was required. All patients showed open-set speech recognition without lipreading, performance varying from 15 to 86 percent correct on sentences and 11 to 57 percent correct on words. Results were noticeably better for patients with

the intracochlear device, 2 of the 3 extracochlear patients scoring markedly and consistently below the remaining 7.

UCSF SINGLE-CHANNEL

After studying a series of patients with single-channel/single-elec-
trode implants (Michelson, 1971a, 1971b; Merzenich et al., 1973), the
group at the University of California, San Francisco (UCSF) experimen-
ted with a 16-electrode array arranged in 8 bipolar pairs, activated by a
single-channel stimulator. It was postulated that the employment of
several electrodes spread along the cochlea would take optimal advantage of the tonotopic cochlear structure, thus providing for pitch differentiation. In practice, only a few of the electrodes, and not always the
same ones, were functional for each patient. Of six patients available for
postimplant evaluation (see Owens, Kessler, & Schubert, 1982), one was
outstanding, achieving open-set recognition on the MAC for 10 of 25
spondees and 33 percent of key words in CID sentences along with well-
above average recognition of consonants, vowels, and other stimuli in
closed-set formats; lipreading scores were markedly higher for device-on
over device-off conditions (lipreading plus auditory versus lipreading
only). Two other patients scored above average on the closed-set tests
with the implant and recognized a few key words on the open-set sentence and spondee tests; their lipreading scores also improved. The remaining three patients identified prosodic stimuli, but could not identify
vowel sounds and showed no improvement in lipreading. No explanation
emerged for the wide differences in performance among the patients.

Dent, Simmons, White, and Roberts (1987) have presented a thorough review and discussion of single-channel implants along with their
findings on four patients who had been implanted with Stanford University single-channel intracochlear systems. A single electrode was used in
two of the patients and multiple electrodes (but one channel of stimulation) in the other two. Three of the patients used their implants regularly
whereas the fourth was a nonuser who nevertheless returned for postimplant evaluations. Although none of the four benefitted from hearing aid
use in daily activities, they wore hearing aids for preimplant testing with
the MAC battery. Except for the Everyday Sounds test, no consistent improvement was demonstrated in the postimplant versus preimplant conditions, and none of the patients identified any of the MAC open-set
speech material. All four showed gains in the lipreading of consonants
and numbers and three of the four achieved noticeable improvement
(device-on over device-off) in a videotaped CID Sentences lipreading
test. The fourth patient (the nonuser) was an excellent lipreader who found
that the implant interfered with her lipreading of connected speech.

EXTERNAL PATTERN INPUT (EPI)

An extracochlear approach to single-channel stimulation has been taken in England (Fourcin et al., 1983; Moore, 1985). An electrode is attached to a conventionally formed earmold, which in turn is attached to an external microphone–transmitter system that extracts the fundamental frequency from ongoing speech. The electrode is adjusted individually to provide secure contact on an appropriate part of the promontory. Patients with no tympanic membrane, usually as a result of a radical mastoidectomy, insert and remove the device by means of the attached earmold. For those with intact tympanic membranes, a surgical procedure excises the incus and handle of the malleus and displaces the membrane so that it is in intimate contact with the promontory. The sound reaching the patient provides voicing and timing information as an aid to lipreading. The investigators state that their patients obtain the same auditory information as those with a single intracochlear electrode while preserving the scala tympani for future generations of more efficient implants.

THE PRELCO SYSTEM

Still another extracochlear device, the PRELCO, in France, has been described by Portmann, Cazals, and Negrevergne (1986) as being used in 20 patients. The aim was to provide for recovery of everyday auditory perceptions and assistance in lipreading. Postimplant abilities, reported for four patients, were restricted to recognition of prosodic cues and a few environmental sounds.

MULTICHANNEL IMPLANTS

Research on the implantation of multichannel devices has been undertaken primarily with the aim of providing the auditory information necessary for the understanding of speech. The general hypothesis has been that several independent channels of auditory stimulation to electrodes spread along the scala tympani can provide the spectral cues that have been largely absent with single-channel stimulation. Five wearable multichannel implants on which published accounts are available are discussed in this section. Major attention is centered on the question whether speech understanding, as reflected by performance on open-set speech recognition tests, has been achieved by the implant recipients.

UTAH/SYMBION INERAID

The Ineraid, manufactured by Symbion, is based largely upon the work of Eddington and colleagues (1978), who demonstrated that a pitch continuum could be produced through multichannel electrode arrays and that the understanding of speech could be a direct result. Although each electrode in a multielectrode array produces rate pitch perception only to 300 Hz, a given frequency is perceived as higher in pitch for electrodes placed toward the base of the cochlea and lower in pitch for those placed toward the apical end. A pitch continuum can therefore be achieved by strategic placement of the electrodes.

The Ineraid provides four channels of monopolar, analog stimulation directed to four of six electrodes placed within the cochlea. The selection of the four electrodes for permanent use is based upon the results of sensitivity and pitch scaling measures in the course of postimplant fitting procedures. This process is made possible by the use of a percutaneous connector permitting direct access to all electrodes.

The most recent report on the Ineraid (Dankowski, McCandless, & Smith, 1988) presented results for 43 patients from several different centers who, at the time of data compilation, had had evaluations at 1 to 3 months and at 6 to 9 months postimplant. The protocol consisted of four tests from the MAC battery, although with different tape recordings than the original ones that were made by Auditec of St. Louis, an independent distributor. For the Ineraid patients, the Four-Choice Spondee and the Spondee Recognition tests were tape-recorded by a female speaker and presented through a speaker system in a sound-treated room. The CID Sentences were given live voice, one list for auditory-only stimulation and two other lists for lipreading in device off, device on conditions. The mean score for the Four-Choice Spondee Test was well above chance at 1 to 3 months and showed a slight increase at 6 to 9 months. On the Spondee Recognition Test (open-set), records were available for 38 patients. At the 1 to 3 months test, 32 of the 38 recognized some of the words, with a mean score of 28.7 percent (range 0-to-84 percent); at 6 to 9 months, 34 of the 38 recognized some of the words, with a mean of 38.1 percent (range 0-to-100 percent). Similarly, on the open-set, auditory-only CID Sentences presented live voice, 23 of 33 patients for whom records were available recognized some key words at 3 to 6 months with a mean score of 26.5 percent (range 0-to-100 percent); at 6 to 9 months, 26 of the 33 recognized some key words, with a mean of 34.4 percent (range 0-to-98 percent). Thus, all auditory tests indicated marked improvement from the 1 to 3 month to the 6 to 9 month visits.

The mean score for Visual Enhancement (lipreading with implant minus lipreading-only) at 1 to 3 months was 28.6 percent; at 6 to 9 months, the mean was 31.8 percent. Of a total 117 patients followed from February, 1984 to December, 1987, 114 (97 percent) were using their devices regularly; one of the three nonusers was not stimulable and the two others disliked the implant for psychological reasons (K. Dankowski, personal communication, November, 1987).

MELBOURNE/NUCLEUS

The basis for the University of Melbourne implant system, manufactured by Nucleus, was described by Tong and colleagues (1982). The externally worn speech processor extracts and encodes estimates of the fundamental frequency ($f0$) and second formant ($f2$) from the speech signal that are picked up by an internal receiver-stimulator and decoded for sequential activation of 22 electrodes, stimulated in pairs, in the scala tympani. The $f0$ information provides prosodic and voicing cues to the listener while the $f2$ information, which depends on electrode position, provides vowel and consonant cues (for further details see Chapter 10). Of 24 Australian patients studied with this device (Brown, Dowell, & Clark, 1987), all but two recognized some key words on a recorded CID Everyday Sentences test, for a mean of 18 percent (range 0-to-58 percent). On a lipreading test with CID sentences, a lipreading-only condition produced a mean score of 53 percent, compared with a lipreading plus implant score of 83 percent. These results were corroborated by speech tracking rates: lipreading alone, 16 words per minute (wpm) versus lipreading with implant, 44 wpm. For a small group of 7 patients, tracking rates in an auditory-only condition averaged 25 wpm.

Patients could also identify recorded environmental sounds in a closed set (chance = 20 percent), attaining a mean score of 75 percent (range 60-to-90 percent). An analysis of 13 patients who had worn the device for a year revealed an open-set CID Everyday Sentences mean score of 37 percent key words on the 12-months test (auditory-only) indicating marked improvement over the three months postimplant mean score, which was 16 percent.

A newer version of the Nucleus implant provides first formant ($f1$) information in addition to the $f0, f2$ information of the earlier version. The most recent report (Beiter, Brimacombe, & Barker, 1987) was based on 88 North American adults using the newer device. The tape-recorded Iowa cochlear implant subtests (Tyler, Preece, & Lowder, 1983), employing a male speaker, were given to the patients preimplant while they wore either a hearing aid or tactile device — and then with their implants at approximately 3-months postsurgery. Mean scores on all closed-set tests (spondees, vowels, and medial consonants) were significantly higher at the 3-months postimplant date. On the open-set NU-6 monosyllable word test the preimplant mean was 0.6 percent and the postimplant mean, 6.5 percent. On the open-set CID sentences the preimplant mean for key words understood was 2.5 percent and the postimplant mean, 20.7 percent (SD 19.5 percent). For the latter test, 76 percent of the patients scored significantly better on the postimplant test than on the preimplant. Mean speech tracking scores, available for 59 of the postimplant patients, were 22 wpm in a lipreading-only condition and 51 wpm in the lipreading plus implant condition, indicating marked improvement with implant activation.

In the same paper, data are presented for a questionnaire survey on telephone use. Of 146 responders, 70.5 percent reported that they used the telephone to some extent, and 51 percent indicated that they used the telephone interactively, the degree of success depending on the familiarity of the person conversing with them.

With respect to long-term use, estimates are based on 660 adults who have received Nucleus implants since September, 1982. As of November, 1987, 9 are nonusers by choice, 2 others were nonstimulable, and 3 experienced mechanical difficulties with the device. In all, the total number of users is 646 (98 percent) (D. Mecklenburg, personal communication, December 1987).

UCSF/STORZ

The postimplant hearing of 15 consecutive patients who received a four-channel implant developed at UCSF and manufactured by Storz Instrument Company has been reported by Schindler and Kessler (1987). Of eight bipolar electrode pairs placed in the cochlea, four are preselected for permanent use. Stimuli from four separate coils on the mastoid are sent transcutaneously to an internal receiver and then to the four intracochlear electrodes. Volume settings can be varied for the four channels separately or combined, and there is an overall compression control. Detailed descriptions were offered by Rebscher (1985) and Schindler and colleagues (1986).

Mean scores for all the MAC closed-set tests were well above chance and, accordingly, well above the mean preimplant scores, which were essentially within the range of chance. The postimplant means for all these tests progressed steadily higher from an initial test at the time of the device fitting (at about 6 weeks postsurgery) through subsequent visits at 6 to 8 weeks and at 6 months after the initial test. For the open-set speech tests, 13 of the 15 patients achieved some measure of speech recognition performance in the process of postimplant testing, compared with preimplant scores of zero. A tabulation of the best postimplant open-set scores achieved by the 15 patients during the course of the test sessions revealed the following: Spondee Recognition, 26 percent (range

0-to-80 percent); CID Sentences, 29 percent (range 0-to-84 percent); and NU-6 Monosyllable Words, 10 percent (range 0-to-34 percent). The latter are especially significant in that they can be compared with conventionally obtained speech discrimination scores. Again, the mean scores improved steadily, showing gradual improvement through the 6-month test date without an intervening aural rahabilitation program.

On the MAC lipreading test (videotaped CID Sentences), mean visual enhancement (device-on minus device-off) at 6 months postimplant was 35 percent, compared with a preimplant enhancement of 0 percent obtained with hearing aids or vibrotactile devices. Speech tracking rates — a device-off mean of 25 wpm versus a device-on mean of 60 wpm — corroborated the CID visual enhancement scores, and the results for a performance scale on which patients rated themselves (Owens & Raggio, 1988) corroborated the overall MAC results.

In a subsequent study of this same patient population, with one additional patient for a total of 16 (Schindler, Kessler, Jackler, & Merzenich, in press), an analysis was undertaken for the first 14 who had completed a 1-year test in addition to the 6 to 8 weeks postoperative test and another test 6-months later. Raw scores showed that only three of the 14 failed to achieve open-set speech recognition in postimplant testing while the remaining 11 showed steady improvement in scores without an intervening rehabilitative program. Recall that all preoperative open-set scores were zero. For these 11 patients on the CID Sentences test postoperatively, the means progressed from 14 percent, to 37 percent, to 50 percent — 6 to 8 weeks, to 6 months, to 1 year; for the NU-6 Monosyllabic Word test, mean scores progressed from 6 percent, to 18 percent, to 22 percent.

Of the 16 patients, all are wearing their devices regularly except for 4 who have experienced difficulties attributed to internal device failures (D. Kessler, personal communication, December, 1987). These 4 patients elected to wait for replacement of the UCSF/Storz system, which has been discontinued, with a new UCSF system being manufactured by MiniMed Technologies of Sylmar, California. The new system will be available for implantation in the winter of 1988. The UCSF/Storz intracochlear electrode is retained, but with the difference that it can be activated either in a monopolar (16-channel) or bipolar (8-channel) mode. The implanted electronics include a multiplexed 8-channel RF receiver. The external RF transmitting antenna is worn on the mastoid process. The speech processor, about the size of a body-worn hearing aid and housing a rechargeable battery pack, can deliver either pulsatile or analog stimuli. The major advantage of the new system is its flexibility in providing a wide range of speech processing strategies that can be tailored to the needs of the individual patient as part of the post-implant device-fitting process.

In summary, the open-set scores for the Symbion, Nucleus, and UCSF/Storz multichannel device groups are most encouraging in representing a marked advance in cochlear implant work. In all three groups an overwhelming majority of the patients achieved open-set speech recognition. According to the results of the studies reported herein, mean scores for the three groups in recognition of spondee words ranged from 25 to 30 percent, and mean scores for CID sentence materials, from 21 to 37 percent. Means for visual enhancement in the lipreading of CID Sentences (device-on over device-off) were between 30 and 35 percent. It seems pertinent to mention that a long-term comparative study of patients with multichannel devices is in progress at the University of Iowa (Gantz, McCabe, Tyler, & Preece, 1987).

EUROPEAN DEVICES

Most of the information available on multichannel devices used in Europe comes from Germany and France. The Cologne-Duren group (Banfai et al., 1987) reported on postimplant results for 100 patients who received a multichannel extracochlear device in which a series of electrodes is inserted into recesses drilled at specific points along the wall of the cochlea without invasion of the membranous labyrinth. Tabled information provides results for mutually exclusive groups, from the best to the worst, as follows: understanding of open speech, 11 percent; ability to participate in conversations with the help of lipreading, 32 percent; improvement in lipreading, 26 percent; awareness of environmental sounds and prosodic cues, 2 percent; dissatisfied patients with demonstrably poor results, 23 percent; and implant removed, 6 percent.

Chouard and colleagues (1986), in France, reported on 105 patients implanted between 1976 and 1986 with the Chorimac 12, a multichannel intracochlear device employing transcutaneous transmission as opposed to percutaneous transmission used in an earlier series of patients. Details of the report are difficult to follow, but evidence from tabled information suggests substantial success of postimplant patients in closed-set vowel recognition. Open-set word recognition was said to have been attained by some patients (number not given) providing that the words are from limited topics such as farm, kitchen, and job. Of the 105 patients, 26 no longer use their implant (details not offered).

Among the multichannel implant devices studied in Europe and the United States by Tyler (in preparation) were the Chorimac, Nucleus, Symbion, and Duren/Cologne. The same two speakers produced recordings of word and sentence tests in French, German, and English languages using the same vocabulary. The patients were selected to be representative of the "better" levels of performance with each device. It was demonstrated that a few patients with each type of implant can achieve some degree of open-set word and sentence recognition.

Interpretation of Implant Reports

Test Materials

With the introduction of cochlear implants came the realization that the conventional audiological tests were too difficult for candidates who are profoundly deaf, obliging audiologists to develop test measures suitable for evaluating the effects of implants. The immediate result was a number of contributions from different centers. The lack of conformity in test materials has impeded realistic comparisons and precise knowledge of implant results. Within centers, moreover, the evaluation process was often complicated by continuous changes in the objects being measured — the implants themselves.

Although the test situation appears to be improving, it must be remembered that the choice of test materials can strongly influence a patient's performance and that comparisons are tenuous unless the same tests are used under the same conditions. Materials may vary in a number of ways. It is fairly well known that spondee words are easier to recognize than monosyllabic words and that sentences rich in context are easier than those spare of context. Probably it is less well known that lists of highly familiar monosyllable words in an open set are more easily understood than lists of those less familiar (Owens, 1961); the same holds true for spondees and for sentences, as can be easily verified clinically during any testing session. Similarly, the test (target) word in closed-set materials is easy or difficult depending on the composition and number of alternative choices available; for example, if the target is a stop consonant in a test of final position consonants in words, it will be easier to identify the word if the alternatives are continuants rather than stops. A patient whose hearing is limited to the detection of durational cues can give a correct response to such an item without actually understanding the target word. In any case, it is inaccurate to refer to the task as *word* identification when it is really *consonant* identification.

Still another example involves guessing behavior by the patient. Although it is obvious that all closed-set items involve guessing, it may not be so obvious that the guessing is seldom random (in the sense that each alternative has the same chance of being chosen). That is, one or two of the alternative choices in an item may be easily eliminated from contention by the listener, through durational or other cues that are not being tested, consequently narrowing the field of choices and enhancing the possibility of a correct guess. Therefore, a large body of items with a range of alternative-choice combinations is necessary for assigning a realistic chance score to any closed-set test.

SUBJECTS

It seems that in the selection of adult subjects for implantation most investigator teams have in general followed guidelines similar to those listed by Dowell, Mecklenburg, and Clark (1986): (1) profound-total bilateral deafness; (2) onset of deafness following the acquisition of language; (3) 18 years of age, or older; (4) no significant benefit from a sensory aid; (5) no contraindications to placement of the electrode array as evaluated through techniques of cochlear imaging; (6) medically suitable for surgery; and (7) appropriate expectations and attitudes. However, it is often difficult to determine from the typical report how subjects were selected for a particular study. Commonly, a series of patients becomes the basis for a study by virtue of having been implanted with the same device, which is appropriate so long as an unbiased sample — such as a consecutive series — has been achieved. Another observation concerning the implant literature is that many of the studies appear to have used the same core of subjects with a few new ones added or subtracted in each of several subsequent reports in other publications, in which case the studies are not independent. In the worst case, a few exceptionally successful patients can contribute to false optimism about overall results, especially if they are included in several reports assumed by the reader to be based on different populations. Finally, regarding test reliability, it is often not stated whether all patients were tested at the same center, whether qualified audiologists were employed, and whether the test materials were carefully chosen and used with calibrated equipment in test suites meeting prescribed standards.

HEARING AIDS

Regarding the criterion of "no significant benefit from a sensory aid," researchers and clinicians involved with implant work agree in general that an implant *not* be recommended for individuals who benefit from hearing aid use. Few define "benefit," however, and fewer describe how benefit, or advantage, derived from a hearing aid is adequately assessed. A hearing aid evaluation for persons with profound hearing loss requires special approaches and materials (Fujikawa & Owens, 1978; 1979). The severity of hearing loss complicates the evaluation process in several ways: the patient typically has a serious communication handicap, being heavily dependent upon lipreading; a zero percent score on any standard speech discrimination test mandates specially adapted materials; the need for high intensity sound in the testing calls for a double-walled, double-windowed sound suite and a high quality speaker system; hearing aids must be selected to ensure extremely high power, excellent compression systems, and highly variable frequency responses; and earmolds must remain comfortable while fitting tightly enough to prevent feedback. Such factors lead, in turn, to the demand for highly qualified audiologists who are experienced and motivated in working with this population. Several sessions are usually necessary unless the patient clearly demonstrates no reponse to various levels of amplification. A rehabilitative program is an important adjunct for offering help to patients in combining amplification with lipreading and in enhancing coping skills for everyday life. Because the requirements for adequate hearing aid evaluations for profoundly impaired patients are unique, they are not commonly fulfilled in audiology clinics and would not be expected in hearing aid sales centers.

If a hearing aid provides sound that can be heard with reasonable comfort in a face-to-face situation, the question arises whether an implant might offer potentially greater benefit. A battery of tests graduated in difficulty, such as the MAC or Iowa batteries, is then in order. At a time when a single-channel implant was the only available choice, Owens, Kessler, and Schubert (1982) suggested that an implant would be contra-indicated for any hearing aid user who recognized any of the MAC open-set materials and whose lipreading score improved in an aid-on over an aid-off condition. It was anticipated that such "yardsticks" would become more tenuous when improved implants with proven records of providing predictable speech understanding (beyond a few open-set spondees) were available. Although that time seems fast approaching, in light of the increasing number of NU-6 scores being reported with implants, research must determine what can be predicted at a given confidence level for a particular implant worn by a specific individual. It is assumed that other aspects including psychological, surgical, and financial will continue to be weighed carefully.

LIVE-VOICE TESTING

Experienced, qualified audiologists are keenly aware of the bias, conscious or unconscious, inherent in live-voice testing. Brandy (1966) has shown experimentally the differences that can occur between scores for live-voice and recorded versions of the same material. An incidental example of score differences that may occur was provided in Brown and colleagues (1987), in which a recorded version of the CID Sentences produced a mean score of 18 percent for 24 patients (range 0-to-58 percent), whereas live-voice presentation to the same patients resulted in a mean of 43 percent (range 0-to-100 percent). Additional examples were provided by Schindler and colleagues (1986). After working with a patient for a time, even in the presentation of materials over a microphone in a standard test suite, a clinician can make changes, perhaps unconsciously, in variables such as rate of speech, intonation, enunciation, duration or stress of fricative consonants, explosion versus implosion of final-position stop consonants, and prolongation of vowels, any of which can produce immediate and marked changes in a patient's test scores. The situation can become extreme in a lipreading test, where exaggerated articulation can permit visualization of lingua-dental sounds, and even some of the velar consonants and vowel sounds, as well as easier identification of the naturally more visible sounds, and where subtle or not so subtle nonverbal cues, also perhaps unconscious, are rife. Live-voice testing that employs any kind of exaggerated delivery can offer some evidence of how a given patient might understand the speech of someone, such as a spouse, who willingly exaggerates in any way that seems helpful, but not the speech of the average person. In any case, live-voice scores are notoriously unreliable, even with the same speaker, and therefore cannot be used legitimately in comparing patients and devices or in measuring changes in ability. Where it is necessary, as with adults who are difficult to test, or with children, its use must be clearly indicated in reports and it must be consciously controlled insofar as possible.

RECORDED TESTS

Problems also arise with recorded materials in that the employment of different speakers (talkers) using different carrier phrases in different levels of noise can render the test more or less difficult, according to Kreul, Bell, and Nixon (1969); these investigators held that only the actual recordings should be thought of as test material. Accordingly, some identification or description of the recordings used in a study is in order.

Given the same tape recording and assuming the use of calibrated equipment in a sound-treated test suite, the level of presentation can also influence the results. The lack of approved standards for calibration of speaker systems has resulted in some centers using a Sound Pressure Level intensity base while others use Hearing Level, presumably following the suggestion of Morgan, Dirks, and Bower (1979). Probably the best solution to this dilemma is to ensure that every patient listens at a most comfortable loudness (MCL), preferably at the everyday "use" setting of the implant system's volume control, and that this be noted in reporting.

TIMETABLE FOR POSTIMPLANT EVALUATIONS

Increasing evidence that some patients with multichannel implants improve in speech reception skills over time suggests that postimplant intervals in weeks, months, or years be specified and related to an identified base, such as the date of surgery, the date of implant fitting (usually after a healing period), or the conclusion of a rehabilitative program. The length of time over which continued improvement can take place, even without a rehabilitative program, is presently unknown, but it appears likely to be longer than a few months.

SINGLE-CHANNEL VERSUS MULTICHANNEL STIMULATION

Despite such limitations in interpreting reported results in the cochlear implant literature, the accumulated evidence seems sufficient to assert that, at present, multichannel stimulation from wearable devices including Nucleus, Symbion, and UCSF/Storz offers substantially greater auditory information than can be expected from single-channel devices. Presumably, the difference lies in spectral information provided by the multichannel systems. A seeming dichotomy exists in which multichannel users have the potential to recognize vowels, usually closed-set, and also open-set materials including spondee words, CID sentences, and even monosyllable words, whereas single-channel users, except those in Vienna, lack this potential. Two studies using the same test materials on two independent, similarly sized samples of implant patients — Edgerton and colleagues (1983) with the House-Urban single-channel, and Schindler and colleagues (1986) with the UCSF/Storz multichannel — bring this dichotomy into sharp focus. The House-Urban single-channel patients (N = 12), all of whom had worn their implants for at least a year, attained mean scores for the closed-set tests of the MAC that were significantly above chance for all but the Accent and Vowel tests. On the open-set tests, attempted by 10 patients, all scores were zero for the Words in Context and NU-6 tests; a few responses on the Spondee Recognition test were said to be generally the result of guessing, and only one patient recognized some key words (4.5 percent) on the CID Sentences. Of the 10 patients in a consecutive series composing the UCSF/Storz multichannel sample, only 7 had completed a 6- to 8-week test following an initial postimplant test, which occurred at about 6 weeks after surgery. Even on the initial test, however, means for the closed-set MAC tests of the 10 patients were well above those of the House-Urban group on all except the Accent Test, on which the means were about equal; the mean for vowel recognition, in contrast to the House/Urban group, was significantly above chance. On the open-set tests, 8 of the 10 patients attained some postimplant speech recognition. For the 7 patients who completed the 6- to 8-week postoperative test, mean open-set scores were 9 percent, 18 percent, 4 percent, and 4 percent for Spondees, CID Sentences, NU-6, and Words in Context, respectively. In short, the UCSF/Storz patients with few exceptions demonstrated speech recognition ability without visual cues, whereas the House-Urban group did not. It may be worth noting in this context that if multichannel stimulation fails to provide some degree of speech recognition, the patient, assuming some response to stimulation, is typically left with the advantages inherent in a single-channel device.

An especially intriguing development with multichannel stimulation is the evidence that increasing numbers of patients improve steadily, sometimes remarkably, with continued use of an implant system; such improvement has not been reported in adults with single-channel systems. Seemingly, the restoration of spectral information, in addition to prosodic cues, serves as a basis for auditory reintegration of speech that fails to occur with only the prosodic cues. In other words, postlingually deafened adults, given basic spectral and prosodic cues, can undergo a learning process maximizing their auditory skills. It should be mentioned, however, that a recent report by Spivak and colleagues (1987) indicated no changes in hearing among their patients using a Nucleus device during the course of postimplant testing.

EFFECTS OF ELECTRICAL STIMULATION UPON SPEECH AND VOICE

A common clinical observation is that most postlingual-loss cochlear implant candidates have retained intelligible speech despite years of complete deprivation in auditory feedback. At the same time, speech-voice usage could scarcely be classified as normal. Leder and colleagues have documented the major speech-voice deviations of postlingually deafened males. Compared with normal male speakers, the deafened have a significantly higher $f0$ (Leder, Spitzer, & Kirchner, 1987a); a significantly slower speaking rate (Leder et al., 1987b); and a significantly increased voice intensity with greater intensity fluctuations (Leder et al., 1987a). Within a day following the fitting of a 3M/House single-channel implant, the $f0$ of the male voice is significantly lowered toward normal-hearing speakers' values, but rate and intensity changes require longer periods of time to assume normal values (Leder, Spitzer, & Kirchner, 1987b). In a case study of one male patient, Leder and colleagues (1986) showed that the patient could produce stress patterns with high accuracy shortly after being implanted with a 3M/House device, whereas he could not perform this task preimplant.

Recently the speech-voice aspects of implant patients have been receiving increased attention, as judged by a series of papers presented at the November, 1987, American Speech-Language-Hearing Association (ASHA) annual convention. Effects of cochlear implants were reported on the following: production of vowels (Braud et al.), articulatory timing (Breaud et al.), oral–nasal coupling (Punch et al.), and overall changes in speech (Medwetsky Boothroyd, & Hanin). All effects were positive — that is, in the direction of improved speech and voice with an implant.

AURAL REHABILITATION

It would seem appropriate that the more recalcitrant aspects of postimplant improvement in speech-voice usage — such as rate, intensity, and articulatory control — be included in a rehabilitative program otherwise directed largely to receptive communicative problems. That continued help is needed for postimplant patients in auditory training and lipreading seems understandable (see Alpiner, 1986), especially in view of the severe speech discrimination problems that are likely to remain. In other words, even the most successful postimplant patients continue to experience significant communication problems, although of a different kind than in their preimplant lives. Only recently, and only in a few instances, has open-set recognition for monosyllable words — specifically on an NU-6 test — been achieved, and in most of these patients the scores have been relatively low. Recognition of monosyllable words is distinctly more difficult than recognition of spondees or of key words in sentences. The achievement of an NU-6 score of 20 percent, say, by an implant user, represents a remarkable recovery from deafness, considering the highly questionable outlook for cochlear implants in the early 1970s. Nevertheless, such an achievement must be tempered by the reality that an NU-6 score of 20 percent, compared with the scores of patients who constitute the usual clinical population, represents a distinct handicap. Persons who can hear a voice fairly easily with or without a hearing aid, but who have such marked reductions in clarity of hearing, experience extreme communicative difficulty in everyday life. They are heavily dependent upon lipreading, which for some seems unaccountably difficult and, in any case, is often unavailable — as in conditions of poor lighting or darkness, or in situations where speakers' lips cannot be seen. They must verify almost everything that is said to them in communicative situations to guard against misunderstandings; they typically cannot hear accurately over the telephone; they usually cannot understand speech on televison; and they are easily lost in commonly occurring situations with other persons in which interruptions, asides, quick changes in topic, and so forth, constitute most of the enjoyable aspects of conversation. Considering such difficulties, it follows that they are apt to experience occupational and everyday communication problems that are out of the ordinary. Moreover, very few persons in ordinary walks of life can grasp the nature of this particular handicap, namely, the seeming paradox that an individual who can talk and who can easily hear a voice may nevertheless be unable to follow what is being said.

Persons with this kind of hearing impairment can become discouraged after wearing an implant for a time, when they fully realize that, despite their gains from the implant, they still experience a substantial amount of communicative difficulty. Special help in understanding and coping with their problems should be invaluable to them.

An extensive literature exists in aural rehabilitation including several recent texts. Programs already functioning for persons who are severely hard of hearing should be appropriate, perhaps with some adjustments, for postimplant patients. Implantees should be encouraged to avail themselves of such help, accepting the reality that the implant has only partially restored them to normal communicative pursuits.

PRELINGUAL LOSS

The term *prelingual* is difficult to define and often remains undefined in implant reports. The term *perilingual* is coming into more frequent use in distinguishing those with congenital loss from those whose loss occurred between birth and around age 5 years. In this chapter the term *prelingual* is retained and will refer to patients whose hearing loss has prevented them from either learning or maintaining speech and language skills through the auditory channel. It includes those who have suffered a profound hearing loss at a very early age as well as those with congenital loss (present at birth). Some have adopted sign as a language modality and others cope through lipreading and through speech that is intelligible to widely varying degrees. With respect to implants, the lack of orientation and memory for sound places these patients in an entirely different situation than the postlingually impaired.

Relatively few adults with prelingual loss have had implants to date. According to Eisenberg (1982), 4 of 12 prelingual patients who received an implant at the House Ear Institute failed to use it. No consistent pattern emerged except that 3 of the 4 were said to have had emotional and personality traits causing difficulty in their lives. The 8 patients who did use the device responded to gross sounds and to music, and the quality of their voices was reported to have changed. Warble-tone thresholds were the same as for the postlingual group. Most of the subjects experienced some unpleasant reactions such as dizziness, pulsation of the eyes, and sensations in the chest and throat upon the introduction of electrical stimulation and, in some cases, several months were required for sound sensation to localize to the ear. No followup reports on the status of the 8 "users" have appeared thus far. Of special interest is the question whether any of them have achieved some skills in speech reception or production.

The Vienna investigators (Burian, Hochmair–Desoyer, & Eisenwort, 1986) included 13 prelingual loss patients in one of their reports, according to an inspection of their tabular data. No specific information was offered on these patients except that all but one were confined to the lowest performing group.

Fugain, Meyer, and Chouard (1985), in France, described 58 patients of whom 36 were congenitally deaf and 22, postlingually deaf. The authors noted a big difference in the test responses of those who were congenitally and postlingually deaf, stating that most of the congenitally deaf patients demonstrate very limited results whereas the postlingual patients can rapidly and without lipreading identify words and sentences.

More recently, Clark and colleagues (1987) described six patients with prelingual loss — three adults, one teenager, and two children — who had received a Nucleus multichannel implant. Only the adults are discussed here. Two of the three adults had profound losses, diagnosed in the one case at 15 months and in the other at 3 years; one of the two was implanted at age 24 years and the other at age 25 years. Both were educated almost entirely by sign and were occasional users of the implant. Both scored poorly on the simplest of auditory tests and their motivation was reported as "questionable." The third adult was diagnosed at the age of 3 years as having a severe–profound loss that over the succeeding 15 years became profound. Educated in an auditory/oral program in a normal school setting, she received an implant at age 22 years and subsequently used the implant regularly. She showed significant speech perception scores for male and female identification, vowels, consonants, open-set monosyllable words, and open-set CID sentences, in addition to a marked improvement in lipreading with the device.

Finally, Brimacombe and colleagues (1987) have reported on three prelingual patients who experienced subjective benefit from the Nucleus implant, which they wear during all waking hours. Except for the tests of prosody and visual enhancement, the MAC was generally too difficult for them, resulting in little or no objectively measured gain from the pre-implant condition. The authors attributed the subjective success of the three patients to their relatively young age, their high motivation, and their use of oral/aural communication in their everyday lives. With respect to the latter, the authors note a consistency in their findings with those of Eisenberg (1982) and of Clark and colleagues (1987).

IMPLICATIONS FOR COCHLEAR IMPLANTS IN CHILDREN

In terms of speech understanding, multichannel stimulation appears superior to that of single-channel. Moreover, multichannel systems continue to improve as newer designs and models are introduced, the improvement being reflected in increasingly higher scores for open-set spondees, sentences, and monosyllable words. In addition, evidence that speech understanding with the same implant may improve steadily over time, even without direct rehabilitative efforts, comes as an exciting development that has not been apparent in adults with single-channel stimulation. A reasonable expectation is that children with profound loss, given multichannel stimulation, would progress much more rapidly than with a single-channel system.

The multichannel devices have been reduced considerably in size over the past few years and are now comfortably wearable, closely corresponding to the body-type hearing aids. As a relatively large proportion of the speech processor space is devoted to batteries, further size reductions may be anticipated as greater efficiency in the power supply is achieved. Although fitting procedures for multichannel systems are more challenging than with single-channel systems, they are doubtless within the capabilities of audiologists experienced in working with hearing impaired children. Surgical aspects may be more complicated than with the simpler single-channel devices, but not forbidding (see Chapter 9), and there seems no reason to believe that long-term considerations would be any different than for single-channel systems.

The evidence at hand suggests, then, that if an implant is to be recommended for a child, the most appropriate choice, in terms of the potential for speech and language acquisition, would be one of the multichannel systems. The premise is that the child would thereby be provided with the most useful auditory information presently available. Recall, however, that the amount and location of stimulable nerve tissue along the cochlea cannot as yet be predicted accurately and, accordingly, neither can the usefulness of the sound that a given individual may receive. Conceivably, the provision of more flexible speech processing strategies with the newer devices, providing wider choices for the patient, might help alleviate this particular limitation.

Nevertheless, the continued reporting of open-set speech recognition, in some cases at high levels, by persons implanted in Vienna with Vienna single-channel devices cannot be ignored, despite lack of published results on any replications that may have been done in other countries. One fairly consistent occurrence is the seeming superiority of the intracochlear device over the extracochlear, although both are treated with the same signal processing scheme. In any event, the opportunity of selecting the best one of four electrodes in the intracochlear device for permanent stimulation, in combination with extensive care in signal processing, bears scrutiny. Hochmair and Hochmair–Desoyer (1985) described the electrode selection process as involving a large dynamic range with adequate input power for comfortable loudness, "proper" frequency equalization with broad band stimulation, and, according to Hochmair–Desoyer, Hochmair, and Stiglbrunner (1985), temporal processing data, notably gap-detection performance. Moreover, Hochmair–Desoyer, Hochmair, and von Wallenberg (1987) found that the addition of second formant information on the same electrode channel can further improve speech recognition postoperatively.

A larger question, of course, concerns whether an implant of any kind should be recommended. It must be stressed that little is known of the long-term effects from electrical stimulation, whether in reference to the auditory system specifically or to general health including psychological well-being. A recent report by Webb and colleagues (1988) was encouraging. On the basis of their studies exploring surgical trauma, otitis media, long-term electrical stimulation, and biocompatibility of materials, they concluded that intracochlear multielectrode stimulation is safe, provided that reasonable care is taken with the procedure.

Some histologic reports were pessimistic about long-term survival of cochlear neural tissue relative to cochlear implants (Lawrence & Johnsson, 1973; Otte, Schuknecht, & Kerr, 1978); others were optimistic (Spoendlin, 1975; Hinojosa & Marion, 1983). The available long-term records on adults suggest that the large majority are continuing to use their implants even after several years, but the estimates must be interpreted cautiously. They are at best subject to the well-known weaknesses of survey and questionnaire methods, and none of the published reports have presented the necessary details for a confident appraisal. What questions were asked, by whom, and how were they posed? How are the numbers of biological failures and mechanical breakdowns being verified? The number of nonusers could well increase at a faster rate after a few years as the inevitable mechanical breakdowns and perhaps biologic complications occur. In short, although reports of long-term adult usage of implants present a generally auspicious picture to date, accurate information in this respect through carefully designed and conducted surveys is needed. It must be realized that the available reports concerning implant usage generally pertain to periods less than 10 years, whereas the question with children may encompass 60 or 70 years.

The outcome of recent work with small numbers of young adult prelingual-loss patients (Brimacombe et al., 1987; Clark et al., 1987; Eisenberg, 1982) suggested that extra care must be exercised in decisions regarding cochlear implants for older children with prelingual loss, particularly those whose education and enculturation have been primarily through sign. For younger children with prelingual loss, little can be offered in the context of this chapter, except that the introduction of cochlear implants, and especially the recent findings on multichannel systems, provide grounds for optimism.

REFERENCES

Alpiner, J. C. (1986). Rehabilitation concepts with the cochlear implant. *Otolaryngologic Clinics of North America, 19,* 259–265.

Banfai, P., Karczaq, A., Kubik, S., Luers, P., Surth, W., & Banfai, S. (1987). Extracochlear eight- and 16-channel cochlear implants with percutaneous and transcutaneous transmission: Experiences with 129 patients. *Annals of Otology, Rhinology, and Laryngology, 96* (Suppl. 128), 118–120.

Beiter, A. L., Brimacombe, J. A., & Barker, M. J. (1987, September). *Speech recognition abilities in profoundly deafened adults using the Nucleus 22-channel cochlear implant system.* Paper presented at the annual meeting of the American Auditory Society, Chicago, IL.

Brandy, W. T. (1966). Reliability of voice tests of speech discrimination. *Journal of Speech and Hearing Research, 9,* 456–460.

Braud, C., Braud, E., Boudreaux, C., Steger, N., Mecklenburg, D. J., & Tobey, E. A. (1987, November). *Influence of cochlear prosthesis upon vowels produced in context.* Paper presented at the annual convention of the American Speech-Language-Hearing Association, New Orleans, LA.

Breaud, J., Hotard, M., Paternostro, J., Tobey, E. A., & Mecklenburg, D. J. (1987, November). *Articulatory timing in persons wearing multichannel cochlear implants.* Paper presented at the annual convention of the American Speech-Language-Hearing Association, New Orleans, LA.

Brimacombe, J. A., Beiter, A. L., Shallop, J. K., Martin, E. L., & Fowler, L. P. (1987, November). *Use of a multichannel cochlear implant by prelinguistically deafened adults.* Paper presented at the annual convention of the American Speech-Language-Hearing Association, New Orleans, LA.

Brown, A. M., Dowell, R. C., & Clark, G. M. (1987). Clinical results for postlingually deaf patients implanted with multichannel cochlear prostheses. *Annals of Otology, Rhinology, and Laryngology, 96* (Suppl. 128), 127–128.

Burian, K., Hochmair–Desoyer, I., & Eisenwort, B. (1986). The Vienna cochlear implant program. *Otolaryngologic Clinics of North America, 19,* 313–328.

Chouard, C. H., Fugain, C., Meyer, B., & Chabolle, F. (1986). The Chorimac 12: A multichannel intracochlear implant for total deafness. *Otolaryngologic Clinics of North America, 19,* 355–370.

Clark, G. M., Busby, P. A., Roberts, S. A., Dowell, R. C., Tong, Y. C., Blamey, P. J., Nienhuys, T. G., Mecklenburg, D. J., & Webb, R. L. (1987). Preliminary results for the Cochlear Corporation multi-electrode intracochlear implant on six prelingually deaf patients. *American Journal of Otology, 8,* 234–239.

Dankowski, K., McCandless, G., & Smith, L. (1988). How does a percutaneous multichannel multielectrode cochlear implant work. *Rocky Mountain Journal of Communication Disorders, 3,* 21–23.

Dent, L. J., Simmons, F. B., White, R. L., & Roberts, L. A. (1987). Speech perception by four single-channel cochlear implant users. *Journal of Speech and Hearing Research, 30,* 480–493.

Dowell, R. C., Mecklenburg, D. J., & Clark, G. M. (1986). Speech recognition for 40 patients receiving multichannel cochlear implants. *Archives of Otolaryngology, 112,* 1054–1059.

Eddington, D. K., Dobelle, W. H., Brackmann, D. E., Mladejovsky, M. G., & Perkin, J. L. (1978). Auditory prostheses research with multiple channel intracochlear stimulation in man. *Annals of Otology, Rhinology and Laryngology, 87* (Suppl. 53), 1–39.

Edgerton, B. J., Prietto, A., & Danhauer, J. L. (1983). Cochlear implant patient performance on the MAC battery. *Otolaryngologic Clinics of North America, 16,* 267–280.

Eisenberg, L. S. (1982). Use of the cochlear implant by the prelingually deaf. *Annals of Otology, Rhinology and Laryngology, 91* (Suppl. 91), 62–66.

Engelmann, L. R., Waterfall, M. K., & Hough, J. V. D. (1981). Results following cochlear implantation and rehabilitation. *Laryngoscope, 91,* 1821–1833.

Fourcin, A. J., Douek, E. E., Moore, B. C. J., Rosen, S., Walliker, J. R., Howard, D. M., Abberton, E., & Frampton, S. (1983). Speech perception with promontory stimulation. In C. W. Parkins & S. W. Anderson (Eds.), Cochlear prostheses: An international symposium. *Annals of the New York Academy of Sciences, 405,* 280–294.

Fretz, R. J., & Fravel, R. P. (1985). Design and function: A physical and electrical description of the 3M House cochlear implant system. *Ear and Hearing, 6* (Suppl.), 14S–19S.

Fugain, C., Meyer, B., & Chouard, C. H. (1985). Speech processing strategies and clinical results of the French multichannel cochlear implant. In R. A. Schindler & M. M. Merzenich (Eds.), *Cochlear implants* (pp. 433–451). New York: Raven Press.

Fujikawa, S., & Owens, E. (1978). Hearing aid evaluations for persons with total postlingual hearing loss. *Archives of Otolaryngology, 104,* 446–450.

Fujikawa, S., & Owens, E. (1979). Hearing aid evaluations for persons with postlingual hearing levels of 90 to 100 dB. *Archives of Otolaryngology, 105,* 662–665.

Gantz, B. J., McGabe, B. F., Tyler, R. S., & Preece, J. P. (1987). Evaluation of four cochlear implant designs. *Annals of Otology, Rhinology and Laryngology, 96* (Suppl. 128), 145–147.

Gantz, B. J., Tyler, R. S., McCabe, B. F., Preece, J. P., Lowder, M. W., & Otto, S. R. (1985). Initial results with two single-channel cochlear implants. In R. A. Schindler & M. M. Merzenich (Eds.), *Cochlear implants* (pp. 539–548). New York: Raven Press.

Hinojosa, R., & Marion, M. (1983). Histopathology of profound sensorineural deafness. In C. W. Parkins & S. W. Anderson (Eds.), Cochlear prostheses: An international sympiosium. *Annals of the New York Academy of Sciences, 405,* 459–483.

Hochmair, E. S., & Hochmair–Desoyer, I. J. (1985). Aspects of sound signal processing using the Vienna intra- and extracochlear implant. In R. A. Schindler & M. M. Merzenich (Eds.), *Cochlear implants* (pp. 101–110). New York: Raven Press.

Hochmair–Desoyer, I. J., Hochmair, E. S., & Stiglbrunner, H.K. (1985). Psychoacoustic temporal processing and speech understanding in cochlear implant patients. In R. A. Schindler & M. M. Merzenich (Eds.), *Cochlear implants* (pp. 291–304). New York: Raven Press.

Hochmair–Desoyer, I. J., Hochmair, E. S., & von Wallenberg, E. L. (1987). Comparative speech results obtained with different speech-coding strategies. *Annals of Otology, Rhinology, and Laryngology, 96* (Suppl. 128), 148.

Hopkinson, N. T., McFarland, W. F., Owens, E., Reed, C., Shallop, J., Tillman, T., Tyler, R. S., Williams, P. S., & Resnick, S. B. (1986). Report of the ad hoc committee on cochlear implants. *ASHA, 28,* 29–52.

House, W. F., Berliner, K. I., Eisenberg, L. S., Edgerton, B. J., & Thielemeir, M. A. (1981). The cochlear implant: 1980 update. *Acta Otolaryngologica, 91,* 457–462.

Kreul, E. J., Bell, D. W., & Nixon, J. C. (1969). Factors affecting speech discrimination test difficulty. *Journal of Speech and Hearing Research, 12,* 281–287.

Lawrence, M., & Johnsson, L. G. (1973). The role of the organ of Corti in auditory nerve stimulation. *Annals of Otology, Rhinology, and Laryngology, 82,* 464–472.

Leder, S. B., Spitzer, J. B., & Kirchner, J. C. (1987a). Speaking fundamental frequency of postlingually profoundly deaf adult men. *Annals of Otology, Rhinology, and Laryngology, 96,* 322–324.

Leder, S. B., Spitzer, J. B., & Kirchner, J. C. (1987b). Immediate effects of cochlear implantation on voice quality. *Archives of Oto-Rhino-Laryngology, 244,* 93–95.

Leder, S. B., Spitzer, J. B., Flevaris–Phillips, C., Milner, P., Kirchner, J. C., & Richardson, F. (1987a). Voice intensity of prospective cochlear implant candidates and normal hearing adult males. *Laryngoscope, 97,* 224–227.

Leder, S. B., Spitzer, J. B., Kirchner, J. C., Flevaris–Phillips, C., Milner, P., & Richardson, F. (1987b). Speaking rate of adventitiously deaf male cochlear implant candidates. *Journal of the Acoustical Society of America, 82,* 843–846.

Leder, S. B., Spitzer, J. B., Milner, P., Flevaris-Phillips, C., Richardson, F., & Kirchner, J.C. (1986). Reacquisition of contrastive stress in an adventitiously deaf speaker using a single-channel cochlear implant. *Journal of the Acoustical Society of America, 79,* 1967–1974.

Medwetsky, L., Boothroyd, A., & Hanin, L. (1987, November). *Objective changes in the speech of cochlear implantees.* Paper presented at the annual convention of the American Speech-Language-Hearing Association, New Orleans, LA.

Merzenich, M. M., Michelson, R. P., Pettit, C. R., Schindler, R. A., & Reid, M. (1973). Neural encoding of sound sensation evoked by electrical stimulation of the acoustic nerve. *Annals of Otology, Rhinology and Laryngology, 82,* 486–503.

Michelson, R. P. (1971a). Electrical stimulation of the human cochlea. *Archives of Otolaryngology, 93,* 317–323.

Michelson, R. P. (1971b). The results of electrical stimulation. *Annals of Otology, Rhinology and Laryngology, 80,* 914–919.

Moore, B. C. J. (1985). Speech coding for cochlear implants. In R. F. Gray (Ed.), *Cochlear implants* (pp. 163–179). San Diego, CA: College-Hill Press.

Morgan, D. E., Dirks, D. D., & Bower, D. R. (1979). Suggested threshold sound pressure levels for frequency-modulated (warble) tones in the sound field. *Journal of Speech and Hearing Disorders, 44,* 37–54.

Otte, J., Schuknecht, H. F., & Kerr, A. G. (1978). Ganglion cell populations in normal and pathological human cochleae. Implications for cochlear implantation. *Laryngoscope, 88,* 1231–1246.

Owens, E. (1961). Intelligibility of words varying in familiarity. *Journal of Speech and Hearing Research, 4,* 113–129.

Owens, E., Kessler, D. K., & Raggio, M. W. (1983). Results for some patients with cochlear implants on the Minimal Auditory Capabilities (MAC) battery. In C. W. Parkins & S. W. Anderson (Eds.), Cochlear prostheses: An international symposium. *Annals of the New York Academy of Sciences, 405,* 443–450.

Owens, E., Kessler, D. K., Raggio, M. W., & Schubert, E. D. (1985). Analysis and revision of the Minimal Auditory Capabilities (MAC) battery. *Ear and Hearing, 6,* 280–290.

Owens, E., Kessler, D. K., & Schubert, E. D. (1982). Interim assessment of cochlear implants. *Archives of Otolaryngology, 108,* 478–483.

Owens, E., & Raggio, M. (1988). Performance inventory for profound and severe loss (PIPSL). *Journal of Speech and Hearing Disorders, 53,* 42–56.

Portmann, M., Cazals, Y., & Negrevergne, M. (1986). Extracochlear implants. *Otolaryngologic Clinics of North America, 19,* 307–312.

Punch, J. L., Stone, R. E., Horii, Y., & Miyamoto, R. T. (1987, November). *Oral-nasal coupling in the speech of cochlear implantees.* Paper presented at the annual convention of the American Speech-Language-Hearing Association, New Orleans, LA.

Rebscher, S.J. (1985). Cochlear implant design and construction. In R. F. Gray (Ed.), *Cochlear implants* (pp. 74–123). San Diego, CA: College-Hill Press.

Risberg, A., Agelfors, E., Ossian–Cook, B., & Lindstrom, B. (1987). Results obtained with the Vienna extracochlear implant. *Annals of Otology, Rhinology and Laryngology, 96* (Suppl. 128), 117–118.

Rose, D. E., Facer, G. W., King, A. M., & Fabry, M. A. (1987). Results using 3M/

Vienna extracochlear implant in five patients. *Annals of Otology, Rhinology and Laryngology, 96* (Suppl. 128), 114–117.

Schindler, R. A., & Kessler, D. K. (1987). The UCSF/Storz cochlear implant: Patient performance. *American Journal of Otology, 8,* 247–255.

Schindler, R. A., Kessler, D. K., Jackler, R. K., & Merzenich, M. M. (In press). Multichannel cochlear implants: Current status and future directions. In Jonas T. Johnson (Ed.), *American Academy of Otolaryngology-Head and Neck Surgery: Introductory course* (Vol. I). St. Louis, MO: C. V. Mosby.

Schindler, R. A., Kessler, D. K., Rebscher, S. J., & Yanda, J. L. (1986). The University of California, San Francisco/ Storz cochlear implant program. *Otolaryngologic Clinics of North America, 19,* 287–305.

Spivak, L. G., Shapiro, W. H., Waltzman, S. B., & Cohen, N. L. (1987, November). *Cochlear implant performance as a function of time.* Paper presented at the annual convention of the American Speech-Language-Hearing Association, New Orleans, LA.

Spoendlin, H. (1975). Retrograde degeneration of the cochlear nerve. *Archives of Otolaryngology, 79,* 266–275.

Thielemeir, M. A. (1985). Status and results of the House Ear Institute cochlear implant project in adults. In R. A. Schindler & M. M. Merzenich (Eds.), *Cochlear implants,* (pp. 455–460). New York: Raven Press.

Thielemeir, M. A., Brimacombe, J. A., & Eisenberg, L. S. (1982). Audiological results with the cochlear implant. *Annals of Otology, Rhinology and Laryngology, 91* (Suppl. 91), 27–40.

Tong, Y. C., Clark, G. M., Blamey, P. J., Busby, P. A., & Dowell, R. C. (1982). Psychophysical studies for two multiple-channel cochlear implant patients. *Journal of the Acoustical Society of America, 71,* 153–160.

Tyler, R. S. (in press). Word recognition with some of the better 3M/Vienna cochlear-implant patients. *Archives of Otolaryngology.*

Tyler, R. S. (in preparation). Open-set word recognition in some of the better cochlear-implant patients.

Tyler, R. S., Lowder, M. W., Gantz, B. J., Otto, S. R., McCabe, B. F., & Preece, J. P. (1985). Audiological results with two single channel cochlear implants. *Annals of Otology, Rhinology, and Laryngology, 94,* 133–139.

Tyler, R. S., Preece, J. P, & Lowder, M. W. (1983). *The Iowa cochlear implant test battery.* Iowa City: University of Iowa, Department of Otolaryngology-Head and Neck Surgery.

Webb, R. L., Clark, G. M., Shepherd, R. K., Franz, B. K-H., & Pyman, B. C. (1988). The biologic safety of the Cochlear Corporation multiple-electrode intracochlear implant. *The American Journal of Otology, 9,* 8–13.

CHAPTER 4

WESLEY R. WILSON

EARLY BEHAVIORAL ASSESSMENT

During the past decade, considerable progress has been made in improving the behavioral methodologies used in assessment of auditory function of infants. A limited database now exists for measurements in the areas of sensitivity and speech–sound discrimination. The same operant procedures can be applied to temporal discrimination, as well as intensity and frequency discrimination tasks. This chapter focuses on the improvements in behavioral methodologies, provides samples of data from normally developing infants and profound hearing impaired infants, and attempts to demonstrate that both electrophysiologic and behavioral approaches are needed in determining auditory function as each approach provides answers to different questions.

Three assumptions are involved. The first assumption is that early intervention is desirable, provided adequate assessment occurs. This assumption underlies the concept that as soon as one can accomplish adequate assessment, all approaches to intervention, including the use of a cochlear prosthesis, should be considered. The basis for this assumption is that there can no longer be any question that normally developing infants are showing learned changes in speech and sound discrimination at least as early as 6 months of age. For example, Eilers, Gavin, and Wilson (1979) have shown that infants reared in Spanish-speaking environments make different discriminations at six months of age as compared to infants reared in English-speaking environments, based on the linguistic rules of the respective language environment. If it is believed that infants must certainly come into the world with the abilities to perceive salient cues in any language (since they do not have information immediately as to which language they will be learning), then evidence of this type suggests that there are substantial learned responses occurring during very early childhood. It is counter-intuitive to believe that witholding auditory stimuli can be beneficial. Thus, the assumption that there is a free period of time during which auditory input makes little difference in later learning is no longer valid.

The second assumption is that the term "assessment" describes some manner of detailed evaluation and description of abilities and must be differentiated from "screening." The purpose of screening procedures is to define a subgroup of a total population that needs more detailed study (i.e., assessment). The more detailed study should facilitate appropriate intervention, complemented by continued assessment. The results of screening evaluations alone usually do not allow appropriate intervention. (A case-in-point is the indiscriminate placement of hearing aids on infants following neonatal screening.) A corollary to this assumption is that assessment should not be limited to sensitivity measures only. In the hearing assessment of adults, the audiologist devotes substantial time to the determination of both air-conduction and bone-conduction hearing sensitivity, based on a medical model of disease. As audiologists have approached the assessment of infants in a clinical setting, the presumption has often been that the primary focus should be on hearing sensitivity. In fact, much of the literature is devoted to discussions of methodologies for determining hearing sensitivity in infants with greater precision. The point of this argument is not to minimize the information available in such assessment, but rather to say that a view of auditory function as being tied predominantly to sensitivity is totally inappropriate. For example, central lesions of the auditory system may not manifest themselves in changes in peripheral hearing sensitivity. Furthermore, it may be realized from the literature available in infant speech perception that infants possess substantially greater auditory abilities than ordinary measurement procedures have assumed.

The third assumption is that the clinical assessment of hearing in infants is a necessary and desirable process, even given the present state of knowledge. Although clinician and researcher alike may be uncomfortable with the many voids in current knowledge concerning the auditory abilities of infants, the reality is that parents of infants with profound hearing loss are making decisions *now* regarding habilitative strategies. They expect informed guidance and have no sympathy for a position that suggests any delay in assessment and intervention for their baby.

Finally, a caveat: the present discussion is based on work over the past 10 years that has focused on infant auditory function and has involved the study of large numbers of normally developing infants. Procedures developed as a part of this work have been used by colleagues at the University of Washington, as well as by the author, in the clinical assessment of both hearing impaired infants and developmentally disabled infants. The work has not been involved directly with infants or young children for whom cochlear implants were being considered and has not been designed to answer the question whether cochlear implants should be used with children. However, it is hoped that data generated over the past few years might be applicable to the cochlear implant as well as to other habilitative measures. (See Thompson & Wilson, 1984, and Wilson & Thompson, 1984, for a detailed review of recent work in the area of behavioral assessment in children. Parts of this chapter are abstracted from these sources.)

AUDITORY THRESHOLDS—AUDIOGRAMS

BEHAVIOR OBSERVATION AUDIOMETRY (BOA)

Behavioral assessment of auditory thresholds of infants is based on observation of overt responses to controlled auditory signals. There are two general approaches that have been used clinically. They can be differentiated by whether or not reinforcement is employed. When no reinforcement is used, the procedure is usually called *behavior observation audiometry* (BOA). As the name implies, this is a passive approach. The examiner observes changes in behavior (responses) that are time-locked to auditory signals, but does not assume an active "teaching" role. As an estimator of hearing sensitivity, the BOA procedure has serious limitations because infant responses are not brought under stimulus control by the examiner. For neonates, suprathreshold stimulation is required to elicit reflexive responses such as startle or eye widening. Older infants demonstrate "awareness" or spontaneous head-turn responses at reasonably low intensity levels (Downs & Sterritt, 1967; Suzuki & Sato, 1961; Thompson & Thompson, 1972), but the probability of obtaining a response is dependent on the nature of the auditory stimulus (Eisenberg, 1976; Hoversten & Moncur, 1969; Ling, Ling, & Doehring, 1970; Thompson & Thompson, 1972); response habituation is likely (Moore, Thompson, & Thompson, 1975) and variability is high (Thompson & Weber, 1974). Because BOA lacks precision as an indicator of hearing status, it is best viewed as a screening procedure, albeit the only available behavioral procedure for some profoundly retarded children, or very young infants who cannot be conditioned to respond to auditory signals. Although Gans (1987) has described procedures for improving the BOA outcome in such cases, alternative electrophysiologic procedures must nonetheless be considered.

VISUAL REINFORCEMENT AUDIOMETRY (VRA)

When reinforcement is employed, the testing approach is a form of operant conditioning in which the auditory signal (discriminative stimulus) cues the availability of reinforcement following the desired response behavior. Among conditioning procedures for very young children, a procedure called *visual reinforcement audiometry* (VRA) has emerged as a successful assessment tool for infants 6 months through 2 years of age. In this procedure, head turns toward a sound source are reinforced by an attractive visual stimulus (animated toy). Suzuki and Ogiba (1960, 1961) first reported on a conditioning procedure involving the localization response, calling the procedure *conditioned orientation reflex* (COR) audiometry. In the initial stages of conditioning, a pure tone was presented through a loudspeaker at an intensity level estimated to be 30 to 40 dB above the infant's threshold. One second later a visual stimulus (illuminated doll) was presented from the same location. The combined tone and light stimulus lasted for about 4 seconds. After a few conditioning trials, the timing sequence was changed so that the visual stimulus followed the auditory stimulus and was presented only if the child had first responded to the tone. The procedure allowed successful threshold estimates for over 80 percent of children in the 1 to 3 year age category, but less than 50 percent for infants under 1 year of age.

Liden and Kankkunen (1969) were the first to use the term *visual reinforcement audiometry* (VRA) to describe a modified COR procedure that they developed. As they accepted any type of response behavior that could be judged (at least for young infants), and always provided "reinforcement," their procedure differed markedly from that described by Suzuki and Ogiba (1960, 1961). Other early studies also reported on the use of VRA procedures for assessment of hearing sensitivity in infants and young children (Haug, Baccaro, & Guilford, 1967; Motta, Facchini, & D'Auria, 1970). Generally, these studies suggested that the lower age limit for widespread use of the procedure was 12 months, although Haug and colleagues (1967) reported clinical success with a small number of infants in the 5- to 12-month range.

While these studies provided support for the use of VRA, there remained a question as to the lower age limit for the procedure as well as to the specific reinforcing value of the visual stimulus because control (no reinforcement) groups were not included for comparison results. Also, it was not clear if the type of visual stimulus employed had any bearing on its effectiveness as a reinforcer. A series of studies conducted at the University of Washington explored auditory localization behavior as a function of reinforcement conditions (Moore, Thompson, & Thompson, 1975; Moore, Wilson, & Thompson, 1977; Wilson & Moore, 1978). The subjects were normally developing infants; the auditory signal was a complex-noise stimulus presented at 70 dB SPL from a loud-speaker located at a 45 degree angle from the infant's front line of vision. Following each appropriate head-turn response, subjects in the experimental groups received reinforcement while the control group received no reinforcement. The test protocol included 30 test trials and 10 control trials randomly mixed; during the control trials, the test-room and control-room examiners recorded whether or not the infant turned toward the loudspeaker in the *absence* of an auditory stimulus. The outcomes of these studies may be summarized as follows: auditory localization behavior of 5- to 18-month old infants is strongly influenced by reinforcement and the type of reinforcement used has a systematic differentiated effect on head-turn response behavior. Visual stimuli containing movement, color, and contour are more apt to be effective reinforcers than less dimensional visual stimuli. This work has been extended to developmentally delayed children with similar results for slightly older children (Greenberg et al., 1978; Thompson, Wilson, & Moore, 1979). Primus (1987), using normally developing 17-month-old infants, also found that an animated reinforcer (as used in the previously described studies) resulted in significantly more responses than did an inanimate reinforcer.

Wilson, Moore, and Thompson (1976) studied soundfield auditory thresholds using VRA. Ninety normally developing infants between 5 and 18 months were divided into groups of 15, according to age. The auditory stimulus was complex noise, and threshold sampling followed a protocol of attenuating the signal 20 dB after each positive head-turn response and increasing the signal 10 dB after each failure to respond. Control intervals were included as before. All appropriate responses were visually reinforced by an animated toy. Threshold was defined as the lowest presentation level at which the infant responded a minimum of three times out of a maximum of six signal presentations. Results are shown in Figure 4–1 and are reported in dB SPL. (Note: Audiometric thresholds and intensity levels are in dB SPL, because no standard exists for converting these values into comparable HL for speaker systems. For comparative purposes, the modal threshold of normal hearing young adults listeners was 20 dB SPL, with a range of 10 dB SPL to 20 dB SPL,

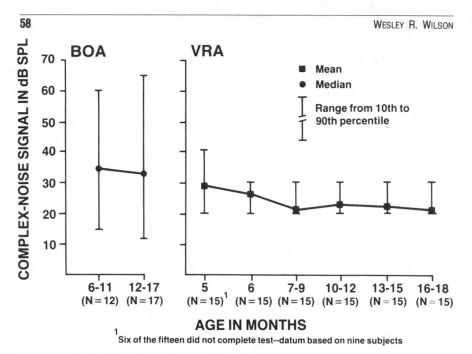

FIGURE 4-1. Auditory thresholds of infants obtained by BOA and VRA methods.From Wilson, Moore, and Thompson (1976). *Soundfield auditory thresholds of infants utilizing visual reinforcement audiometry (VRA)*. Paper presented at the annual convention of the American Speech and Hearing Association, Houston.

under the same signal and measurement-step conditions.) As can be noted, the average response levels improved slightly with age, ranging from 21 to 29 dB SPL. The 10th and 90th percentile points were 20 and 40 dB SPL for the 5-month old infants and 20 and 30 dB SPL for the 6-to 18-month old infants. Compared to thresholds obtained by BOA for the same ages (from Thompson & Weber, 1974), the VRA thresholds are lower. But of far greater importance is the reduced variability of response associated with the VRA procedure. For infants 6 months old and above, the range between the 10th and 90th percentile is reduced from the 45 to 50 dB reported for BOA to 10 dB (or one measurement step) for VRA. The clinical implications of this study are substantial: (1) thresholds obtained from infants do not vary dramatically as a function of age and are elevated only slightly from those obtained from adults using the same test protocol; (2) even more importantly, the range of thresholds for the population of presumed normal hearing infants was very small, indicating that the values obtained can serve a usable function as clinical norms — a finding in direct contrast to the very wide dispersion demonstrated for BOA procedures; and (3) the procedure is economical of time and highly applicable to infants 6 months of age and older.

Whereas the above study used a broad-band signal, Wilson and Moore (1978) investigated the use of VRA with pure-tone stimuli in a soundfield. Two groups of 15 normally developing infant subjects — 6 to 7 months of age and 12-to-13 months of age — were selected by the same criteria as in previous studies. Pure tones of 500, 1000, and 4000 Hz with a 5-percent warble served as the auditory stimuli. Because obtained thresholds did not vary systematically as a function of infant age (at least, given the 10-dB step size used in this experiment), the results for the two groups of infants were collapsed and compared to a group of young adults (N = 20), tested with the same protocol and step size, as shown in Figure 4–2. The difference in obtained thresholds is from 5 to 12 dB, depending on frequency, with the range of responses similar for

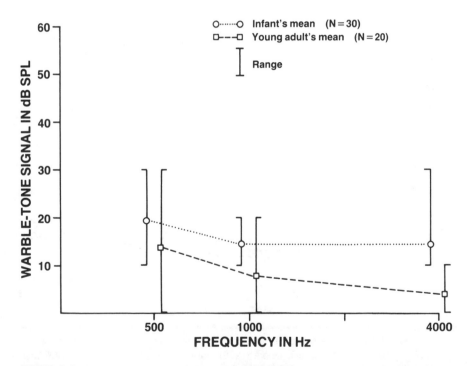

FIGURE 4–2. VRA pure-tone soundfield thresholds for infants and adults. From Wilson and Moore (1978). *Pure-tone earphone thresholds of infants utilizing visual reinforcement audiometry (VRA).* Paper presented at the annual convention of the American Speech and Hearing Association, San Francisco.

both the infant and the adult groups. In a study similar to that of Wilson and Moore but accomplished in a different laboratory, Goldman (1979) also used VRA with infants 6- to 12-months of age. His mean thresholds for infants were 17 dB SPL at 500 Hz, 14 dB SPL at 1000 Hz, 17 dB SPL at 2000 Hz, and 15 dB SPL at 4000 Hz. Figure 4–3 provides a comparison of the Goldman (1979) and Wilson and Moore (1978) data, with both data sets plotted relative to young adult thresholds for the same signal and protocol conditions. There is excellent agreement across studies accomplished in two different settings with both studies demonstrating that a pure-tone signal can be used successfully with infants.

Thompson and Folsom (1985) and Primus and Thompson (1985) have also studied the effectiveness of various signals in the VRA paradigm. Both studies found that whereas stimulus characteristics play an important role in eliciting spontaneous responses, they do not appear to influence response behavior after conditioning has been established.

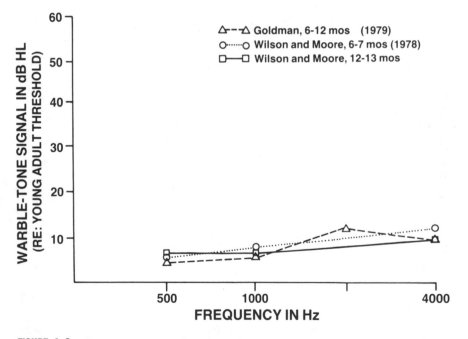

FIGURE 4–3. VRA pure-tone soundfield threshold agreement across studies using a clinical protocol. Adapted from Wilson and Moore (1978). *Pure-tone earphone thresholds of infants utilizing visual reinforcement audiometry (VRA).* Paper presented at the annual convention of the American Speech and Hearing Association, San Francisco; and Goldman (1979). *Response of infants to warble-tone signals presented in soundfield using visual reinforcement audiometry.* Unpublished master's thesis, University of Cincinnati, Ohio.

This means that the examiner may select signal type based on the clinical exigencies of the case and not be restricted because of a fear of degrading response behavior.

Because many clinical and research questions dealing with auditory sensitivity and perceptual abilities of infants demand individual ear data as well as greater signal specificity, Moore and colleagues (1976) developed a headband and harness made of elastic and Velcro to hold a standard TDH-39 earphone and MX-41/AR cushion in place. Twenty infants between 6 and 8 months of age were selected as in the previous studies. The auditory signal was the same as was the threshold protocol. Thresholds were obtained for both ears and soundfield; mean thresholds were 35 dB SPL for earphones and 28.5 dB SPL for the soundfield. Comparing the infant results to a small sample of young, normal-hearing adults, using the same signal and test protocol, the adult thresholds were approximately 10 dB better than the infant thresholds for each condition. The difference between the minimum audible field (MAF) and minimum audible pressure (MAP) values was the same — 6 dB for both groups.

Wilson and Moore (1978), as part of the study on VRA with puretones in the soundfield, also investigated the use of VRA with pure-tone stimuli under earphones using two groups of normal infant subjects, one group 6- to 7-months of age and the other 12- to 13-months of age. The headband and harness made of elastic and Velcro, or a modified child's headset, held a standard TDH-39 earphone and MX-41/AR cushion in place on the left ear of each subject. Average thresholds were 33 dB SPL at 500 Hz and 24 dB SPL at 1000 and 4000 Hz. At 500 Hz, the younger infants are set apart from the older infants with poorer mean thresholds. Figure 4–4 groups the infant data and provides a comparison with a group of normal-hearing young adults run under the same conditions, including the 10-dB step size. Whereas the infant/adult soundfield differences were 5 dB at 500 Hz and 12 dB at 4000 Hz in the same study, the infant/adult earphone differences were on the order of 16 dB at 500 Hz and 11 dB at 4000 Hz. These findings first led to the question of the possible effect of leakage around the earphone cushion as one cause of the elevated low-frequency earphone thresholds for the infants. However, a study by Hesketh (1983) utilized a subminiature microphone mounted in the MX-41/AR cushion to record acoustic energy in the canal during testing of infants, children,and young adults. Her results do not support a finding of differential energy in the canal. In a recent study, Berg and Smith (1983) reported pure-tone threshold values quite similar to those of Wilson and Moore (1978) including elevated low-frequency thresholds for infants tested with an earphone. Further study is needed to determine the cause of these apparent differences.

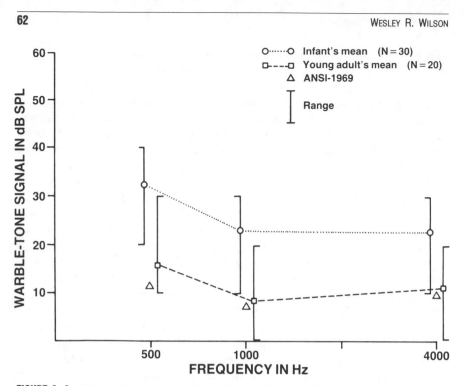

FIGURE 4–4. VRA pure-tone earphone thresholds for infants and adults. From Wilson and Moore (1978). *Pure-tone earphone thresholds of infants utilizing visual reinforcement audiometry (VRA).* Paper presented at the annual convention of the American Speech and Hearing Association, San Francisco.

Nozza and Wilson (1984), as a part of a study on critical ratios in infants, used a computer-controlled adaptive procedure to develop earphone auditory thresholds in quiet and in noise. Their procedure employed a 5-dB step size with threshold defined as the mean of the intensity levels of the last 8 turn-around points. Of interest here is the fact that the infants were able to accomplish this psychophysical procedure and yielded pure-tone thresholds in quiet of 19 dB SPL at 1000 Hz and 15 dB SPL at 4000 Hz under earphones.

TANGIBLE REINFORCEMENT OPERANT CONDITIONING AUDIOMETRY (TROCA)

Another example of an operant conditioning paradigm makes use of a bar-press response coupled with edible reinforcement and is called *tangible reinforcement operant conditioning audiometry* (TROCA). In 1968, Lloyd, Spradlin, and Reid described the use of TROCA with three normally developing infants 7, 15, and 18 months of age. Fulton, Gorzycki, and Hull (1975), using pure-tones and earphone presentation, studied 12 children between 9 and 25 months of age with a median age of 12 months and found the procedure to be successful with 7 of the children. Of the remaining 5, 2 were withdrawn by their parents and 3 did not demonstrate stimulus control. All of the subjects who successfully completed the task were 12 months of age or older. A second study using TROCA and VROCA (bar-press response coupled with visual reinforcement) followed 32 infants between the ages of 7 and 20 months (Wilson & Decker, 1977). Threshold was determined by a bracketing procedure using 10-dB measurement steps. The signals were warbled pure-tones of 0.5, 1.0, 2.0, and 4.0 kHz, presented in a soundfield. The procedure was successful with 64 percent of the infants under 12 months of age, and with 82 percent of those 13 to 20 months of age. Multiple test sessions were required.

PREDICTABILITY OF LATER TESTS FROM EARLY TEST RESULTS

A question of interest relates to how accurately early behavioral audiograms predict degree of impairment as determined by later testing. Talbott (1984) followed 25 infants who were moderately to profoundly hearing impaired and found that differences in serial audiograms were no greater than 15 dB at any single frequency and most typically were on the order of 0 to 5 dB. VRA was used as the first test procedure and the results were very predictive of later test results at 3-, 4-, and 5-years of age, using play and standard audiometry.

Throughout the progress of the recent studies of auditory thresholds of infants, comparisons between adult and infant results have been provided. One reason for the comparison is that the clinician needs to know the adult/infant threshold relationships in terms of assignment of "normal" threshold to obtained results as a function of age. Specific to this point is the important fact that, although the studies reported provide very tight groupings of obtained threshold values, caution must be exercised in generalizing these values to other clinics. Differences in signal, soundfield test environments, and VRA test protocol may lead to differences in individual clinic normative values. Each clinic should see a small sample of normally developing infants to establish normative data for that setting. The sample need not be large, based on the findings that infant dispersion data in these procedures are equal to that of young adults in the same conditions.

In terms of clinical utility, it has been the experience of Wilson and colleagues that the VRA procedure is equally as robust as the TROCA/

VROCA procedure and far less time consuming. Normally developing infants make head turns toward a sound source in the first few months of life. The localization response represents a behavioral "window" through which many aspects of auditory behavior can be studied. If an infant's localization behavior deviates markedly from the normal developmental pattern, there is strong reason to suspect the presence of either hearing loss or other problems, such as mental retardation. While there is a decided tendency for infants to turn initially toward "interesting" or "novel" auditory stimuli, there is a limit to the number of times head turns will occur to repeated stimuli (Moore et al., 1975; 1977). Proper use of operant conditioning procedures greatly reduces this habituation of response.

SUMMARY STATEMENTS ON THRESHOLD ASSESSMENT

The following list summarizes statements on threshold assessment:

1. Appropriate procedures include VRA and TROCA.
2. Pure-tones (warble), noise (broadband or passband), and speech may be used as auditory signals.
3. Test stimuli may be presented with earphones, a bone oscillator, or in a soundfield.
4. The earliest ages at which pure-tone behavioral audiograms can be obtained are as follows: normally developing infants — 6 months; infants with hearing loss — 6 to 12 months; infants with multiple handicaps — 6 to 18 months.
5. Intrasubject variability of pure-tone behavioral audiograms from infants is equal to or greater than in adults; intersubject variability is smaller than in adults. Regarding test–retest reliability, results are repeatable within one measurement step (10 dB). With respect to validity, obtained thresholds show no change or *slight* improvement with age that is signal specific and on the order of 10 dB.
6. Limited research results to date suggest high predictability of later test results from early behavioral audiograms.

ASSESSMENT OF SUPRA-THRESHOLD AUDITORY ABILITIES

Whereas the VRA threshold task involves detection of the presence or absence of a signal, supra-threshold tasks involve detection of a change in the signal. Eilers, Wilson, and Moore (1977) developed a procedure called the *Visually Reinforced Infant Speech Discrimination* (VRISD) paradigm to study developmental changes in discrimination as a function of age. All details of the VRA paradigm remained the same, except that one syllable of a recorded contrastive pair was presented at a repetition rate of 1 syllable per second at 50 dB SPL. While the infant was entertained at midline, the syllable was changed during a 4-second interval, with the temporal pattern of repetitions held constant. The infant was reinforced for a head turn to the change in signal by the activation of an animated toy. Three studies using the VRISD procedure (Eilers, Wilson, & Moore, 1977,1979; Eilers, Gavin, & Wilson, 1979) have shown that a high percentage of infants 6- to 14-months of age can be tested for discrimination of subtle speech contrasts. Furthermore, it has been demonstrated that the VRISD paradigm can provide data on individual infants on a repeated basis in order to obtain information concerning discrimination of a variety of contrasts over time. Some infants have been tested on as many as 10 speech contrasts in as few as three 20-minute sessions. The possibilities for applying this procedure to disordered populations are exciting. For example, because this discrimination procedure does not require receptive language abilities, as other tests of auditory discrimination for children do, testing of discrimination function can occur at a very early age. Further, as more information about the discrimination abilities of normal infants becomes available, a normative guide against which to compare performance of youngsters who are developmentally delayed will evolve. Resnick, Bookstein, and Talkin (1982) have described the results of preliminary work in this direction.

Diefendorf (1981) made use of the basic VRISD paradigm to study binaural fusion with infants 6- to 8-months old. Binaural fusion is the capacity of the auditory system to integrate separate inputs to the two ears into a single auditory percept. When the two ears are stimulated by dichotic speech signals (signals differing with respect to each other in one or more signal parameters), a listener perceives one central image and is incapable of separating the individual speech signals. When the left ear-only or right ear-only is stimulated, no centrally fused subjective image is formed. In his study, Diefendorf used two computer-generated speechlike vowels made up of a high and low passband each. The four waveforms (two vowels × two passbands) could be instrumentally presented with the low passband of vowel one combined with the high passband of either vowel one or vowel two. Likewise, the low passband of vowel two could be combined with the high passband of either vowel two or vowel one. The resultant four signals could be presented in diotic or dichotic mix. His results indicated that 6- to 8-month-old infants demonstrate fusion of auditory information in the central auditory system.

Three studies (Bull, Schneider, & Trehub, 1981; Trehub, Bull, & Schneider, 1981; Nozza & Wilson, 1984) have explored the topic of masking with infants using head-turn procedures. Masking studies not only provide information relative to the effect of noise (or other masking signals) on thresholds, but also on the basic frequency selectivity of the ear. Masking is a consequence of the ear's limited frequency selectivity; that is, as the energy in a masking stimulus approaches a test stimulus in frequency, there is an increase in the masking effect. Collectively these studies indicate that the use of a masking signal in a clinical paradigm should produce similar results in infants and adults. In another approach to the study of frequency resolution, Olsho and colleagues (1982) have utilized the reinforced head-turn procedure to study frequency discrimination in infants.

BEHAVIORAL AND ELECTROPHYSIOLOGIC TESTING

Behavioral testing may be described as a learned response to an auditory signal, whereas evoked response testing involves a measurement of the responsivity of the neural system. Both behavioral and electrophysiologic procedures should be used, along with tests of middle-ear function, in assessing the auditory function of children. The three approaches complement one another and provide answers to different questions.

CONCLUSION

It would seem unconscionable to consider an implant procedure with young children unless the most careful pre- and postoperative assessments of auditory function possible occur. This need for study goes beyond the normal need for proper patient care, because so little data are available to guide further development of the devices, the assessment and candidate selection protocols, and the training regimens.

ACKNOWLEDGMENT

Research at the Child Development and Mental Retardation Center, University of Washington, has been supported in part by grants from the Deafness Research Foundation; the National Foundation — March of Dimes; Maternal and Child Health Services; and the National Institute of Child Health and Human Development.

REFERENCES

Berg, K. M., & Smith, M. C. (1983). Behavioral thresholds during infancy. *Journal of Experimental Child Psychology, 35,* 409–425.

Bull, D., Schneider, B. A., & Trehub, S. E. (1981). The masking of octave-band noise by broad-spectrum noise: A comparison of infant and adult thresholds. *Perception and Psychophysics, 30,* 101–106.

Diefendorf, A. O. (1981). *An investigation of one aspect of central auditory function in an infant population utilizing a binaural resynthesis (fusion) task.* Unpublished doctoral dissertation, University of Washington, Seattle.

Downs, M. P., & Sterritt, G. M. (1967). A guide to newborn and infant hearing screening programs. *Archives of Otolaryngology, 85,* 15–22.

Eilers, R. E., Gavin, W., & Wilson, W. R. (1979). Linguistic experience and phonemic perception in infancy: A crosslinguistic study. *Child Development, 50,* 14–18.

Eilers, R. E., Wilson, W. R., & Moore, J. M. (1977). Developmental changes in speech discrimination in infants. *Journal of Speech and Hearing Research, 20,* 766–780.

Eilers, R. E., Wilson, W. R., & Moore, J.M. (1979). Speech discrimination in the language-innocent and the language-wise: A study in the perception of voice onset time. *Journal of Child Language, 6,* 1–18.

Eisenberg, R. B. (1976). *Auditory competence in early life — The roots of communicative behavior.* Baltimore: University Park Press.

Fulton, R. T., Gorzycki, P. A., & Hull, W. L. (1975). Hearing assessment with young children. *Journal of Speech and Hearing Disorders, 40,* 397–404.

Gans, D. P. (1987). Improving behavior observation audiometry testing and scoring procedures. *Ear and Hearing, 8,* 92–100.

Goldman, T. M. (1979). *Response of infants to warble-tone signals presented in sound-field using visual reinforcement audiometry.* Unpublished master's thesis, University of Cincinnati, Ohio.

Greenberg, D. B., Wilson, W. R., Moore, J. M., & Thompson, G. (1978). Visual reinforcement audiometry (VRA) with young Down's syndrome children. *Journal of Speech and Hearing Disorders, 43,* 448–458.

Haug, O., Baccaro, P., & Guilford, F. R. (1967). A pure-tone audiogram on the infant: The PIWI technique. *Archives of Otolaryngology, 86,* 435–440.

Hesketh, L. J. (1983). *Pure-tone thresholds and ear-canal pressure levels in infants, young children, and adults.* Unpublished master's thesis, University of Washington, Seattle.

Hoversten, G., & Moncur, J. (1969). Stimuli and intensity factors in testing infants. *Journal of Speech and Hearing Research, 12,* 687–702.

Liden, G., & Kankkunen, A. (1969). Visual reinforcement audiometry. *Acta Otolaryngologica, 67,* 281–292.

Ling, D., Ling, A. H., & Doehring, D. G. (1970). Stimulus response and observer variables in the auditory screening of newborn infants. *Journal of Speech and Hearing Research, 13,* 9–18.

Lloyd, L. L., Spradlin, J. E., & Reid, M. J. (1968). An operant audiometric pro-

cedure for difficult-to-test patients. *Journal of Speech and Hearing Disorders,*
33, 236–245.

Moore, J. M., Thompson, G., & Thompson, M. (1975). Auditory localization of
infants as a function of reinforcement conditions. *Journal of Speech and*
Hearing Disorders, 40, 29–34.

Moore, J. M., Wilson, W. R., Lillis, K. E., & Talbott, S. A. (1976, November).
Earphone audiometry thresholds of infants utilizing visual reinforcement audi-
ometry (VRA). Paper presented at the annual convention of the American
Speech and Hearing Association, Houston, Texas.

Moore, J. M., Wilson, W. R., & Thompson, G. (1977). Visual reinforcement of
head-turn responses in infants under 12-months of age. *Journal of Speech and*
Hearing Disorders, 42, 328–334.

Motta, G., Facchini, G. M., & D'Auria, E. (1970). Objective conditioned-reflex
audiometry in children. *Acta Otolaryngologica, Suppl. 273,* 1–49.

Nozza, R. J., & Wilson, W. R. (1984). Masked and unmasked pure-tone thresholds of infants and adults: Development of auditory frequency selectivity
and sensitivity. *Journal of Speech and Hearing Research, 27,* 613–622.

Olsho, L. W., Schoon, C., Sakai, R., Turpin, R., & Sperduto, V. (1982). Preliminary
data on frequency discrimination in infancy. *Journal of the Acoustical Society*
of America, 71, 509–511.

Primus, M. A. (1987). Response and reinforcement in operant audiometry. *Jour-*
nal of Speech and Hearing Disorders, 52, 294–299.

Primus, M. A., & Thompson, G. (1985). Response strength of young children in
operant audiometry. *Journal of Speech and Hearing Research, 28,* 539–547.

Resnick, S. B., Bookstein, E. W., & Talkin, D. (1982, November). *Clinical measure-*
ment of nonsense syllable discrimination in infants. Paper presented at the
annual convention of the American Speech-Language-Hearing Association,
Toronto.

Suzuki, T., & Ogiba, Y. (1960). A technique of pure-tone audiometry for children
under three years of age: Conditioned orientation reflex (COR) audiometry.
Revue de Laryngologie, 81, 33–45.

Suzuki, T., & Ogiba, Y. (1961). Conditioned orientation reflex audiometry.
Archives of Otolaryngology, 74, 192–198.

Suzuki, T., & Sato, I. (1961). Free field startle response audiometry. *Annals of Otol-*
ogy, Rhinology, and Laryngology, 70, 998–1007.

Talbott, C. B. (1984). *A longitudinal study comparing infants' responses to pure tones*
and speech using two behavioral test paradigms. Paper presented at the Audiology Update 1984: Pediatric Audiology Conference, Newport, Rhode Island.

Thompson, G., & Folsom, R. C. (1985). Reinforced and nonreinforced head-turn
responses of infants as a function of stimulus bandwidth. *Ear and Hearing, 6,*
125–129.

Thompson, M., & Thompson, G. (1972). Response of infants and young children
as a function of auditory stimuli and test methods. *Journal of Speech and*
Hearing Research, 15, 699–707.

Thompson, G., & Weber, B. A. (1974). Responses of infants and young children
to behavior observation audiometry (BOA). *Journal of Speech and Hearing*

Disorders, 39, 140–147.

Thompson, G., & Wilson, W. R. (1984). Clinical application of visual reinforcement audiometry. In T. Mahoney (Ed.), *Seminars in hearing: Early identification of hearing loss in infants* (pp. 85–99). New York: Thieme-Stratton, Inc.

Thompson, G., Wilson, W. R., & Moore, J. M. (1979). Application of visual reinforcement audiometry (VRA) to low-functioning children. *Journal of Speech and Hearing Disorders, 44,* 80–90.

Trehub, S. E., Bull, D., & Schneider, B. A. (1981). Infants' detection of speech in noise. *Journal of Speech and Hearing Research, 24,* 202–206.

Wilson, W. R., & Decker, T. N. (1977). [Auditory sensitivity in infants using TROCA]. Unpublished raw data.

Wilson, W. R., & Moore, J. M. (1978, November). *Pure-tone earphone thresholds of infants utilizing visual reinforcement audiometry (VRA).* Paper presented at the annual convention of the American Speech and Hearing Association, San Francisco.

Wilson, W. R., Moore, J. M., & Thompson, G. (1976, November). *Soundfield auditory thresholds of infants utilizing visual reinforcement audiometry (VRA).* Paper presented at the annual convention of the American Speech and Hearing Association, Houston.

Wilson, W. R., & Thompson, G. (1984). Behavioral audiometry. In J. Jerger (Ed.), *Pediatric audiometry: Current trends* (pp. 1–44). San Diego,CA: College-Hill Press.

THOMAS J. FRIA
JON K. SHALLOP

APPLICATION OF EVOKED POTENTIAL AUDIOMETRY TO CHILDREN WITH COCHLEAR IMPLANTS

n view of the substantial contribution that auditory evoked potentials have made to clinical audiology and otology, it seems natural to expect that these evoked potentials might play a role in cochlear implantation. However, the present and future utility of evoked potential audiometry in the assessment and management of cochlear implant patients is speculative in some respects. Accordingly, a re-examination of the topology and clinical application of evoked potential audiometry as well as an appraisal of the technique's strengths and limitations seems in order.

Operationally defined, auditory evoked potentials involve the use of scalp-derived responses that determine the presence or absence of an auditory impairment. If the estimation is consistent with an impairment, the purpose expands to include an approximation of the type, degree, laterality, and configuration of the loss. Extensive reviews of evoked potential audiometry have been presented by Fria (1980), Moore (1983), and Jacobson (1985).

ACOUSTICALLY DERIVED EVOKED POTENTIALS

THE RESPONSE ARRAY

The evoked responses (detected with scalp electrodes) that are typically used in audiometry occur in a 600 msec time period following stimu-

Schematic of Human Auditory Potentials

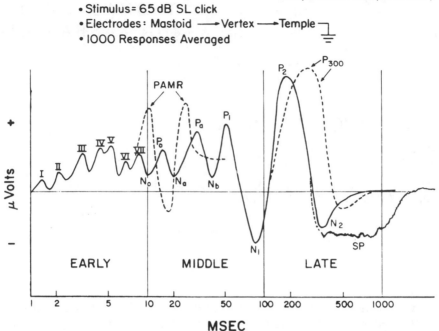

FIGURE 5-1. Auditory evoked potentials from an adult with normal hearing are depicted schematically. Stimulus was an unfiltered click presented at a rate of 1/sec. Unaveraged responses were recorded on FM tape and processed off-line to optimize the various responses by changing the bandpass filtering prior to signal averaging. The postauricular muscle response (PAMR), which occurs in some persons during evoked response audiometry, can be used as a response index even though it may cause problems by overshadowing other evoked response potentials, particularly those in the middle-latency category. Adapted from Picton, T. W., Woods, D. L., & Baribeau-Braun, J. (1977). Evoked response audiometry. *Journal of Otolaryngology, 6,* 90–119.

us onset, as shown by Shallop, Fria, and Kunov (1978) (Figure 5-1). The array of responses includes early latency, middle latency, and late components. The early components span the first 10 msec following stimulus onset. The auditory brainstem response (ABR), elicited with broad-band clicks and high frequency, brief tonebursts, is the most widely used member of this category. The scalp negative response at 10 msec, referred to as the SN10 (Davis & Hirsh, 1979), is also representative of the early latency responses. When high-pass filtering that extends downward to 20 to 30 Hz is employed during response acquisition, the SN10 consists of a slow negative wave which at high stimulus intensities occurs at approximately 10 msec. The SN10 has thus been directed to hearing loss estimations that incorporate low-frequency tonebursts as stimuli (Stapells et al., 1985).

The audiometric response array also includes the Pa/Na waves and the N1–P2 complex. The Pa wave occurs at approximately 25 msec and is the most prominent member of the middle latency components. Investigators have recently demonstrated that its derivation can be enhanced by stimulating with tone bursts or clicks at a rate of 40 per second. The resulting 40 Hz sinusoidal response, as with the SN10, has been directed to obtaining frequency specific information (Shallop, Osterhammel, & Tubergen, 1984; Stapells et al., 1985).

The N1–P2 complex constitutes the so-called "cortical" (late) response that predates all other components in terms of the estimation of hearing loss. This response, usually elicited with tone bursts, was first observed in the third decade of the 20th century, and, unfortunately, has been nearly forgotten as a viable component of evoked potential audiometry.

When considered on an individual basis, a given child might be assessed with any of the above components of evoked potential audiometry. The ABR response is the favored member of the array for providing an indication of the status of the subcortical auditory tract and is popular because of its relative ease of derivation and comparatively constant parameters; moreover, it is unaffected by various stages of sleep, natural or sedated, for achievement of a quiet state required of the patient in all evoked response testing. Unfortunately, the frequency specificity of ABR threshold estimations remains tenuous. The middle and late components, which can be elicited with frequency specific stimuli, constitute useful audiometric tools in awake, vigilant, and neurologically intact patients who can voluntarily maintain the necessary quiet state. However, the vulnerability of these components to sedated or natural sleep jeopardizes their widespread audiometric use in pediatric populations (Osterhammel, Shallop, & Terkildsen, 1985).

CLINICAL INDICATIONS AND APPLICATIONS

In most clinical situations, evoked potential audiometry should serve as a supplement to conventional, behaviorally based audiometric procedures. In other words, whenever conventional test results cannot clearly determine the presence or absence of impairment and the type, degree, laterality, and configuration of impairment, then evoked potential audiometry is indicated. The technique may also play a role in assessing the need and suitability of amplification (Mahoney, 1985). These issues obviously pertain to the management of the child with suspected hearing loss, and evoked potential audiometry may contribute to the information vital for such management.

Although these management issues are always important, they are essential for certain groups of children, including high risk newborns (Swigonski et al., 1987), post-meningitic children, and others whose severity of hearing loss may suggest their consideration for a cochlear implant. Hearing loss is an uncomfortably likely event in the first two groups, and it needs to be identified, characterized, and managed at the earliest opportunity. Because the issue is whether the child's residual auditory response is inadequate for conventional amplification and management, the preoperative evaluation of prospective implant candidates must include the ultimate and most extensive means available. For all children who are implant candidates, the clinician is obligated to explore both the behavioral and the electrophysiological indicators of the child's auditory integrity.

ADVANTAGES AND LIMITATIONS

The most obvious advantage of evoked potential audiometry is that it provides a reasonably accurate, ear-specific estimation of hearing loss in the very young child. It therefore lowers the age at which hearing loss can be objectively identified and quantified, leading to an earlier initiation of appropriate management. The technique is noninvasive and does not require the overt response of the child. Evoked potential audiometry cannot mimic the audiogram, but the procedure can give a reasonable estimation of auditory impairment. Thereby, it provides a strong impetus for close followup until the hearing loss can be defined more specifically.

Evoked potential audiometry does not constitute a test of hearing in the perceptual sense of the word. Rather, it tests the ability of auditory neurons to respond in roughly synchronous fashion to the most primitive (in perceptual terms) stimuli; that is, clicks and brief tonebursts. The results provide no indication of the child's ability to integrate auditory information at a higher level.

A related limitation pertains to the interpretation of a no-response result. This situation continues to challenge the accuracy of evoked potential audiometry, particularly when corroborating evidence from behavioral or acoustic immitance tests is not available. For example, the absence of a response in ABR testing can mean severe or profound impairment, a precipitous loss limited to the higher test frequencies, or an inability of the auditory system to respond synchronously in the context of relatively good hearing. A no-response result warrants particular caution when interpreting results. Another limitation is that many chil-

dren need to be sedated for evoked potential audiometry. Because sedation is not without risk, it should only be given at centers having the
facilities and personnel for appropriate administration and monitoring
of the procedures. The need for sedation thus restricts the full utilization
of evoked potential audiometry as a standard clinical tool.

Perhaps the most serious limitation of evoked potential audiometry
as it exists today is the lack of standardization in terms of the training of
personnel, test protocols, interpretation of results, and equipment specifi-
cations. Without such standards, the clinical application of the technique is dangerously susceptible to error. As the use of the procedure
becomes more widespread and this diversity expands from clinic to
clinic, the possibility for error continues to increase.

These limitations serve to emphasize the need for corroboration of
evoked potential audiometry by behavioral testing in the context of
habilitative planning.

EVOKED POTENTIALS AND THE COCHLEAR IMPLANT

Regarding the application of evoked auditory potentials to cochlear
implantation, one possibility is the ruling out of conventional amplification for the child who is a candidate for an implant. A review by
Mahoney (1985) has suggested that ABR data can be applied to the
assessment of the need for and suitability of amplification for children
who are hearing impaired. This is an important area, especially if the
cochlear implant candidate is a very young child for whom the question
of conventional amplification cannot be addressed with standard audiometric tests. However, the reliability and validity of the ABR in this
context is still uncertain. The most immediate advantage of evoked
potential audiometry lies in its role of assisting with the complete assessment of children who are being considered for a cochlear implant.
Again, the most judicious position to adopt is that it be integrated with
behavioral testing.

THE ELECTRICAL AUDITORY BRAINSTEM RESPONSE (EABR)

The electrical auditory brainstem response (EABR) employs an
electrical stimulus rather than the acoustic stimulus of the typical ABR.
Stypulkowski, van den Honert, and Kvistad (1986) and Miyamoto (1986)
have reported on recordings from subjects with single-channel cochlear
implants. Stimuli were transmitted directly to the implant in the cochlea
via the subcutaneously implanted coil. For preimplant measurement, how-

ever, cochlear stimulation was achieved with electrodes placed in the round window via an exploratory tympanotomy.

The waveform morphology and magnitude of the EABR are similar to those of the acoustic ABR except for the shorter absolute latency of the EABR and the typical absence in EABR of Wave I, obscured by stimulus artifact. Although EABR recordings are susceptible to contamination by electromyographic and vestibular responses, specific criteria for waveform morphology, magnitude, and latencies can be brought to bear in distinguishing auditory from nonauditory signals.

Stypulkowski and colleagues (1986) discuss several possible applications for EABRs to cochlear implantation on the basis of present knowledge: (1) for assessment of neural survival within the cochlea; (2) as an objective measure for loudness growth in the fitting of devices; (3) as a possible prognostic indicator for performance of future patients; and (4) for long-term tracking of cochlear or CNS functional integrity. The first application would depend primarily on Wave I responses, because of their known relation to auditory nerve activity. The frequent obliteration of Wave I from stimulus artifact, however, has been a discouraging factor. Application 2 is tenuous because there seems no clear relationship between EABR elicitation and subjective loudness of the stimulus. This application must be investigated more extensively. Application 3 holds more promise because of the likely relation between EABR waveform definition and the preservation of neural firing synchrony within the brainstem. Thus, the EABR may reflect the degree to which fine temporal structures in a stimulus can be perceived. The greatest promise for EABR at present probably rests with the fourth application, in which EABR might track changes in the auditory system resulting from long-term electrical stimulation. For example, any prevention or reversal of CNS degeneration with the restoration of peripheral input from an implant might be monitored with sequential EABRs.

In addition it might be mentioned that EABRs provide an objective method for assessing device function and failure. Regarding the second application, it must also be noted that the stimulus duration and pulse rate for EABR testing differs from the stimulation mode of the speech processor when the latter is used in its intended capacity, namely, the reception of speech.

Recent work employing multichannel implant stimulation by EABR has been done by Shallop and Beiter (unpublished data, 1988). Examples of EABRs recorded in an adult patient with a Nucleus multichannel cochlear implant are shown in Figure 5–2. The waveform morphology is similar to single-channel recordings. With a multichannel implant, however, it is possible to stimulate various portions of the cochlea (e.g., basal

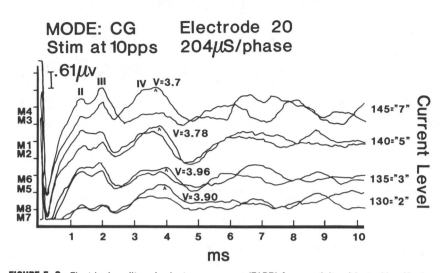

FIGURE 5-2. Electrical auditory brainstem respones (EABR) for an adult subject with a Nucleus multichannel cochlear implant. The cochlear implant was activated directly by software control through an interface unit connected to the speech processor. The stimulus was delivered using the standard transmission coil for the implant system. Current level was adjusted based on a subjective loudness scale (1 to 10 points) in which a value of 1 is threshold (120) and 8 is maximum comfort level (150). Values of 9 and 10 are avoided in any behavioral or EABR testing. Current level units (for 120, 150, and those on the ordinate) are based on a formula by Nucleus Corporation relating to microamperes.

versus apical regions) independently. In this example, the electrode is apical (electrode 20 or E20) and the patient had a behavioral current level threshold of 120 (see note in the figure legend regarding current level units). The waveform morphology does not include a Wave I because it is obscured by stimulus artifact.

Another example of multichannel EABRs, in this case from a child aged 2 years 5 months, is given in Figure 5-3. These tracings were obtained intraoperatively immediately after the surgeon had placed the 22 active bands of the Nucleus electrode array into the cochlea. The responses for electrode 20 demonstrate the apparent activation of the cochlear implant as well as an adequate neural population to produce a synchronous evoked potential. The response is obvious at a current level of 180 and seems to be absent at a current level of 160. Although not illustrated in the figure, responses on electrode 12 were also obtained for this child.

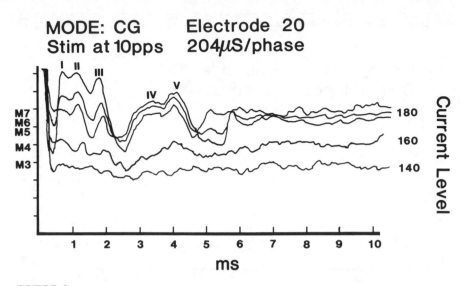

FIGURE 5-3. The EABR tracings, from a child of 2 years 5 months, were obtained intraoperatively.

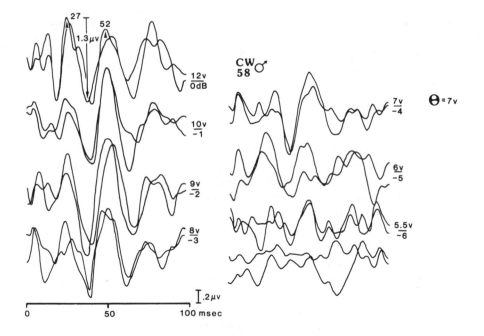

FIGURE 5-4. Electrically evoked middle latency responses (EMLRs) for an adult male who uses a single-channel cochlear implant. From Young, K. B., Miyamoto, R. T., & Shallop, J. K. (1982, October). Middle-latency responses in cochlear implant patients. Paper presented at the International Evoked Potential Symposium–II. Cleveland, Ohio.

THE ELECTRICAL MIDDLE LATENCY RESPONSE (EMLR)

Middle latency responses elicited with electrical stimulation (EMLRs) have been obtained by Young, Miyamoto, and Shallop (1982), as shown in Figure 5-4. These tracings were from an adult male who utilizes a single-channel cochlear implant. The middle latency waves Pa, Pb, and Pc can be clearly identified down to this patient's professed subjective threshold of 7 volts (peak-to-peak). This individual failed to respond behaviorally until he was "certain" that the signal was present, and thus his threshold may have been elevated. His EMLR was measurable below 7 volts at 5.5 to 6 volts.

In short, the feasibility of EABR and EMLR measurements has been established today despite the technical difficulties inherent in the recording processes. Although these difficulties have impeded the use of electrically stimulated evoked responses of the auditory neural tract as a routine clinical measure, future research can be expected to improve and simplify recording techniques and to reveal further direct clinical applications.

REFERENCES

Davis, H., & Hirsh, S. K. (1979). A slow brainstem response for low frequency audiometry. *Audiology, 18,* 445–461.

Fria, T. J. (1980). The auditory brainstem response: Background and clinical applications. *Maico Monographs in Contemporary Audiology, 2,* 1–44.

Jacobson, J. T. (Ed.). (1985). *The auditory brainstem response.* San Diego: College-Hill Press.

Mahoney, T. M. (1985). Auditory brainstem response hearing aid applications. In J. T. Jacobson (Ed.), *The auditory brainstem response* (pp. 349–370). San Diego: College-Hill Press.

Miyamoto, R. T. (1986). Electrically evoked potentials in cochlear implant subjects. *Laryngoscope, 96,* 178–185.

Moore, E. J. (Ed.). (1983). *Bases of auditory brain-stem evoked responses.* New York: Grune & Stratton.

Osterhammel, P. A., Shallop, J. K., & Terkildsen, K. (1985). The effect of sleep on the auditory brainstem response (ABR) and the middle latency response (MLR). *Scandinavian Audiology, 14,* 47–50.

Shallop, J. K., Fria, T. J., & Kunov, H. (1978). *School for electric response audiometry.* (Workbook, 2 vols.) Toronto, Canada: Madsen Electronics, Ltd.

Shallop, J. K., Osterhammel, P. A., & Tubergen, L. B. (1984). Comparative measurements of SN-10 and the 40/sec MLRs in newborns. In R. Nodar & C. Barber (Eds.), *Evoked potentials II* (pp. 548–552). Boston: Butterworth.

Stapells, D.R., Picton, T.W., Perez-Abalo, M., Read, D., & Smith, A. (1985). Frequency specificity in evoked potential audiometry. In J. T. Jacobson (Ed.),

The auditory brainstem response (pp. 147–177). San Diego: College-Hill Press.

Stypulkowski, P., van den Honert, C., & Kvistad, S. D. (1986). Electrophysiological evaluation of the cochlear implant patient. *Otolaryngologic Clinics of North America, 19,* 249–257.

Swigonski, N., Shallop, J., Lemons, J., & Bull, M. (1987). Hearing screening of high risk newborns. *Ear and Hearing, 8,* 26–30.

Young, K. B., Miyamoto, R. T., & Shallop, J. K. (1982, October). Middle-latency responses in cochlear implant patients. Paper presented at The International Evoked Potential Symposium-II. Cleveland, Ohio.

CHAPTER 6

ARTHUR BOOTHROYD

HEARING AIDS, COCHLEAR IMPLANTS, AND PROFOUNDLY DEAF CHILDREN

The mid-1980s have seen increasing use of cochlear implants in the treatment of childhood deafness (e.g., see Berliner, Eisenberg, & House, 1985). This development has made it more important than ever that the nature and potential value of residual hearing assisted by hearing aids be understood. In theory, cochlear implants are used only with children who are unable to benefit from hearing aids — that is, with children who are totally deaf. It is unusual, however, for a child who is hearing-impaired to be totally without a sense of hearing. Most of the children who are typically classified as *profoundly deaf* possess hair cells that are capable of stimulating the auditory nerve in response to loud sound. With modern hearing aids and appropriate educational management, this residual sense of hearing can often be used to great advantage. Unfortunately, there is considerable misunderstanding about the nature and possibilities of residual hearing, and it is often difficult even to measure the amount of residual hearing in a young child.

There are at least three ways in which information about residual hearing is of potential relevance to cochlear implants:

1. *Candidacy.* Without adequate information on what can be expected from different amounts of residual hearing, there is an ever-present possibility that implants will be placed in children who could have gained more benefit from hearing aids.

2. *Performance.* As we accumulate data on the performance of implanted children, it is important that these data be related to equiva-

lent data on the performance of children who use hearing aids. Only with such comparisons can the objectivity of future clinical decisions be increased.

3. *Training:* The success of any form of prosthetic assistance for children who are hearing-impaired depends very much on the adequacy of educational management. Many years of experience have been gained in the use of hearing aids and residual hearing to enhance development and learning. This experience should be applied to the management of implanted children.

The goals of this chapter are (1) to review current knowledge of the auditory capabilities of hearing-impaired children who have been fitted with hearing aids, and in whom hearing has played a major role in development; and (2) to compare this information with that obtained from implanted subjects.

TERMINOLOGY

Before presenting research data, it is important to define terms. Much of the confusion in this field arises from inconsistencies in the use of terminology. One person, for example, may use *hearing-impaired* synonymously with *hard-of-hearing* while another may use it as a generic term, relating to any disorder of hearing, regardless of type or severity. Similarly, one person's *profound hearing loss* may be another person's *total deafness.*

Some of this confusion is due to the imperfect correlation between relatively objective measures, such as pure tone threshold, and nebulous, but important, criteria such as the potential contribution of hearing to spoken language development. Because there is a correlation between threshold and potential performance, the procedure of defining hearing impairment on the basis of pure tone threshold has merit, especially when dealing with group data, or when estimating the probable results of specific types of intervention. But because the correlation is less than perfect, such definitions should only be applied to individual children with what might be called "informed caution."

For the purposes of this chapter, the following definitions will be used. Each definition is accompanied by an indication of the kind of relationship that exists between the objective measure and the probable results of intervention (see also Boothroyd, 1982).

A *hearing impairment* is any disorder of hearing, regardless of cause, type or severity. This definition encompasses mild hearing losses, total deafness, and auditory attention deficits without change of threshold. The corresponding adjective is *hearing-impaired.*

A *hearing loss* is a subnormal ability to detect sound. Hearing loss is measured as a shift of threshold in dB re ANSI standards for normal threshold. Unless ear and frequency are specified, the magnitude of a hearing loss is defined by the average of the pure tone thresholds at 500, 1000, and 2000 Hz in the better ear. Qualifiers may be added as follows:

MILD. Refers to a hearing loss of 15 through 30 dB. A *stable* mild hearing loss need not have a significant effect on development, and a hearing aid is seldom called for.

MODERATE. Refers to a hearing loss of 31 through 60 dB. Without intervention, moderate hearing losses affect and delay, but do not prevent, speech and language development. With hearing aids and modest intervention efforts, children with moderate hearing losses can develop almost normally.

SEVERE. Refers to a hearing loss of 61 through 90 dB. Without intervention, a severe hearing loss can *prevent* the development of speech and language. With hearing aids, good early intervention, and continued special training, hearing can become the *principal* avenue for speech and language development, and most children with severe hearing losses can be expected to develop almost normally.

PROFOUND. Refers to a hearing loss in excess of 90 dB. Without intervention, speech and language development will not occur. With intense intervention, speech and language development can occur, but slowly and with difficulty. The role of hearing will seldom be that of the principal avenue for such development. Rather, hearing will become a *complement to lipreading.* The exact contribution of hearing can vary widely among profoundly deaf children. The profoundly deaf category can be roughly subdivided into three:

1. *Those with considerable residual hearing.* These children have hearing losses from 91 through 100 dB HL with thresholds above 1000 Hz of 105 dB HL or less. Hearing can usually play a major role in development, giving excellent information about intonation and vowel articulation, and some information about consonant articulation. With high quality intervention, some profoundly deaf children with good residual hearing can develop like severely deaf children (e.g., see Ling & Milne, 1981).

2. *Those with a little residual hearing.* These children have hearing losses from 101 through 110 dB HL with thresholds above 1000 Hz of 110 dB or more. Hearing can play an important role in development, providing information on intensity, duration, rhythm, and perhaps some intonation and vowel cues.

3. *Those with no residual hearing.* These children are *totally deaf.* They can, however, respond to sound through the sense of touch and, when tested under headphones, may appear to have hearing. In such cases, the measured average threshold is usually well in excess of 110 dB (Boothroyd & Cawkwell, 1970). Hearing will obviously play no role in development, regardless of the type or intensity of intervention or the application of hearing aids. This is not to imply that speech and language development are impossible. It does, however, require remarkable teachers and a remarkable child for speech and language to be learned by vision only, and the results will be far from perfect.

The expressions *severely, profoundly,* and *totally deaf* will be used as qualifiers to describe children who have severe, profound, and total hearing losses. In making the foregoing statements about relationships between hearing loss and performance, certain conditions are assumed. These include:

1. *A purely sensorineural hearing loss.* In the case of a mixed hearing loss, the potential use of hearing is determined by the sensorineural component, but the pure tone threshold is determined by the sum of the sensorineural and the conductive components. Note also that a conductive component overlaid on a severe or profound sensorineural loss can make it very difficult to provide suitable amplification.

2. *The fitting and fulltime use of appropriate amplification equipment.* Such equipment is not limited to personal hearing aids, but may include special classroom amplification systems with wireless microphones. Children with severe and profound hearing losses have a particular need for such systems in order to insure an adequate signal level and a tolerable signal-to-noise ratio (see Bess, Freeman, & Sinclair, 1981).

3. *Appropriate educational management.* One of the strengths of normal children is that they can develop well in spite of any inadequacies of educational management. The mark of a hearing impaired child is that progress becomes directly related to the quality and suitability of management.

4. *An otherwise intact child.* The presence of impairments in addition to those of hearing can seriously compromise the goals of

management as they relate to the use of residual hearing in development.

5. *An insightful and supportive family.* The potential contribution of the child's family can never be overstated.

The inability to control, or even define, these variables is one of the reasons for the imperfect correlations that are found between hearing loss and performance.

SPEECH CONTRAST PERCEPTION AND DEGREE OF HEARING LOSS

When asking about the auditory capabilities of hearing-impaired children with various degrees of hearing loss, the first question to be addressed is "How sensitive are they to those differences among the acoustic patterns of speech that are used to define word meaning and sentence structure?"

Figure 6–1 shows results obtained by hearing-impaired teenagers on a test requiring the perception of phonologically significant speech pattern contrasts. These subjects had all been educated in a high quality auditory–oral program in which personal and classroom hearing aids were in fulltime use, organized speech instruction was provided, and face-to-face communication was by spoken language only.

The test called for subjects to identify words and phrases from small closed sets in which the response alternatives differed by one or two features such as consonant voicing or vowel height. For increased face validity, the test contrasts were presented in a phonetic context that changed from item to item. The test was administered under headphones to the better ear, using linear, nonfrequency-selective amplification at the highest comfortable level. Group means are shown as a function of three-frequency-average pure tone threshold. Data points were obtained by interpolation and extrapolation from two studies (Boothroyd, 1984). Forced-choice scores have been adjusted so that 0 percent represents chance performance.

The results, illustrated in Figure 6–1, show that auditory access to all speech contrasts decreases with increasing hearing loss, but at a rate that changes from contrast to contrast. While place of consonant articulation, for example, becomes virtually inaccessible for losses of 90 dB or more, vowel height and syllabic (or temporal) pattern remain partially accessible for losses as high as 120 to 130 dB. Contrasts of vowel height are accompanied by changes of intensity, and the perception of syllabic pattern merely requires access to variations of intensity over time. It may, therefore, be inferred that children with sensorineural hearing losses in

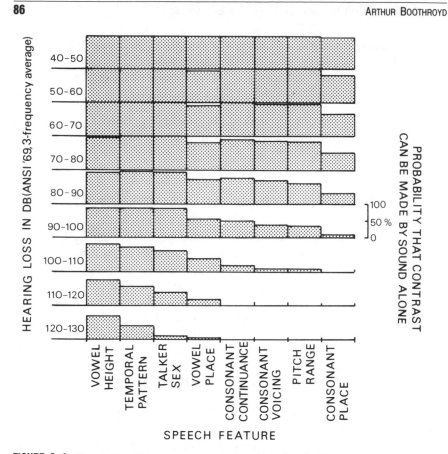

FIGURE 6–1. Probability of the perception of phonologically significant speech pattern contrasts by children with sensorineural hearing losses. Group mean values on the Speech Pattern Contrast (SPAC) test (Boothroyd, 1986) are shown as a function of pure tone threshold (hearing loss) and speech contrast (feature). The data were obtained by interpolation and extrapolation from 2 studies involving teenage subjects who had been educated in a high quality auditory–oral program (Boothroyd, 1984). Note that a probability value of 0 percent represents chance performance on a forced-choice test. Note also that *temporal pattern* refers to the number of syllables in a word or phrase; *pitch range* refers to the difference between speech produced with constant fundamental frequency and speech produced with natural intonation; and consonant continuance, voicing, and place contrast were tested only in word-initial position. From Boothroyd, A. (1985). Residual hearing and the problem of carry over in the speech of the deaf. *ASHLA Reports, 15,* 8–14. Copyright 1985 by ASHA. Reprinted with permission.

excess of 120 dB have access to time and intensity cues only. Such access could be provided by the sense of touch, or by rudimentary residual hearing whose performance is indistinguishable from that of the sense of touch. Children with losses in the range of 90 to 120 dB, however, give evidence of at least partial access to frequency-dependent contrasts such as talker sex and vowel place, and to contrasts that are dependent on fine temporal cues, such as initial consonant voicing and continuance.

One of the puzzling aspects of the data shown in Figure 6–1 was the poor performance of profoundly deaf subjects on the test of sensitivity to intonation patterns, labelled *pitch range*. This test required only that subjects decide whether a short phrase was spoken with constant pitch or naturally rising and falling intonation. The two response alternatives were labelled "sad" and "happy," and subjects were given examples before the test began. Nevertheless, subjects with hearing losses in excess of 90 dB generally performed close to chance levels, even though the intonation patterns of their own speech indicated that many of them had auditory access to this acoustic feature. One obvious implication was that the poor performance was task-dependent rather than capacity-dependent. This interpretation was supported by a subsequent study in which an imitative task was used (Most, 1985).

The results of Most's study are shown in Figure 6–2. The task of the 40 subjects (aged 3 to 10 years) was to imitate a series of falling, rising, and flat intonation contours carried by one or two syllable utterances. The test stimuli were computer generated to avoid the confounding of

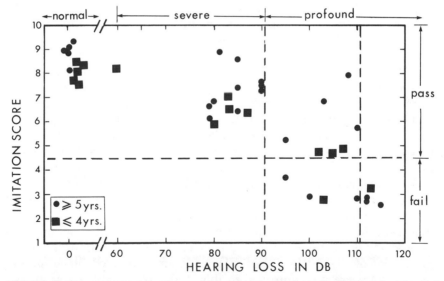

FIGURE 6–2. Scores obtained by 10 normal hearing, 15 severely deaf, and 15 profoundly deaf children on a test involving the imitation of synthetic intonation contours. Imitations were rated on a 10-point scale by 5 experienced judges. Each data point is the average of the judges' ratings of 72 imitations. From Most, T. (1985). *The perception of intonation by severely and profoundly hearing-impaired children.* Unpublished doctoral dissertation, City University of New York, NY. Reprinted with permission.

frequency, intensity, and duration. Each child imitated 24 models on each of 3 test sessions, for a total of 72. Recordings of the children's imitations were played, along with the relevant models, to a group of 5 experienced listeners. The listeners were asked to rate the similarity between the model and the imitation on a 10-point scale. The vertical axis of Figure 6–2 shows the mean rating for each child collapsed across the 72 utterances and the 5 judges. A rating of 4 or less indicates that the child was not able to change pitch in the direction of the model. Children with ratings of more than 4 may be assumed to exhibit some sensitivity to changes of fundamental frequency. (This assumption was supported in a second study in which the same test stimuli were used in a three-interval oddity task).

It will be seen from Figure 6–2 that all of the 15 children with severe hearing losses were able to perceive intonation contours, though, on average, their performance was not as good as that of the 10 normal children. Among the profoundly deaf, however, only 7 of the 15 subjects with profound hearing losses received passing scores. Four of the subjects in the profoundly deaf group had hearing losses in excess of 110 dB. Not one of these gave evidence of being sensitive to pitch changes. Of the subjects whose losses were greater than 90 dB, but not greater than 110 dB, 7 of 11 obtained passing scores.

On average, the younger children in Most's study performed less well than the older ones at all hearing-loss levels, but it is clear from Figure 6–2 that age was by no means the most important variable.

What is not apparent from Figure 6–2 is the possible role of educational management. Of the subjects who were hearing-impaired, 15 came from an oral program that places strong emphasis on the development and use of auditory skills. The other 15 came from a total communication program in which this particular aspect of management receives much less emphasis. Among the severely deaf children, performance on the imitative task was unrelated to educational program. Among the profoundly deaf children with losses in the 91 to 110 dB range, however, the type of program was an almost perfect predictor of performance. With only one exception, the children in this group who obtained passing scores on the imitative task were from the auditory-oral program. This observation does not necessarily imply a cause–effect relationship, as the placement of a child in a particular program depended on numerous factors that were not controlled in this study. What these data do confirm, however, is that a profound hearing loss in the range 90 to 110 dB does not preclude the possibility of auditory access to the intonation patterns of speech.

Phoneme Recognition and Degree of Hearing Loss

The second question to be asked is "How well can children with various degrees of sensorineural hearing loss learn to recognize the phonemes of English?" Figure 6–3 shows data on phoneme recognition ability as a function of 3-frequency average pure tone threshold in a large group of hearing-impaired children ranging in age from 11 through 19 years. All had sensorineural hearing losses, prelingually acquired, and all had been educated in the same auditory-oral program as the subjects reported in Figure 6–1. These data are taken from routine clinical records.

The phoneme recognition scores of Figure 6–3 are the percentage of phonemes correctly recognized in lists of meaningful consonant-vowel-consonant (CVC) words. The lines show mean values and the upper and lower quartiles. Previous research has shown that, although

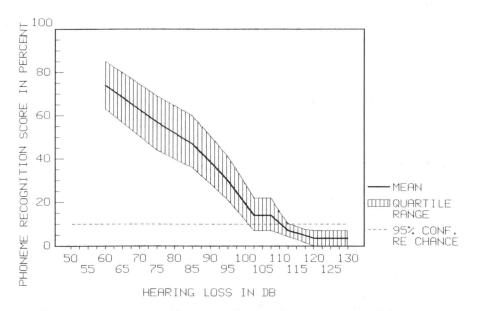

FIGURE 6–3. The percentage of phonemes recognized, in the context of CVC words, by hearing-impaired subjects aged 11 through 19 years. All had been educated in a high quality auditory-oral program. The heavy line shows group means as a function of three-frequency average pure tone threshold. The shaded area shows the interquartile range, estimated from the standard deviations of group data. Subjects who responded with randomly selected CVC words were expected to score 7 to 10 percent on this test.

the phoneme recognition score is affected by subjects' knowledge of vocabulary, the effect is relatively small, and phoneme scores obtained by auditorally experienced subjects may be taken as fairly valid indicators of auditory and phonetic, rather than lexical, capability (Boothroyd & Nittrouer, 1987).

Examination of Figure 6–3 shows that the typical child with a 90 dB hearing loss may be expected to recognize between 30 and 50 percent of the phonemes in CVC words. The score for the average subject does not drop to chance levels (approximately 10 percent) until a hearing loss of 110 dB is reached. Even here, however, 50 percent of the children recognize more than 10 percent of the phonemes. These results show convincingly that the contrast perception data illustrated in Figure 6–1 are predictive of genuine open-set recognition ability at the phoneme level.

It should be noted that when the results of word recognition tests are reported as the percentage of *whole words* recognized, the typical subject with a hearing loss of 90 to 110 dB scores close to zero. It is unfortunate that standard clinical practice calls for whole-word scoring of such tests. The results often lead to the conclusion that subjects have "no open-set recognition ability" when they can, in fact, recognize a high percentage of the phonemic elements within words.

COMPARATIVE PERFORMANCE OF SINGLE CHANNEL IMPLANTEES

Bilger's (1977) data on adults showed that single-channel stimulation of the auditory nerve provides access to amplitude–envelope cues and to periodicity pitch. Similar findings have been obtained by Berliner and Eisenberg (1987) of the House Ear Institute (HEI), using an expanded version of the Speech Pattern Contrast (SPAC) test (Boothroyd, 1986). Using data collected at HEI, Figure 6–4, illustrates the means of eight ears implanted with the 3M/House single-channel device. It will be seen that subjects gave evidence of good access to contrasts of stress (location of the stressed word in a three-word phrase), intonation (pitch rise versus pitch fall), talker sex (male versus female), and final consonant voicing. They also showed some access to vowel height (high versus low) and place (front versus back) contrasts. This list includes not only contrasts that can be perceived on the basis of time versus intensity cues (stress, vowel height, and final voicing) but also contrasts that presumably require access to fundamental frequency (talker sex), variations of fundamental frequency over time (pitch rise and fall), and spectrum (vowel place). The results are similar to those obtained by profoundly deaf children with losses in the range 100 to 110 dB, shown in Figure 6–1.

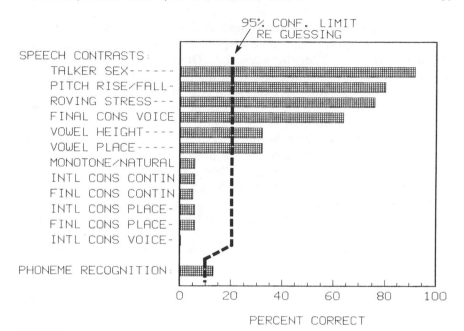

FIGURE 6–4. Mean scores of 8 adult ears, implanted with the 3M/House single-channel implant, on the various subtests of the SPAC test (Boothroyd, 1986), by hearing alone (see also Boothroyd, 1987). Note that there are two extra suprasegmental contrasts compared with Figure 6–1. *Roving stress* refers to the ability to locate the stressed word in a 3-word phrase; *pitch rise/fall* refers to the ability to identify whether a short phrase is spoken with a rising or a falling intonation contour. Note also that separate scores are reported for word-initial and word-final consonant contrasts. The contrast scores have been corrected for guessing, using the formula: $p_c = 2 (p_u - 50)$; where p_c and p_u are the corrected and uncorrected scores, respectively, in percent. At the bottom of the figure will be found the mean score for the recognition of phonemes in CVC word context. The vertical broken line shows the upper 95 percent confidence limits for scores that would be expected on the basis of guessing alone. These data were kindly supplied by Laurie Eisenberg of the House Ear Institute.

This conclusion is supported by the phoneme recognition data of the eight subjects shown in Figure 6-4, whose average score is 13 percent phonemes correct. This score is just above chance levels and is equal to the expected mean score for subjects with 105 dB losses (see Figure 6-3).

On the basis of the data just reported, and of similar data reported from post-lingually deafened adults, one would be justified in concluding that the 3M/House single-channel device should be capable, at best, of converting a totally deaf child into the equivalent of a profoundly deaf child with a little residual hearing — that is, a child with a hearing loss in the 100 to 110 dB range and no useful hearing above 1000 Hz.

More recent results, however, have shown that a limited number of child implantees have been able to perform considerably better than would be predicted from the adult data (Berliner & Eisenberg, 1987). Twelve of these children are described in some detail in Chapter 11 of this text. In terms of contrast perception and phoneme recognition, they behave like children who are severely deaf. Phoneme recognition scores, for example, range from 34 to 85 percent, as assessed using the CVC items from the Auditec PBK word list recordings. When these results are compared with the mean data for the orally-trained, prelingually deaf subjects illustrated in Figure 6–3, it will be seen that the phoneme recognition scores of the 12 implanted children are equal to the mean scores of aided children with hearing losses in the range of 50 to 93 dB (see Figure 6–5). Exactly how the implanted children are extracting the necessary temporal and spectral detail from the single-channel input is not clear. Nevertheless, in terms of the ability to recognize phonemes in CVC

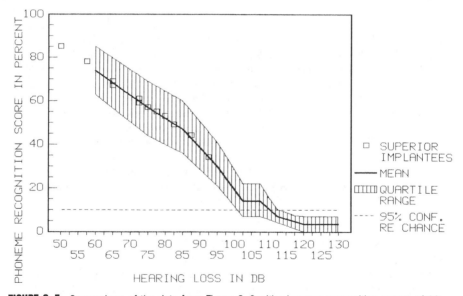

FIGURE 6–5. Comparison of the data from Figure 6–3 with phoneme recognition scores of 12 highly successful child users of the 3M/House single-channel implant. Scores for the implantees were obtained using only the CVC items from the Auditec recordings of the PBK monosyllabic word lists. Children's imitations of the words, presented by hearing alone, were recorded and then phonetically transcribed by 2 independent judges. The data shown here are the means of the judges. By placing the implantees' data on the mean curve for the amplified children, it is possible to convert the phoneme scores into equivalent hearing loss values. These data were kindly supplied by Lisa Tonokawa of the House Ear Institute.

words by hearing alone, these 12 children offer proof that a single-channel device may be capable of providing as much auditory capacity as is possessed by a child with a severe hearing loss in the 60 to 90 dB range.

Encouraging as these new data are, it is important to keep them in context. Children who demonstrate this level of performance represent only about 10 percent of the current total population of single-channel child implantees. Moreover, they have a common etiology, namely, meningitis. Even among post-meningitic child implantees, they represent only about 30 percent of the population. In contrast, the data in Figures 6–1 and 6–3 show *average* performance for children with a wide range of etiologies, and almost exclusively congenital acquisition. It is only with such data, however, that it will become possible to assess for individual subjects, the a priori probabilities of various levels of success with amplification and implantation.

COMPARATIVE PERFORMANCE OF MULTICHANNEL IMPLANTEES

At this time, the most widely used multichannel implant is the Nucleus 22-electrode system. This is also the only multichannel system approved for investigational use in deaf children. The results obtained by adults with the Nucleus device have varied widely from individual to individual. Roughly 50 percent have attained quite good open-set recognition of words by implant alone, and dramatic improvements of lip-reading performance when the implant is used as a supplement to vision. The other half have obtained results similar to those of single-channel adult implantees.

Figure 6–6 shows mean speech contrast perception data for three very successful and three less successful adult subjects. These are data from work in progress. It will be seen that the more successful subjects demonstrate at least some access to every phonetic contrast tested except that of final consonant place. The less successful group, however, gives evidence of access to only a few contrasts, these being the ones conveyed by time versus intensity cues and, perhaps, gross spectral cues. The contrast perception data are well supported by phoneme recognition results, which show scores as high as 50 or 60 percent (i.e., equivalent to the mean 70 to 80 dB loss data of Figure 6–3) in the more successful subjects, but at chance levels in the less successful ones.

Comparing these results with the data in Figures 6–1 and 6–3, tentative conclusions are that, for a subject implanted with the Nucleus device, there is roughly a 50 percent chance that he or she will acquire auditory capabilities similar to those of a subject who is severely deaf. At this time, however, too few data are available on the results of multichan-

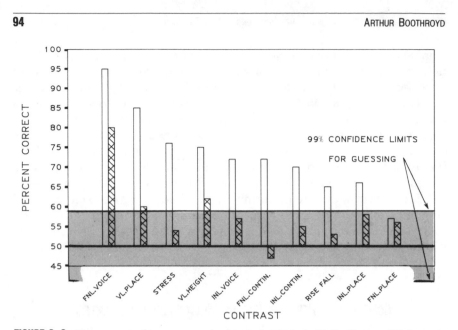

FIGURE 6–6. Mean scores of two groups of subjects, implanted with the Nucleus 22-electrode system, on various subtests of the SPAC test, by hearing alone. The successful group, shown by open bars, consisted of 3 subjects who had open-set sentence perception by implant alone, and over 90 percent recognition of words in sentences by lipreading plus implant. The less successful group, shown by shaded bars, consisted of 3 subjects who did not have open-set sentence recognition by implant alone and whose lipreading scores were barely enhanced with the use of the implant.

nel implantation in children to indicate whether they perform better or worse, on average, than post-lingually deafened adults with the Nucleus device.

Auditory Management of Children With Profound, Prelingually Acquired Sensorineural Hearing Loss

Hearing is so well suited to its role as input and feedback modality during the acquisition of spoken language that any sensory alternative that can be presently provided pales by comparison. Moreover, it has become clear that profound, sensorineural hearing loss need not prevent hearing from playing its natural role, at least for some aspects of speech perception and production (Boothroyd, 1985).

There are, however, two major prerequisites: one is the provision of suitable amplification; the other is the provision of suitable training. It is not easy to provide profoundly deaf children with suitable amplification.

Full access to the spectrum of speech, when it is produced at a distance of 5 or 6 feet from the microphone of the hearing aid, requires gains in excess of 60 dB. This requirement is seldom met, partly because of the problem of acoustic feedback. Even with sufficient gain the child often cannot distinguish between the speech signal and the environmental noises that are also rendered audible by the aid. These problems have been partially solved for classroom situations by the use of wireless microphones that are placed close to the mouth of the talker (Bess, Freeman, & Sinclair, 1981), but a solution for the self-contained personal hearing aid is still lacking.

It should be noted that one of the unplanned advantages of a cochlear implant for the profoundly deaf is freedom from acoustic feedback. The problem of signal-to-noise ratio, however, is as serious for the implantee as it is for the hearing aid user because the ability to distinguish speech from noise is impaired in both groups.

The second prerequisite, that of suitable training, presents even more serious problems. The fact that residual hearing in the 90 to 100 dB range can be used with dramatic effect in the acquisition of spoken language skills has been demonstrated by numerous educators and researchers (e.g., see Ling & Milne, 1981). There is, however, a serious lack of knowledgeable and qualified personnel to provide the kind of training that can convert auditory potential into communicative performance, and a shortage of educational programs within which such training is accorded high priority. One reason for these shortages is the limited availability of suitable personnel preparation programs (Hochberg, Levitt, & Osberger, 1983). Another is the wholesale abdication, on the part of teachers of the deaf, of responsibility for the development of spoken language skills in deaf children (Scott, 1983). These problems will negatively affect the training of implanted children just as they have negatively affected the training of profoundly deaf children who wear hearing aids.

Circumstantial evidence of the need for suitable training has already been presented in the summary of Most's (1985) study, in which the type of training program was an almost perfect predictor of the performance of profoundly deaf children on a task requiring the imitation of intonation contours. More direct evidence came from a study by Nittrouer, Devan, and Boothroyd (1976), in which a group of seven preteenagers with severe and profound hearing losses were given 45 min/day of "listening skills" training. The hearing losses of these students ranged from 85 to 103 dB. The program was instituted because the students, though educated in an auditory–oral program, were performing at a level that was considered by teachers to be below their auditory potential. The evidence cited was their failure to respond when called by name, their frequent failure to wear their personal hearing aids, and their frequent failure to report dead batteries or broken aids.

Figure 6–7 shows group mean scores obtained on three speech perception tests administered before, during, immediately after, and 7 months after an 8-week training period. The first test was of contrast perception, and the mean scores showed no significant changes during this study. The second test was of phoneme recognition. On this test, the mean score rose from 55 to 75 percent during training, but returned to 55 percent after 7 months without training. The third test was of the recognition of words in unknown sentences. The subjects refused to take this test at the beginning of training, believing themselves incapable of perceiving sentences by hearing alone. After 4 weeks, their confidence improved and they recognized about 70 percent of the words in the sentences. By the end of training, their mean score rose to over 90 percent words correct,

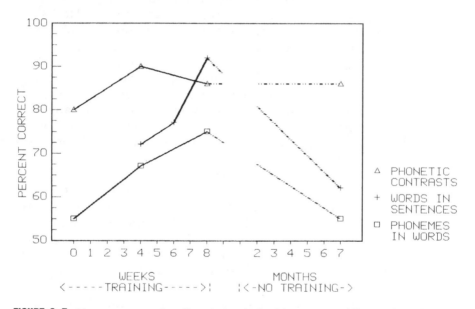

FIGURE 6–7. Mean scores, on 3 auditory tests, obtained by a group of 7 severely and profoundly hearing-impaired children during an 8-week training period and after a 7-month period with no special training. Changes in the perception of phonetic contrasts were not statistically significant. The subjects did, however, show significant improvements, during training, in the recognition of phonemes in CVC words and in the recognition of words in unfamiliar sentences. These improvements vanished when special training was discontinued. The training consisted of a 45-minute period in each school day during which all spoken language reception was via hearing alone.

but after 7 months without the special class the score fell to 63 percent. It should be added that the phoneme and word recognition scores rose again when the special class was reinstated.

These data, which were in keeping with informal observations of subjects' attitudes and behavior, underline the need for a communicative environment that continuously challenges and reinforces auditorally based spoken language skills once they have been acquired. There is no reason to believe that this need will be any less for implanted children than it is for children wearing hearing aids.

Conclusion

In conclusion, data presented show that:

1. A profoundly deaf child, with a hearing loss in the 90 to 110 dB range, may well be capable of perceiving a variety of frequency-dependent speech pattern contrasts and of using this capacity to acquire phoneme recognition skills.

2. A totally deaf child, with a hearing loss in excess of 110 dB, fitted with a single-channel implant, may reasonably be expected to acquire an auditory capacity similar to that of a profoundly deaf child with a little residual hearing. There is a limited chance that he or she will acquire an auditory capacity similar to that of a child who is severely deaf. At the time of writing, however, only children who are post-meningitic implantees, and only about one-third of this group, have demonstrated such good results.

3. There is, perhaps, a 50 percent chance that a totally deaf child fitted with a Nucleus implant, will acquire an auditory capacity similar to that of a child who is severely deaf, but the data on this point are scant and none has yet come from child implantees.

4. The limited auditory capacity of severely and profoundly deaf children can, if properly used, make a significant, and sometimes dramatic, difference to the acquisition of spoken language skills. There is every reason to expect that totally deaf children, if they are effectively transformed into severely and profoundly deaf children by cochlear implants, will have similar potential.

5. In order for this potential to be realized, the implanted children should be enrolled in quality programs in which special emphasis is placed on the use of audition for the acquisition and application of spoken language skills.

These conclusions carry three major implications for the continued evaluation of the potential role of cochlear implants in the management of childhood deafness: (1) Children's implant programs should incorporate, or be affiliated with, quality intervention programs in which appropriate diagnostic and rehabilitative therapy can be provided; (2) Such programs should have a strong commitment to empirical research so that future developments can be guided by more data, and more objective data, than currently exist; and (3) At the present time, the evidence, though limited, favors multichannel implants as being likely to provide a more successful outcome than single-channel implants, but definitive evidence on this point must await the results of further, carefully designed, performance evaluations.

ACKNOWLEDGMENT

This work was partially supported by National Institutes of Health grant number 17764.

REFERENCES

Berliner, K. I., & Eisenberg, L. S. (1987). Our experience with cochlear implants: Have we erred in our expectations? *American Journal of Otology, 8,* 222–229.

Berliner, K. I., Eisenberg, L. S., & House, W. F. (Eds.). (1985). The cochlear implant: An auditory prosthesis for the profoundly deaf child. *Ear and Hearing, 6* (Suppl.), 1S–69S.

Bess, F., Freeman, B., & Sinclair, J. (Eds.). (1981). *Amplification in education.* Washington, DC: Alexander Graham Bell Association for the Deaf.

Bilger, R. C. (Ed.). (1977). Evaluations of subjects presently fitted with implanted auditory prostheses. *Annals of Otology, Rhinology, and Laryngology, 86* (Suppl. 38), 3–176.

Boothroyd, A. (1982). *Hearing impairments in young children.* Englewood Cliffs, NJ: Prentice Hall.

Boothroyd, A. (1984). Auditory perception of speech contrasts by subjects with sensorineural hearing loss. *Journal of Speech and Hearing Research, 27,* 134–144.

Boothroyd, A. (1985). Residual hearing and the problem of carry over in the speech of the deaf. *ASLHA Reports, 15,* 8–14.

Boothroyd, A. (1986). *SPAC test version II: A test of the perception of speech pattern contrasts.* New York: City University.

Boothroyd, A. (1987). Perception of speech pattern contrasts via cochlear implants and limited hearing. *Annals of Otology, Rhinology, and Laryngology, 96* (Suppl. 128), 58–62.

Boothroyd, A., & Cawkwell, S. (1970). Vibrotactile thresholds in pure-tone audiometry. *Acta Otolaryngologica, 69,* 381–387.

Boothroyd, A., & Nittrouer, S. (1987). *Mathematical treatment of context effects in phoneme and word recognition.* Manuscript submitted for publication.

Hochberg, I., Levitt, H., & Osberger, M. (Eds.). (1983). *Speech of the hearing impaired: Research, training, and personnel preparation.* Baltimore, MD: University Park Press.

Ling, D., & Milne, M. (1981). The development of speech in hearing-impaired children. In F. Bess, B. Freeman, & J. Sinclair (Eds.), *Amplification in education* (pp. 98–108). Washington, DC: Alexander Graham Bell Association for the Deaf.

Most, T. (1985). *The perception of intonation by severely and profoundly hearing-impaired children.* Unpublished doctoral dessertation, City University of New York, NY.

Nittrouer, S., Devan, M., & Boothroyd, A. (1976). *It's never too late: An auditory approach with hearing-impaired pre-teenagers* (SARP report No. 24). Northampton, MA: The Clarke School for the Deaf.

Scott, P. (1983). Have the competencies needed by teachers of the hearing impaired changed in 25 years? *Exceptional Children, 50,* 48–53.

CHAPTER 7

ROSS J. ROESER

TACTILE AIDS: DEVELOPMENT ISSUES AND CURRENT STATUS*

T he majority of individuals who are hearing impaired benefit from conventional amplification. In such cases, acoustic signals are amplified to an intensity within that person's range of residual hearing to make them perceptible to the impaired ear. In cases of profound or total deafness, however, amplification through the use of conventional hearing aids may provide only limited benefit, or virtually no benefit at all. It is estimated that in the United States alone, there are between 292,000 and 367,000 deaf individuals aged 3 years and above who receive little or no benefit from amplified sound (Ries, 1982). For these individuals, increasing the amplitude of the acoustic signal does not provide enough additional information to improve communication.

For those patients who cannot benefit from conventional amplification, alternative methods must be considered to provide assistance in the two primary areas germane to spoken communication: the reception of speech from others and the production of speech by the person who is hearing impaired. Two techniques that are currently available to assist patients with profound hearing loss are cochlear implants and tactile aids. Tactile aids for the profoundly deaf are considered in this chapter.

With tactile aids, acoustic signals are transduced into vibratory or electrical patterns that are presented on the skin in a manner that opti-

---

* Portions of the material in this chapter appeared in Roeser, R. J. (1985). Tactile aids for the profoundly deaf. *Seminars in Hearing, 6* 279–298. Reprinted with permission.

mizes the skin's capacity to receive sound. The goal of a tactile communication system is to extract relevant information from the acoustic signal and present it to the individual in a tactile mode as a means of supplementing or replacing the auditory reception of the acoustic signal, with the successful reception of speech as the ultimate challenge. In this chapter, issues surrounding tactile stimulation in deaf individuals are explored. In addition, performance variables for tactile aids and cochlear implants are compared and a description of six wearable tactile aids now available commercially is presented.

THE SKIN AS A RECEPTOR OF SOUND

Before addressing the development of tactile aids, it is of critical importance to review current knowledge on the capability of the skin as a receptor of acoustic stimulation. The basic philosophical approaches applied in the development of tactile aids and the techniques used to evaluate their efficacy are considered when addressing this issue.

The designated biological function of the skin in humans is not to act as a receiver of acoustic information. As a result, the skin's receptive characteristics to sound are highly limited compared to the ear. Gault (1924), the undisputed pioneer in tactile aid research, was unaware of the limited characteristics of the skin. He centered his work around the question, "Can a subject learn to interpret vibrations against the skin in a situation when hearing is out of the question?" (p. 157) With this basic hypothetical construct, he was attempting to develop a sensory *substitute* for the defective ear, rather than a sensory *supplement* to visual cues to assist the hearing-impaired person in the communication process. Since this early work, a valid question has emerged: Is it appropriate to expect that a tactile aid can act as a sensory substitute for the auditory mode? That is, can the skin replace the ear as a receptor of sound?

Table 7–1 provides a comparison between the auditory and vibrotactile systems in sound reception. These data indicate that, compared with the ear, the skin has severe limitations as a sensory receptor of acoustic information. For example, the normal auditory system has a dynamic range of 130 dB, but the range for the vibrotactile system is only about 30 to 35 dB. Moreover, the auditory system is responsive to frequencies ranging from 20 to 20,000 Hz and has an optimum frequency range between 300 and 3000 Hz; the upper limit of the efficient vibrotactile system is only 400 to 500 Hz and the vibratory receptors are best stimulated by frequencies in the 40 to 400 Hz range. Also, the vibrotactile mode is inferior to the ear in the time it requires for the full development of sen-

TABLE 7-1
Comparison of Auditory and Vibrotactile Modes in the Reception of Sound

Acoustic Variable	Auditory Mode	Vibrotactile Mode
Dynamic range	0–130 dB	0–35 dB
Frequency range	20–20,000 Hz	10–500 Hz
Optimal frequency range	300–3,000 Hz	40–400 Hz
Time for full development of sensation	0.18 sec	1.2 sec
Difference limen for frequency	0.2%	5–10%

* Adapted from Keidel, W. D. (1974). The cochlear model in skin stimulation. In F. A. Geldard (Ed.), *Cutaneous communication systems and devices* (pp. 62–73). Austin, TX: Psychonomic Society.

sation and difference limen for frequency. In addition to these psychoacoustic variables, Keidel (1974) reported that the vibrotactile system has poor memory compared with the highly developed one for the auditory system. That is, there is poorer ability to retain images that are displayed on the skin either on a short-term or long-term basis.

The ideal tactile aid would stand alone as a substitute for hearing. However, with the limitations of the skin as a receptor of sound, it is quite probable that the tactile mode may not be an appropriate substitute for the ear. Sherrick (1984) recently addressed the issue of whether it is possible to represent speech successfully by visual or tactile means alone. He states that there are two philosophies on this issue. The first is that speech is represented by a special code that only the auditory system can interpret. Support for this is apparent from the psychophysical data presented in Table 7-1 and from the very modest gains that have been realized in experiments using relatively complex tactile systems. Proponents of this view believe that a tactile (or visual) display should serve as a supplement to communication, rather than a substitute for the ear.

The opposing philosophy is that it will be possible to communicate successfully with a tactile system without supplemental visual input. Those holding this philosophy contend that gains have been minimal in communicating speech with tactile or visual modes because of inappropriate training strategies, limited training time, and inadequate experimental devices. They believe that hearing can be replaced by either the tactile or visual modes alone if proper instruments are developed. At present, it is unclear whether highly sophisticated tactile aids will be able to substitute for a defective auditory system. With the rapid technological advancements being made, the answer to this question should be forthcoming in the near future.

HEARING AIDS AS TACTILE DEVICES

Nober (1964, 1967) was among the first to caution clinicians that acoustic signals presented at high intensities in the low frequencies may be felt by the ear rather than heard. He demonstrated that pure tone air conduction thresholds in the 125 to 1000 Hz range, obtained from the ears and hands of 94 subjects with profound deafness, were identical once the levels reached 75 to 105 dB HL (Nober, 1964). For bone conduction thresholds the levels were between 25 and 55 dB HL, respectively. This observation explains why those with severe to profound deafness have air-bone gaps in the low frequencies in the absence of conductive pathology. It also explains why the profoundly deaf benefit minimally from conventional amplification, despite their documented improvement in speech and warble tone awareness; the high intensity acoustic stimuli delivered through the hearing aid may be providing tactile, rather than acoustic stimulation.

Providing tactile stimulation through hearing aids has adverse consequences. Whereas the individual with some residual hearing will be able to obtain spectral and temporal cues through the hearing aid signal, the profoundly deaf individual who relies on tactile sensations will receive only rudimentary awareness and some temporal information from the low frequencies delivered by the hearing aid (Sweetow, 1979). This concept is illustrated in Figure 7–1, in which a comparison is made between the frequency sensitivity of the ear and the skin measured at the forearm and fingertips. Two relevant points are demonstrated in this figure. First, the sensitivity of the skin varies as a function of body location. This observation raises the question of where the ideal place for tactile stimulation is located, an issue that is extensively discussed in a later section of this chapter. As detailed in Table 7–1, a more significant point shown in this figure is that the frequency response of the skin is limited to the low frequencies. As hearing aids do not faithfully amplify low frequencies, it becomes clear why they are of limited help to those with profound deafness who are dependent on low frequency tactile stimulation. Most likely, this is the primary reason why the majority of individuals with profound deafness obtain little benefit from hearing-aid use, and as many as 23 percent of the profoundly deaf school-aged population choose not to wear hearing aids (Karchmer & Kirwin, 1977). With tactile aids, the acoustic signals within the frequency range of the normal ear are changed into vibratory or electrical patterns and presented to the skin in the low frequency region at which the skin is most sensitive. In this way, the maximum potential of the skin can be realized.

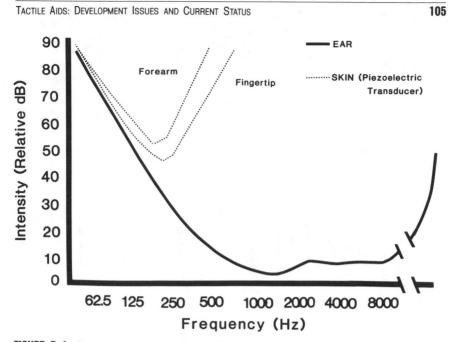

FIGURE 7-1. Frequency response of the skin measured at the forearm and fingertip compared with the frequency response of the normal ear. From Roeser, R. J. (in press). Cochlear implants and tactile aids for the profoundly deaf student. In R. J. Roeser & M. R. Downs (Eds.), *Auditory disorders in school children* (2nd ed.). New York: Thieme-Stratton Inc. Reprinted with permission.

ISSUES WITH TACTILE AIDS

Table 7-2 outlines the major attempts that have been made to develop and evaluate tactile aids. Issues regarding tactile aids can be addressed by reviewing each of the major areas listed in this table.

TYPE OF STIMULATION AND CONFIGURATION OF ARRAY

There are two types of stimulation that have been used with tactile devices: *vibrotactile* in which the acoustic signal is presented as a vibration to the skin using bone conduction vibrators, small solenoids, or other types of mechanical transducers; and *electrotactile* (or electrocutaneous) in which the acoustic signal is presented to the skin as an electrical current. A combination of the two has been attempted (DeFilippo, 1984), but only limited data are available on this approach.

TABLE 7-2
Summary of Major Studies Developing or Evaluating Tactile Aids

Investigators	Name or Description	Configuration and Type of Display*	Location of Stimulation	Primary Training Procedure	Subjects†	Training Period†
Pickett and Pickett (1963)	Tactile vocoder	10 (V) channels	Fingertips	Discrimination and identification of consonants/vowels	(n = 2)NH,A	26 hr
Kringlebothn (1968)	Tactile	5 (V) channels	Fingertips	Speech identification and speech correction	(n = ?)HI,A	N/A
Kirman (1974)	Formant code	15 by 15 (V) matrix	Fingers	Word identification	(n = 6)NH,A	17–25 hr
Englemann and Rosov (1975)	Tactile vocoder	23 (V) channels	Arms and legs	Word identification	(n = 4)NH,HI,C	20–80 hr
Goldstein and Stark (1976)	Tactile vocoder	24 by 6 (V) matrix	Fingers and hand	CV production	(n = 12)HI,C	2½ hr
Traunmuller (1977)	Sentiphone	1 (V) channel	Jawbone and hand	Word and phoneme identification	(n = 1)NH,A	N/A
Yeni-Komshian and Goldstein (1977)	Optacon	24 by 6 (V) matrix	Fingers and hand	Vowel and word recognition	(n = 10)NH,A	15 hr
Sparks et al. (1978, 1979)	Multipoint, Electrotactile Speech Aid (MESA)	36 by 8 (E) matrix	Abdomen	Vowel and consonant recognition and speech tracking	(n = 7)NH,A	15–20 hr

Reference	Device	Channels	Location	Task	Subjects	Duration
Scott (1979)	Speech Recognition Aid (SRA-10)	3 (V) channels	Abdomen	Speech tracking	(n = 4)NH,A	8 hr
Saunders (1973), Saunders et al. (1979)	Telector	2,20, or 32 (E) channels	Forehead or abdomen	Word recognition	(n = 2)HI,C	N/A
Goldstein et al. (1983)	Hybrid Tactaid I	1 (V) channel	Sternum	Speech and language therapy	(n = 1)HI,C	Daily for 9 mo
Oller et al. (1980)	Tactile vocoder	24 (V) channels	Left arm	Word discrimination	(n = 8)HI,C	N/A
Brooks and Frost (1983)	Tactile vocoder	16 (V) channels	Forearm	Word and phoneme recognition	(n = 2)NH,A	41–55 hr
Friel–Patti and Roeser (1983)	Speech Recognition Aid (SRA-10)	3 (V) channels	Abdomen	9 mo of language interaction therapy	(n = 4)HI,C	Daily for 4 mo
Gentile (1984)		1 (V) channel	Fingertip	Speech reading sentences	(n = 30)NH,A	N/A
Franklin (1984)	Tactaid I	1 (V) channel	Wrist or sternum	Subjective	(n = 3)NH,A	1 hr to 11 mo

* V: vibrotactile; E: electrotactile.
† NH: normal hearing; HI: hearing impaired; n: number; C: children; A: adults; N/A: not available.
From Roeser, R. J. (1985). Tactile aids for the profoundly deaf. *Seminars in Hearing, 6,* 279–298. Reprinted with permission.

Because of the availability of vibrators for experimental use and the inherent difficulties experienced in applying an electrical current to the skin, the vibrotactile approach has been preferred over the electrotactile. However, until recently, serious drawbacks with commercially available mechanical transducers have placed severe restrictions on vibrotactile aids, namely, their poor frequency response characteristics and their high power requirements. The presence of harmonic frequencies can generate audible noise, producing an echo-like effect when the acoustic signal activates the device. Moreover, high power requirements of many of the available mechanical transducers make them inefficient. These factors have prevented vibrotactile aids from being developed into efficient wearable units.

A relatively new type of electro-mechanical vibrotactile transducer uses the piezoelectric properties of certain alloys. When a small pulse voltage is applied to this material, a displacement occurs and the amplitude and frequency of the pulses can control the amplitude and frequency of vibration. The most common form of material used in this type of transducer is the reed bender Bi-morph. Reed bender Bi-morphs can generate adequate displacements with small power inputs, thereby making it possible to develop an efficient, small wearable vibrotactile aid (Sherrick, 1984).

Gentile (1984) reported one of the few studies using a reed Bi-morph. She administered a videotaped speechreading sentence test to three groups of 10 hearing subjects each. One group used lipreading alone, one listened to the fundamental speech frequencies ($f0$) while lipreading, and one used a single piezoelectric reed Bi-morph stimulating the fingertip while lipreading. Findings clearly showed that the $f0$ information acquired through tactile cues using the Bi-morph provided the same prosodic characteristics of speech (stress and syllabification) as in the $f0$ listening–lipreading group. This type of tactile aid is promising.

Several researchers have preferred using electrotactile stimulation. Saunders (1973) and Saunders, Hill, and Easley (1978–1979) developed the first electrotactile aid, the Teletactor, now called the Tacticon. Originally, the instrument was a two-channel device providing stimulation to the forehead. Later versions of the instrument contained 20 and then 32 electrodes applied to the abdomen through a linear array. Although a concern with electrotactile stimulation is the adverse effects of applying electrical currents to the skin, it was reported that the electrical stimuli could be tolerated for an extended period of time without side effects and that intensity level was unaffected by perspiration and other changes in skin resistance. Sparks, Kuhl, Edmonds, and Gray (1978) also developed and evaluated an electrotactile unit, the Multipoint Electrotactile Speech

Aid (MESA), a highly complex array of 288 electrodes in a 36 × 8 array presented to the abdomen. They reported no problems with painful stimuli or untoward side effects.

Blamey and Clark (1985) describe a wearable multiple-electrode electrotactile device with two electrodes on each finger located between the palm and first knuckle (see Figure 7–2). A common electrode is placed on the underside of the wrist. The sensations produced are described as being similar to those experienced if a vibrating object were placed against the side of the finger. Psychophysical testing indicated that stimuli from electrodes placed on either side of each finger were identified easily by all subjects and showed similar findings to electrical stimulation of more peripheral nerve structures (Blamey & Clark, 1987). Based on these encouraging results, Blamey and Clark have proposed the development of an electrotactile speech processor that codes speech amplitude as pulse width, $f0$ as pulse rate, and second formant frequency as electrode position.

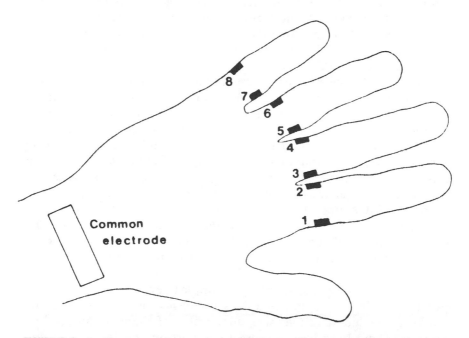

FIGURE 7–2. Configuration of an 8-channel electrotactile aid described by Blamey and Clark (1985). The electrodes are held in place by springy plastic clips (not shown) which insulate the electrodes from one another. From Blamey, P. J., and Clark, G. M. (1987). Psychophysical studies to the design of a digital electrotactile speech processor. *Journal of the Acoustical Society of America, 82,* 116–125. Reprinted with permission.

Comparison of vibrotactile and electrotactile devices suggests that the mechanical vibrotactile devices are more efficient in the lower frequencies and electrotactile devices are more efficient for higher intensities (Sachs, Miller, & Grant, 1980). Although each type of stimulation has advantages and disadvantages, comparative longitudinal clinical research is needed to determine which will be the most efficient form of stimulation. It is possible that a combined approach will yield the most favorable form of stimulation. DeFilippo (1984) compared the performance of a single-channel vibrotactile aid with that of a combined vibrotactile and electrotactile aid on the hand and found that the combined system produced superior scores. This isolated report should encourage further comparative investigations.

With respect to configuration of array, devices range from very simple one-channel units to extremely complex multichannel systems. With a single-channel device, the available information is restricted to awareness of environmental sounds and temporal cues (stress patterns and prosody). For speech, the single channel device is severely limited and is capable of displaying only rudimentary fundamental frequency information. However, although extremely limited, single-channel devices have proven to be beneficial as a supplement to speechreading (Reed, Durlach, & Braida, 1982).

Multiple channel aids can present tactile information using a one dimensional (linear) or two dimensional approach. With a one dimensional multiple channel system, spectral cues are presented in a linear fashion in a manner that attempts to simulate the cochlea. Frequency is coded by place of stimulation, similar to a piano keyboard, and intensity is coded by vibration amplitude. For example, if the abdomen is being used as the place of stimulation, low frequencies might be presented on the right, mid-frequencies in the center, and high frequencies on the left (Saunders, Hill, & Franklin, 1981). Two dimensional arrays code speech frequency along one spatial axis and intensity along another. In this way it is theorized that additional information makes it possible for the skin to extract both frequency and intensity cues from the complex speech signal.

Although a number of simple and complex devices have been developed (see Table 7-2), optimum values for basic features are yet to be established, including display size, the number of channels, and coding strategies. There have been no direct comparisons made between one and two dimensional displays, so it is not known which of these is actually superior (Sherrick, 1984). A flexible wearable multichannel tactile instrument capable of changing coding parameters so that longitudinal field trials can be conducted is needed.

LOCATION OF STIMULATION

Different body locations, including the hands, arms, abdomen, jaw, thorax, forehead, and thighs, have been studied to investigate the efficacy of tactile stimulation. As a sensor for vibrations, the hand has structural and functional characteristics that are unmatched by other body parts. Geldard and Sherrick (1983) have recently shown that the fingertips, compared with the arm, thigh, and thorax, have the best resolving power for vibratory patterns.

Although several studies have failed to document an apparent advantage of one body location over another, there are a limited number of comparative tactile studies using different body parts. Englemann and Rosov (1975) trained their subjects using the forearms and fingers. When the transducers were relocated to the thighs of their subjects, transfer was reported to be immediate. This finding suggests that performance was a function of pattern recognition, rather than increased sensitivity of a particular body part or neurological adaptation. Similarly, Yeni-Komshian and Goldstein (1977) transferred tactile patterns from the right hand to the left and from the fingers to the palm of the same hand; no performance differences were found.

One recent study provided direct evidence that the fingertips, compared to the wrist, thorax, abdomen, and thigh, are superior for recognizing vibratory speech patterns. Spens (1985) used a variety of different tactile arrays on seven different body locations of one subject (himself) in a number identification task. Results from his study are shown in Figure 7–3. Performance ranged from a low of 46 percent for a single vibrator placed on the wrist to a high of 77 percent for a 6×16 vibrator placed on the index finger. From these results, as well as the observations of Geldard and Sherrick (1983), it is clear that to achieve maximum discrimination consideration should be given to the fingertips in tactile stimulation. However, one major problem with the fingertips is that using them for tactile stimulation would affect manual dexterity.

One clinical approach might be to use the fingers and hands to learn patterns initially and then to transfer the patterns to another less conspicuous part of the body, such as the abdomen. Sherrick (1984) described a "double-barreled" approach in which the hands could be used for fine discrimination by grasping a tactile display, while a second body part, the abdomen or thigh, could be used for constant monitoring and alerting. This system takes advantage of the superiority of the hands in sensing tactile information, allows for freedom of the hands for manipulations, and provides for constant monitoring of the sound environment.

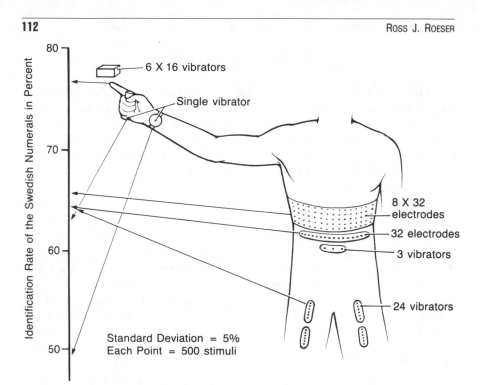

FIGURE 7-3. Identification rate of Swedish numbers in percent as a function of stimulating place, the method of stimulation, and the number of stimulators. Data adapted from Spens (1985). From Roeser, R. J. (in press). Cochlear implants and tactile aids for the profoundly deaf student. In R. J. Roeser and M. R. Downs (Eds.), *Auditory disorders in school children* (2nd ed.). New York: Thieme-Stratton Inc. Reprinted with permission.

An interesting idea is to stimulate the skin close to the ear, perhaps the pinna or outer ear canal itself. This may have a psychological advantage; after all, sound reception is not associated with the hands, abdomen, or other body parts. No direct data are readily available on the tactile sensitivity of the skin on the ear (Sherrick, 1984), but indirect evidence from Nober (1964, 1967) suggests that the vibrotactile thresholds of the pinna and ear canal are within 5 dB of those for the hand. These data indicate that the ear may be an excellent location for stimulation.

No matter what body location is chosen for a particular tactile aid, clinicians must be sensitive to the issue that each patient is different and, just as hearing aids are individually fit, tactile aids should be evaluated to identify a suitable location for each patient. The evaluation consists of obtaining sound field warble tone thresholds with the instrument on the body locations under consideration. Typically, clinical experience (Roeser and colleagues, unpublished observations) indicates that thresholds are within 5 to 10 dB for most body locations. It has also been observed, however, that some subjects have little or no sensitivity at certain body locations. For example, one 64-year-old man who was profoundly deaf could not detect any vibrotactile sensation on his abdomen, even at intense levels, despite being able to perceive sensations on his sternum, clavicle, and forearm at levels between 45 to 55 dB HL. This finding emphasizes the need for a prefitting evaluation of tactile aids.

TRAINING PROCEDURE

The procedures used to evaluate tactile aids depend largely on the ability of the subjects under investigation. Age, linguistic ability, and hearing status are important factors in determining the procedures that will be most adequate. Regardless of the subjects, two basic questions are considered: are the procedures designed to assess the reception of sound by the wearer, or will they assess the speech production of the wearer? Of course, both questions can be addressed simultaneously.

For the most part, investigations evaluating tactile devices have studied speech reception rather than speech production. The majority of these studies have investigated how a particular tactile aid functions with isolated consonants and vowels (Sparks et al., 1978), isolated words (Brooks & Frost, 1983; Englemann & Rosov, 1975; Kirman, 1974; Oller, Payne, & Gavin, 1980), and words or phonemes embedded in sentences or surrounded by other phonemes (Pickett & Pickett, 1963). All of these studies showed that benefits can be derived from tactile aids, and each provides valuable data on the capability of the skin in the reception of certain acoustic properties of sound. However, these results cannot be generalized to tactile reception of ongoing speech. To date, there have been only a few attempts to quantify the benefits that can be derived through tactile aids in the reception of ongoing speech (Roeser, Friel-Patti & Scott, 1983; Scott, 1979; Sparks et al., 1979).

A procedure designed specifically as an objective measure of the ability to process ongoing speech is "tracking" (DeFilippo & Scott, 1978). In this technique, the term tracking describes an objective measure of speechreading using continuous text. A talker, reading from a text, presents material to a receiver who then attempts to repeat the text verbatim. Performance is measured according to the rate of verbatim repetition by the receiver, or as a correct wpm score. As a guide, normal-hearing subjects average about 100 to 120 wpm when neither ear plugs nor noise is used.

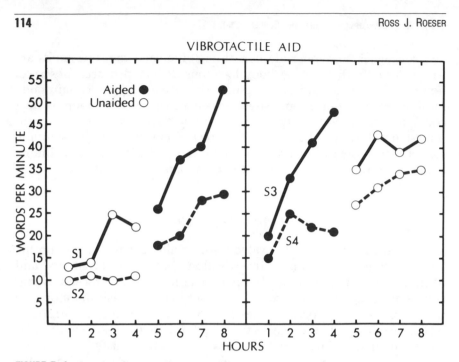

FIGURE 7–4. Tracking performance in words per minute from four subjects using a 3-channel vibrotactile aid. S1 and S2 began with unaided lipreading (open circles, left panel). S3 and S4 began lipreading with the tactile aid (filled circles, right panel) and changed to unaided lipreading (open circles, right panel). From Scott, B. L. (1979). Development of a tactile aid for the profoundly hearing impaired: Implication for use with the elderly. In M. Henoch (Ed.), *Aural rehabilitation for the elderly* (pp. 83–103). New York: Grune & Stratton. Reprinted with permission.

Scott (1979) used speech tracking to evaluate a 3-channel vibrotactile aid with very promising findings. Results from this experiment with four young adult, normal hearing subjects who were functionally deafened with ear plugs and white noise, are shown in Figure 7–4. Two conditions, lipreading alone (open circles) and lipreading with a tactile aid (closed circles), are depicted. Two of the subjects began lipreading-only for 4 hours without the use of the vibrotactile aid, then switched to the aided lipreading condition for 4 more hours. For the other two subjects, the order was reversed, beginning in the aided condition and switching to the unaided condition. As evidenced by the change in mean scores and the slopes of the learning curves, subjects 1 and 2 clearly demonstrated improvement from the unaided to the aided condition. Subject 4 shows slight improvement in the aided condition, but to a lesser extent than subjects 1 and 2. With subject 3, however, a slight decrease in performance was found in the aided condition. In addition, subject 3 complained of feeling nauseous when receiving vibrotactile stimulation. Significantly, although these subjects had no previous experience or training with the aid, three of the four benefitted almost immediately from its use. The clinician is also cautioned that some individuals may not benefit from tactile stimulation and, perhaps, may deteriorate in their performance.

Other studies using the tracking procedure to evaluate tactile aids have shown benefits, but to a lesser degree than Scott's (1979) experiment. DeFilippo (1984) found that tactile stimulation yielded higher tracking scores than did a nonaided condition. Sparks and colleagues (1979), using the MESA, found that tactile stimulation gave an initial advantage in tracking, but this advantage was eliminated after extensive training.

When attempts are made to assess the effects of any type of sensory aid with young deaf children, difficulty is encountered because of their severely limited speech and language abilities and a lack of standardized tests. Recognizing these difficulties, Friel-Patti and Roeser (1983) developed a computer-based procedure to assess the efficacy of one vibrotactile aid applied to profoundly deaf children. The method was similar to the assessment of ongoing speech in adults with the tracking procedure.

In their study, an attempt was made to quantify objectively changes in socially directed, purposeful communication that could be attributed to the use of the vibrotactile aid under investigation. Subjects were four profoundly deaf children. Each was enrolled in a preschool program for the deaf and in language therapy, during which they were seen for 30-minute, tri-weekly individual sessions. During these sessions, trained observers monitored targeted communication behaviors and recorded their occurrence.

In the study-design, each subject served as his or her own control; the subjects were evaluated when wearing the vibrotactile aid (aid-on) and then compared to the unaided (aid-off) condition. In the aid-on period (Phase I), subjects wore the vibrotactile aid in the tri-weekly language sessions and in the classroom. Mean wearing time was 10.5 hours per week. In the aid-off condition (Phase II), subjects did not use the vibrotactile aid in the individual therapy sessions or in the daily classroom program.

The measure used to assess the efficacy of the vibrotactile aid was termed the Communication Index, which was defined as the total amount of time each child used some form of communication, including vocalization only, sign language only, or combined vocalization and sign. This measure was obtained using a custom-designed, computer-based observation system.

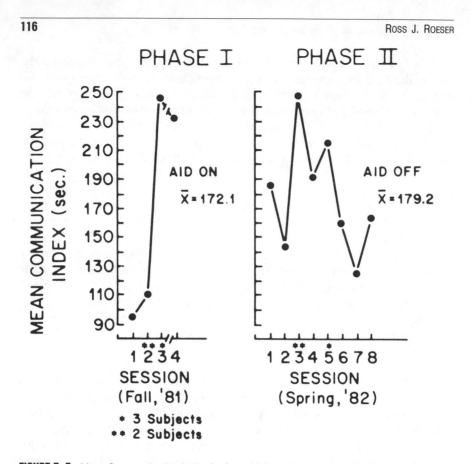

FIGURE 7–5. Mean Communication Index for four children who were hearing-impaired for aided (Phase I) and unaided (Phase II) conditions. From Friel–Patti, S., and Roeser, R. J. (1983). Evaluating changes in the communication skills of deaf children using vibrotactile stimulation. *Ear and Hearing, 4,* 31–40. Reprinted with permission.

Figure 7–5 displays the mean data obtained by Friel-Patti and Roeser. In the aid-on condition (Phase I), there was a very clear increase in the Communication Index which could have been a result of the use of the vibrotactile aid, a result of the intervention program, or perhaps a combination of both. However, following this very clear increase in performance in the aid-on condition, there was a definite decrease in performance in the eight evaluation sessions in the aid-off condition (Phase II). This decrease in performance would strongly indicate that the tactile aid alone was responsible for providing the increase in the Communication Index, as all conditions remained essentially the same except that the aid was removed for Phase II.

In order to further analyze the nature of the changes that occurred in the aid-on (Phase I) and aid-off (Phase II) conditions, the component responses of the Communication Index were analyzed separately. During Phase I, vocalization-only and sign-only appeared to show little change over the four evaluation sessions. However, the use of vocalization-plus-sign increased noticeably during this phase, changing from 48.3 seconds for evaluation session 1 to 183.7 seconds for session 4. During Phase II, greater variability was present. However, sign-only showed a gradual increase and vocalization-plus-sign decreased sharply. This study provides encouragement for improving communication through the vibrotactile mode for the young profoundly deaf population.

The effect of tactile aids on speech production was the primary question addressed by Goldstein and Stark (1976). Three groups of four profoundly deaf children were given training to produce consonant–vowel (CV) syllables using tactile, visual, and nonspeech displays. Results showed a significant increase in CV production for the two experimental groups (tactile and visual) and no significant change for the control group, providing evidence that the tactile and visual displays were essential in changing CV production.

Kringlebothn (1968) and colleagues (1983) also reported clear improvements in speech production with tactile stimulation. Kringlebothn (1968) showed that, compared with the conventional method of teaching the /s/ phoneme, more efficiency is gained with tactile stimulation. Goldstein and associates (1983) reported that with one deaf child who wore a tactile aid for 9 months, production of vocalizations increased in frequency within the first week, and the production of a variety of CV and CVC combinations improved greatly. Moreover, rate of production, breath control, and voice quality (loudness) all were improved by using the tactile aid.

In addition to these studies, investigators have commented on improved speech production even though the studies were not specifically designed for its measurement. For example, Oller, Payne, and Gavin (1980) stated that several of their subjects manifested important improvements in pronunciation of both fricative and nasal consonants while using the tactile aid they investigated. Similar improvements have been observed by Friel-Patti and Roeser (1983). Thus, clinical investigations support the notion that tactile aids should benefit not only speech reception, but also speech production.

SUBJECTS

Investigators assessing tactile aids can employ either normal hearing subjects who are functionally deafened with bilateral ear plugs and white noise introduced through earphones or subjects with hearing loss. Normal hearing subjects are readily available and have been used extensively in tactile aid research. As shown in Table 7–2, 9 of the 17 studies summarized were done with normal hearing subjects. Although this is a recognized practice, a potential problem exists because direct generalization of findings from normal hearing to hearing impaired subjects may lead to inaccuracies.

Few studies have been conducted with both normal hearing and hearing-impaired subjects using the same training procedures. Englemann and Rosov (1975) found that their subjects who were deaf initially learned to recognize single words more slowly than their hearing subjects, although the differences appeared to diminish with extended practice periods. Roeser, Friel-Patti, and Scott (1983) used speech tracking with four adult subjects, two with normal hearing and two with acquired profound deafness. Results from one of the normal hearing subjects showed that the vibrotactile aid provided benefit. Neither of the hearing impaired subjects, however, showed any gains with the same vibrotactile aid. Although these investigations are not definitive, they support the use of deaf subjects in experiments on tactile aids and exemplify why caution must be exercised in generalizing from normal hearing to hearing impaired subjects.

TRAINING

Most studies fail to provide specific information regarding the total amount of time subjects wear their tactile aids during the experimental procedures, but estimations are usually possible. Although several recent longitudinal studies have been reported, in the majority of investigations the total amount of wearing time ranges from as little as 2.5 hours to about 26 hours. In view of the time required for the normal auditory system to learn to process sound, it seems unreasonable to expect a subject to learn the complicated processing of tactile patterns in these relatively short periods. For those studies failing to show benefits from tactile stimulation, an important question is raised: was there sufficient training time allowed? Studies by Englemann and Rosov (1975) and Brooks and Frost (1983) indicated that only by using a tactile aid on a long-term basis will its total potential be realized.

Longitudinal studies provide very encouraging findings. Goldstein and colleagues (1983) and Friel-Patti and Roeser (1983) studied young profoundly deaf subjects with vibrotactile aids for 9 and 4 months respectively; significant gains in language skills and speech production were observed. These gains were related directly to the use of the aid.

Now that wearable tactile aids are commercially available, longitudinal studies are possible.

COMPARISON OF TACTILE AIDS AND COCHLEAR IMPLANTS

The goals of tactile aids and cochlear implants are essentially the same: (1) to provide wearers with increased auditory contact with their environment, including awareness of their own voice; (2) to improve their ability to speechread; and (3), ultimately, to provide the ability to discriminate connected discourse. Because the two devices have common goals, it would be logical to assume that numerous research studies have compared tactile aid and cochlear implant performance. Unfortunately, this is not the case. Apparently, most cochlear implant research teams do not feel compelled to study tactile aids, and those working with tactile aids often do not have populations of subjects with implants available for study. However, comparisons between tactile aid and cochlear implant performance are possible by reviewing functional differences, detection thresholds, and the available limited research data.

FUNCTIONAL DIFFERENCES

Table 7–3 compares functional differences between hearing aids, cochlear implants, and tactile aids on six performance factors. Hearing aids are usually recommended for daily use. In the case of children,

TABLE 7–3.

Functional Differences Between Hearing Aids, Cochlear Implants, and Tactile Aids

Factor	Hearing Aids	Cochlear Implants	Tactile Aids
Daily usage	Yes	Probably	?
Trial period	Yes	No	Yes
Initial cost	$550–$1200	$10,000–$25,000	$450–$3000
Risk	None	Yes	None
Long-term sequelae	Minimal	?	None
Effectiveness	Depends on type of loss and amount of residual hearing	Depends on residual neural population and coding/ processing technique	Depends on skin's ability to process sound and processing technique

teachers and classroom assistants are encouraged to check hearing aids on a regular basis to ensure proper function. A similar philosophy is present for cochlear implants. On the other hand, the issue of daily use is equivocal with tactile aids. Unquestionably, tactile aids provide maximal benefit in face-to-face conversation, where the signal-to-noise ratio is favorable and the use of visual cues is maximized. Tactile aids can also provide alerting signals to inform the wearer of the presence of warning or functional acoustic signals. However, whether the available wearable tactile systems can provide information in a sophisticated enough manner to be useful in a normal environment with the variety of signal-to-noise conditions that are present, has not been demonstrated. Trial period, initial cost, and long-term sequelae need no discussion, and risks are noted by Jackler and Bates (Chapter 9) and Loeb (Chapter 8). The issue of effectiveness is of major importance. With conventional amplification, effectiveness depends on the type of loss and the amount of residual hearing. With cochlear implants, the range in performance is very wide. Some patients perform extremely well, demonstrating open-set speech recognition and even communicating by telephone; others are unable to understand speech without lipreading. Why this variation in results occurs remains a mystery; it is still only speculative that the residual neural population is a factor. With tactile aids, both the limitations of the skin and the coding strategy are major factors in effectiveness.

SOUND DETECTION

Sound awareness is the ability to detect the presence of auditory stimuli in the environment. Detection of sound is important in providing alerting signals and must be present if discriminations are to be made. However, simple detection of sound does not imply discrimination. Table 7–4 compares sound awareness thresholds for the two systems when the instruments were set at their typical use gain settings. The data for cochlear implants are from a summary of findings from a large number of children using the 3M/House single-channel device (Thielemeir et al., 1985) and the data for tactile aids are from four children fit with a three-channel vibrotactile aid (Friel-Patti & Roeser, 1983). As indicated, awareness thresholds for the two devices are similar, being within 0 to 4 dB for the frequencies 500 through 4000 Hz. Speech awareness thresholds were slightly better for the tactile aid than for the cochlear implant, at 47 dB compared to 55 dB respectively. Overall, the data indicate that on measurements of sound awareness the same performance is possible for tactile aids and single-channel cochlear implants.

Comparable findings for sound awareness thresholds with single-channel cochlear implants and tactile aids are not surprising, because

TABLE 7–4.

Comparison of Mean Aided Awareness Thresholds for Single-channel Cochlear Implants and Tactile Aids (dB SPL)*

	Warbled Pure Tones						Speech Awareness Thresholds
	250	500	1000	2000	3000	4000	
Cochlear implants at 24 months†	59	56	57	57	59	64	55
**Tactile aids‡	68	58	60	61	59	63	47

   * Data were obtained at user-level volume settings.

   ** Thresholds converted from dB HL to dB SPL.

   † Adapted from Thielemeir, M. A., Tonokawa, L. L., Peterson, B., and Eisenberg, L. S. (1985). Audiological results in children with a cochlear implant. *Ear and Hearing, 6* (Suppl.), 27S–35S.

   ‡ Adapted from Friel-Patti, S., and Roeser, R. J. (1983). Evaluating changes in the communication skills of deaf children using vibrotactile stimulation. *Ear and Hearing, 4,* 31–40.

the amplitude of the stimulating signal, whether an electrical signal delivered to the cochlea or a tactile signal delivered to the skin, is determined by the gain setting of the amplifier. It is possible to increase the gain setting of either a cochlear implant or a tactile aid and significantly reduce the levels at which the patient responds to sound. However, the negative effect of increasing the gain of an amplifier with either device is a corresponding and increasing difficulty with background noise. That is, the background sounds will increasingly disrupt the processing of the primary signal. The application of microprocessing techniques, such as automatic noise suppression circuits, should significantly improve sound detection thresholds for both cochlear implants and tactile aids while reducing the effects of background noise.

RESEARCH STUDIES

Pickett and McFarland (1985) addressed several issues on cochlear implants and tactile aids and present a thorough review of the literature. In this paper, they provided a cross-comparative analysis of data from numerous studies. Performance with cochlear implants and tactile aids were compared in investigations using speech tracking, consonant identification, PB monosyllabic word recognition, and recognition of CID Everyday Sentences. Among the conclusions pertinent to this chapter were that (1) "the best implant performance is not substantially better, at this time, than for practiced subjects with multichannel tactile speech

systems" (p. 145); and that (2) "the current evidence on childrens' performance, all with single-channel implants, indicates that they are receiving the
same information as adults with single-channel implants: time and intensity information" (pp. 145–146). Pickett and McFarland warned that their
cross-comparative technique had inherent problems. However, the fact that
their research did not overwhelmingly demonstrate the superiority of
cochlear implants gives significant support for the use of tactile aids.

Additional data were also presented by Geers and Moog (1986) and
Miyamoto, Myers, and Punch (1987). Geers and Moog (1986) observed
performance on two large samples of profoundly deaf children with hearing aids, 10 children with single channel vibrotactile aids, and 2 children with single channel cochlear implants. Included in their analysis
was a comparison of their findings with results reported by the House
Ear Institute for 54 implanted children. Performance was compared on a
number of audiological tests and on measures of speech production and
language development. Children were placed in one of four categories
based on their test performance: category 1, No Pattern Perception; category 2, Pattern Perception; category 3, Some Word Identification; and
category 4, Consistent Word Identification. Their results indicated that
single-channel devices, both tactile and cochlear implant, provided only
pattern information (category 2), not spectral information. For children
in category 2 who had learned to categorize words according to stress
pattern and monitor their vocalizations through hearing aids, the single-
channel vibrotactile aids and single-channel cochlear implants provided
similar information with no apparent advantage from either device. (See
Chapters 10 and 11 for recent information on implanted children who
achieve higher perceptual categories.) These authors encourage the development of multichannel devices, both tactile aids and cochlear implants.

Miyamoto, Myers, and Punch (1987) incorporated vibrotactile aids
into their cochlear implant program, allowing their patients to experience tactile stimulation prior to receiving an implant. They report this
experience to be highly favorable. Basic stress differentiation and temporal concepts can be taught preoperatively with vibrotactile devices and
the ability of the subject to apply these cues to speech identification tasks
can be assessed. Because this training can be incorporated into the initial phases of cochlear implant rehabilitation, the probability of postimplant success is greatly enhanced. As part of their report, Miyamoto
and colleagues present vibrotactile data from one adult and one child
and compare these results to their implant scores. From these limited
data, it was concluded that the tactile aid provided notable benefit on
most of the suprasegmental tasks and on some of the segmental tasks,

with little difference in performance observed between the two types of stimulation.

An additional factor to be considered is patient acceptance. Is there a preference for one type of device over the other? No formal efforts have been made to address this question, although anecdotal reports are available. In a study by Cummins and Roeser (1987), two patients who had been fitted with cochlear implants were allowed to use wearable tactile aids. When given the option of using either of the instruments, both subjects indicated a preference for the cochlear implant; apparently implant stimulation was associated with "hearing," whereas tactile stimulation was not. It is difficult to factor out patient preference in subjects who have already received cochlear implants due to the "aura" and expectations surrounding the procedure. However, the concept of hearing restoration appears to be favored over replacement or substitution of hearing with tactile sensations.

Expected performance from single-channel cochlear implants and tactile aids on a number of different tasks can be predicted by retrospective analysis of available research studies. Table 7-5 compares expected performance between the two devices on eight different auditory tasks, six of which are time and intensity discriminations. For seven of these tasks, no differences between the two systems are observed. For differentiation of environmental sounds, however, it appears that cochlear implant stimulation provides superior input compared with tactile aids. Regarding open-set speech discrimination, recent evidence (see Chapter 10) indicates that a few children with the 3M/House single-channel device are outstanding in that they obtain some auditory-only, open-set speech recognition. In addition, recent reports on postlingually deafened adults with multichannel implants indicate that an increasing number are receiving some degree of auditory speech understanding (see Chapter 3). For the most part, however, open-set speech recognition with single-channel cochlear implants has not been documented in either children or adults.

Generally, the data available fail to show major performance differences between single-channel cochlear implants and tactile aids. Clearly, the need for comprehensive intrasubject comparisons of performance with cochlear implants and tactile aids is born out by this review. An important over-riding conclusion from the available data is that tactile aids appear to provide as much benefit as single-channel cochlear implants. When the costs, risks, and benefits are considered, there appears to be questionable justification for single-channel implants when wearable tactile aids are available.

TABLE 7–5
Comparison of Single-Channel Cochlear Implant and Tactile Aid Expected Performance (Courtesy of A. Proctor, 1986)*

Task	Cochlear Implant	Tactile Aid
Discriminate loud and soft sounds	Yes	Yes
Discriminate continuous and interrupted sounds	Yes	Yes
Discriminate long and short sounds	Yes	Yes
Discriminate number of sounds	Yes	Yes
Differentiate number of syllables in words	Yes	Yes
Differentiate number of syllables in sentences	Yes	Yes
Differentiate different types of sounds in the environment	Yes	Yes
Open-set speech recognition	No	No

*Adapted from the following sources: Geers, A., Miller, J., and Gustus, C. (1983, November). *Vibrotile stimulation — case study with a profoundly deaf child.* Paper presented at the annual convention of the American Speech-Language-Hearing Association, Cincinnati, OH. Geers, A., & Moog, J. S. (1986, November). *Long-term benefits from single-channel cochlear implants.* Paper presented at the annual convention of the American Speech-Language-Hearing Association, Detroit, MI. Thielemeier, M. A., Tonokawa, L. L., Petersen, B., and Eisenberg, L. A. (1985). Audiological results in children with a cochlear implant. *Ear and Hearing, 6 (Suppl.), 27S–35S.*

COMMERCIALLY AVAILABLE TACTILE AIDS

The lack of commercially available tactile aids and the large size of those that have been available experimentally, precluding easy wearability, have until recently adversely affected their widespread application. However, several wearable instruments for tactile stimulation have now been introduced. Table 7-6 lists the commercially available tactile aids and Appendix I contains addresses for those who wish to obtain additional information about these devices.

TACTAID

The Tactaid (Franklin, 1984) was originally a single channel device (Tactaid I), but recent developments have expanded the device to two channels (Tactaid II). The instruments were based on the work of Goldstein and colleagues (1983). In appearance and use, this aid is similar to a conventional body-type bone conduction hearing aid (see Figure 7-6). Tactaid I consists of a signal processing unit containing the microphone,

TABLE 7–6
Commercially Available Tactile Aids

Name of Instrument	Company	Type of Stimulation	Number of Channels	Approximate List Price
Tactaid I	Audiological Engineering	Vibrotactile	1	$ 435.00
Tactaid II	Audiological Engineering	Vibrotactile	2	825.00
Mini-Fonator	Siemens	Vibrotactile	1	895.00
Tacticon	Tacticon Corporation	Electrotactile	16	3300.00
Minivib	AB Special Instruments	Vibrotactile	3	n/a
KS 3/2	Telex	Vibrotactile	2 or 3	1600.00
Silent Page	Quest Electronics	Vibrotactile	1 to 15	348.00

cord, bone conduction transducer, and harness that mounts the transducer on the sternum. The aid can also be equipped with an optional wrist-strap or head-band to hold the vibrator.

Although Tactaid I is similar in appearance to a standard body-type bone conduction hearing aid, it has three important signal processing differences to accomodate presentation of signals to the skin. First, since the skin is less sensitive to vibrations than the ear, more power is incorporated into the unit. Second, due to the limited frequency response of the skin above 600 to 800 Hz, a frequency lowering (transposing) system is used to reduce frequencies to 250 Hz. Finally, because of the very limited ability of the skin to process information with background signals present, an automatic noise suppressing network is incorporated into the system.

Geers, Miller, and Gustus (1983) reported results from a 9 month longitudinal study using Tactaid I with a 2-year-old child who was profoundly deaf. Initially the child wore the tactile aid only in her nursery class, but after 2 months she began wearing it at home also. They found very impressive gains in expressive and receptive vocabulary that were related directly to the use of Tactaid I, as well as clear improvements in speech production.

Tactaid II (Figure 7–6) is similar in appearance and has similar operating characteristics as Tactaid I, but it is a 2 channel device. The

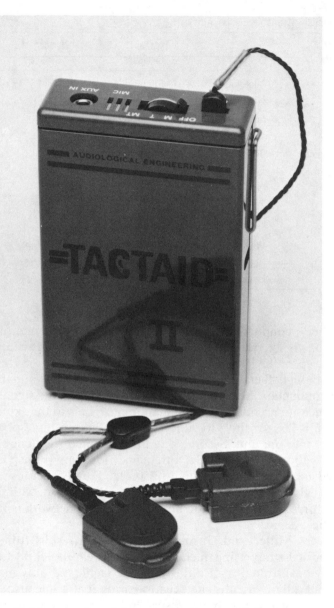

FIGURE 7-6. Tactaid II is a two-channel device with two bone conduction transducers and a three-way telepone (T) coil and microphone selector switch. Courtesy of Audiological Engineering Corp.

frequency spectrum is divided into two segments, with the lower channel covering the range 100 Hz to 1.8 kHz and the upper channel covering the range 1.5 kHz to 10 kHz. The unit includes a built-in microphone, a built-in telephone (T) coil, and a three-way T coil and microphone selector switch. The addition of the T coil option allows the user to carry out coded telephone communication, and opens up a new dimension in the use of tactile aids. The addition of the second channel should also provide enriched information to the wearer.

MINI-FONATOR

The Mini-Fonator is a single-channel device consisting of a wrist-worn vibrator and an external microphone that attaches to a signal processor by cords (see Figure 7-7). With the Mini-Fonator, acoustic signals are transposed to a peak frequency of 250 Hz before delivery to the wrist-worn transducer. At present no studies have been conducted in the United States with the Mini-Fonator, although informal studies have been carried out in Germany.

TACTICON

The Tacticon aid, a 16 channel device, is the only commercially available instrument based on electrotactile presentation. The unit consists of a sound processor, a stimulator belt with 16 electrodes worn on the waist, a microphone, and a battery charger (see Figure 7-8). The Tacticon was developed over a period of more than 15 years (Saunders, 1973; Saunders & Collins, 1971). Recent field studies reported by Saunders, Hill, and Franklin (1981) with profoundly deaf children aged 5 through 9 years using a nonportable prototype of the Tacticon showed that the electrotactile sensation was acceptable; the subjects reportedly enjoyed vocalizing to create the electrotactile sensation. In individual training sessions, the deaf children were reported to improve in their speech recognition, auditory awareness, and speech production. Now that this electrotactile aid is available as a wearable unit, the benefits of this novel form of tactile stimulation can be assessed on a long-term basis.

MINIVIBRATOR 3

The Minivibrator 3 (MINIVIB 3), developed in Sweden, is about the size of a small body-worn hearing aid (see Figure 7-9). The vibrator is usually attached to the wrist by a band, but can also be held in the hand or attached to other parts of the body with surgical tape. A noise rejection circuit is used to reduce unwanted background signals.

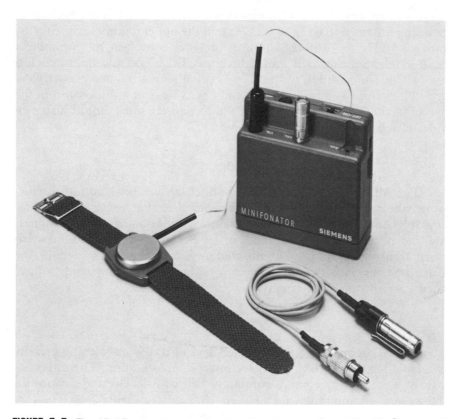

FIGURE 7–7. The Mini-Fonator is a single channel wrist-worn vibrotactile aid. Courtesy of Siemens Hearing Instruments.

Only limited data are available on this instrument. Spens (1985) reported that through 1985, over 200 units had been placed on wearers who were profoundly deaf. A survey of 14 users revealed very positive comments. Negative reactions and comments related to the cosmetics and size of the device have also been reported by some users; it should be pointed out, however, that these two problems plague virtually all of the available devices.

KANIEVSKI SOUND TACTILE AID (KS)

The KS device consists of two electromechanical vibrators, a miniature microphone, the electronics package and a battery (see Figure 7–10). The components together are small enough to fit into the palm of an adult's hand. The device has three channels: one for voiced speech

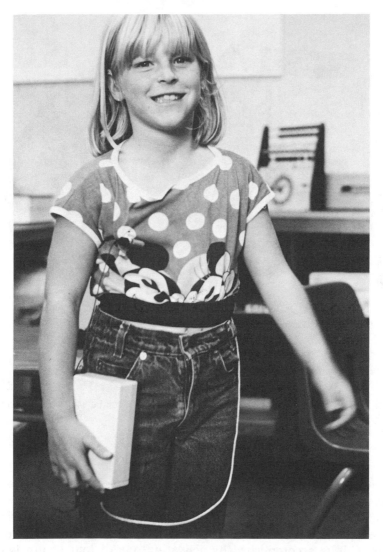

FIGURE 7–8. The Tacticon electrotactile aid provides electrical stimulation to the abdomen. Courtesy of Tacticon Corp.

sounds, one for voiceless speech sounds, and one for "partial" voiced sounds. A noise suppression circuit is built into the electronics package. Although there are no published reports on the KS device to date, the manufacturer reports that over 1400 units are in daily use throughout the world. Several U.S. clinics and laboratories are investigating this instrument and data are forthcoming.

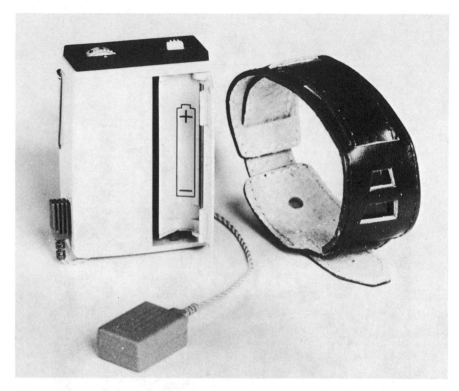

FIGURE 7–9. The Minivibrator 3 aid has a single vibrator that can be wrist worn or hand held. Courtesy of AB Special Instruments.

SILENT PAGE

This instrument serves a purpose quite different from the other commercially available and wearable tactile aids. Rather than attempting to improve communications by transposing airborne acoustic signals directly to the skin, the Silent Page notifies the wearer when specific sounds occur. This is accomplished by activating one of four channels on a wrist-worn vibrator and receiver whenever the specified sound occurs.

The instrument package consists of from 1 to 4 sensor-transmitters and a 4-channel wrist-worn vibrator and receiver (see Figure 7–11). Placed near a sound source to be monitored (e.g., telephone, doorbell, baby, fire alarm), the sensor-transmitter sends a coded radio signal to the vibrator and receiver upon receiving the acoustic signal. The wearer, who perceives the tactile vibrations, can identify the sound source by looking at the coded light on the receiver. With this system, the profoundly deaf individual can monitor up to 15 different sound sources, activating the

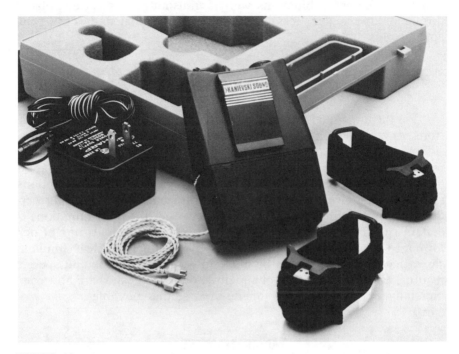

FIGURE 7-10. The Kanievski Sound Tactile Aid has two wrist-worn vibrators. Courtesy of Telex.

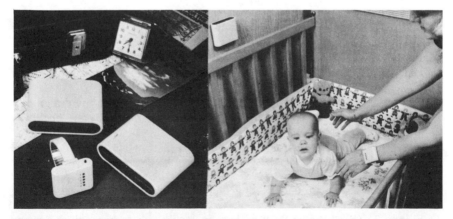

FIGURE 7-11. Silent Page notifies the wearer of acoustic stimuli by a wrist-worn vibrator after it is activated by a sensor-transmitter. Courtesy of Quest Electronics.

lights in different combinations, with 15 transmitters strategically placed throughout the wearer's residence or office. No formal studies are available on this system.

SUMMARY

For the individual who is profoundly deaf and who does not benefit from conventional amplification, the use of a tactile aid should be considered. In this chapter, the development of tactile aids is discussed with an emphasis on the type of configuration, location of stimulation, training procedures, subjects, and training period. With few exceptions, studies have shown that tactile aids provide benefits in both the reception of sound (sound awareness, and gross and fine discriminations of certain speech elements) and speech production. Comparisons of performance between tactile aids and single-channel cochlear implants show that similar gains can be made in sound awareness and speech-reading. Single and multiple channel wearable tactile aids are now commercially available, making longitudinal studies possible.

ACKNOWLEDGMENT

Portions of this work were supported by NIH Grant number R01 NS15982–01A1.

REFERENCES

Blamey, P. J., & Clark, G. M. (1985). A wearable multiple-electrode electrotactile speech processor for the profoundly deaf. *Journal of the Acoustical Society of America, 77,* 1619–1620.

Blamey, P. J., & Clark, G. M. (1987). Psychophysical studies to the design of a digital electrotactile speech processor. *Journal of the Acoustical Society of America, 82,* 116–125.

Brooks, P. L., & Frost, B. J. (1983). Evaluation of a tactile vocoder for word recognition. *Journal of the Acoustical Society of America, 74,* 34–39.

Cummins, C. C., & Roeser, R. J. (1987, March). Tactile aids: A case report. Paper presented at the annual meeting of the Texas Speech-Language-Hearing Association. Ft. Worth, TX.

DeFilippo, C. (1984). Laboratory projects in tactile aids to lipreading. *Ear and Hearing, 5,* 211–227.

DeFilippo, C. L., & Scott, B. L. (1978). A method for training and evaluating the reception of ongoing speech. *Journal of the Acoustical Society of America, 63,* 1186–1192.

Englemann, S., & Rosov, R. (1975). Tactual hearing experiments with deaf and hearing subjects. *Exceptional Children, 41,* 243–253.

Franklin, D. (1984). Tactile aids: New help for the profoundly deaf. *Hearing Journal, 37,* 20–24.

Friel-Patti, S., & Roeser, R. J. (1983). Evaluating changes in the communication skills of deaf children using vibrotactile stimulation. *Ear and Hearing, 4,* 31–40.

Gault, R. H. (1924). Progress in experiments on tactual interpretation of oral speech. *Social Psychology, 14,* 155–159.

Geers, A., Miller, J., & Gustus, C. (1983, November). *Vibrotactile stimulation —case study with a profoundly deaf child.* Paper presented at the annual convention of the American Speech-Language-Hearing Association, Cincinnati, OH.

Geers, A., & Moog, J. S. (1986, November). *Long-term benefits from single-channel cochlear implants.* Paper presented at the annual convention of the American Speech-Language-Hearing Association, Detroit, MI.

Geldard, F. H., & Sherrick, C. E. (1983). The cutaneous saltatory area and its presumed neural basis. *Perception and Psychophysics, 33,* 299–304.

Gentile, F. E. (1984). *Speech perception through the skin: Design and testing of a single channel tactile aid to supplement lipreading.* Unpublished senior independent project, Princeton University, NJ.

Goldstein, M. H., Proctor, A., Bulle, L., & Shimizu, H. (1983). Tactile stimulation in speech reception: Experience with a non-auditory child. In I. Hochberg, H. Levitt, & M. Osberger (Eds.), *Speech for the hearing impaired* (pp. 147–166). Baltimore, MD: University Park Press.

Goldstein, M. H., & Stark, R. E. (1976). Modifications of vocalizations of preschool deaf children by vibrotactile and visual displays. *Journal of the Acoustical Society of America, 59,* 1477–1481.

Karchmer, M. A., & Kirwin, L. (1977). *The use of hearing aids by hearing impaired students in the United States* (Series No. 4). Washington, DC: Office of Demographic Studies.

Keidel, W. D. (1974). The cochlear model in skin stimulation. In F. A. Geldard (Ed.), *Cutaneous communication systems and devices* (pp. 62–73). Austin, Texas: Psychonomic Society.

Kirman, J. H. (1974). Tactile perception of computer driven formants from voiced speech. *Journal of the Acoustical Society of America, 55,* 163–169.

Kringlebothn, M. (1968). Experiments with some visual and vibrotactile aids for the deaf. *American Annals of the Deaf, 113,* 311–317.

Miyamoto, R. T., Meyers, W. A., & Punch, J. L. (1987). Tactile aids in the evaluation procedure for cochlear implant candidacy. *Hearing Instruments, 38,* 33–37.

Nober, E. H. (1964). Pseudoauditory bone conduction thresholds. *Journal of Speech and Hearing Disorders, 29,* 469–476.

Nober, E. H. (1967). Vibrotactile sensitivity of deaf children to high intensity sound. *Laryngoscope, 77,* 2128–2148.

Oller, D. K., Payne, S. L., & Gavin, W. J. (1980). Tactual speech perception by minimally trained deaf subjects. *Journal of Speech and Hearing Research, 23,* 769–778.

Pickett, J. M., & McFarland, W. (1985). Auditory implants and tactile aids for the profoundly deaf. *Journal of Speech and Hearing Research, 28,* 134–150.

Pickett, J. M., & Pickett, B. H. (1963). Communication of speech sounds by a tactual vocoder. *Journal of Speech and Hearing Research, 6,* 207–222.

Reed, C. M., Durlach, N. I., & Braida, L. D. (1982). Research on tactile communication of speech: a review. *ASHA Monographs, 20,* 1–23.

Ries, P. W. (1982). *Hearing abilities of persons by socio-demographic and health characteristics: United States* (Series 10, Number 140). Washington, DC: National Center for Statistics.

Roeser, R. J. (1985). Tactile aids for the profoundly deaf. *Seminars in Hearing, 6,* 279–298.

Roeser, R. J. (in press). Cochlear implants and tactile aids for the profoundly deaf student. In R. J. Roeser & M. R. Downs (Eds.), *Auditory disorders in school children* (2nd ed.). New York: Thieme-Stratton Inc.

Roeser, R. J., Friel-Patti, S., & Scott, B. L. (1983). Development and evaluation of a tactile aid for the reception of speech. *Audiology, A Journal for Continuing Education, 8,* 79–94.

Sachs, R. M., Miller, J. D., & Grant, K. (1980). Perceived magnitude of electrocutaneous pulses. *Perception and Psychophysics, 28,* 255–262.

Saunders, F. A. (1973). An electrotactile sound detector for the deaf. *IEEE Transactions on Audio Electronics, 21,* 285–387.

Saunders, F. A., & Collins, C. C. (1971). Electrotactile stimulation of the sense of touch. *Journal of Biomedical Systems, 2,* 27–37.

Saunders, F. A., Hill, W. A., & Easley, T. A. (1978–1979). Development of a PLATO-based curriculum for tactile speech recognition. *Journal of Educational Technology Systems, 7,* 19–27.

Saunders, F. A., Hill, W. A., & Franklin, B. (1981). A wearable tactile sensory aid for profoundly deaf children. *Journal of Medical Systems, 5,* 265–270.

Scott, B. L. (1979). Development of a tactile aid for the profoundly hearing impaired: Implication for use with the elderly. In M. Henoch (Ed.), *Aural rehabilitation for the elderly* (pp. 83–103). New York: Grune & Stratton.

Sherrick, C. E. (1984). Basic and applied research on tactile aids for deaf people: Progress and prospects. *Journal of the Acoustical Society of America, 75,* 1325–1342.

Sparks, D. W., Ardell, L. A., Bourgeois, M., Wiedmer, B., & Kuhl, P. (1979). Investigating the MESA (Multipoint Electrotactile Speech Aid): The transmission of connected discourse. *Journal of the Acoustical Society of America, 65,* 810–815.

Sparks, D. W., Kuhl, P., Edmonds, A. E., & Gray, G. P. (1978). Investigating the MESA (Multipoint Electrotactile Speech Aid): The transmission of segmental features of speech. *Journal of the Acoustical Society of America, 63,* 246–257.

Spens, K. E. (1985). *Experiences of a tactile "hearing" aid.* Paper presented at the

International Congress on the Education of the Deaf, Stockholm, Sweden.

Sweetow, R. W. (1979). Amplification and the development of listening skills in deaf children [Audio Cassette]. *Audiology, A Journal for Continuing Education, 4.*

Thielemeir, M. A., Tonokawa, L. L., Petersen, B., & Eisenberg, L. S. (1985). Audiological results in children with a cochlear implant. *Ear and Hearing, 6* (Suppl.), 27S–35S.

Traunmuller, H. (1977). *The sentiphone, a tactual speech communication aid.* Paper presented at the Research Conference on Speech Processing Aids for the Deaf, Gallaudet College, Washington, DC

Yeni-Komshian, G. H., & Goldstein, M. H. (1977). Identification of speech sounds displayed on a vibrotactile vocoder. *Journal of the Acoustical Society of America, 62,* 194–198.

APPENDIX
SOURCES FOR ADDITIONAL INFORMATION ON
COMMERCIALLY AVAILABLE TACTILE AIDS

KANIEVSKI SOUND TACTILE AID

Telex
9600 Aldrich Avenue
Minneapolis, MN 55420

MINI-FONATOR

Siemens Hearing Instruments
685 Liberty Avenue
Union, NJ 07083

MINIVIBRATOR 3

AB Special Instruments
Box 27 066
S-102 51 Stockholm
Sweden

SILENT PAGE

Quest Electronics
510 S. Worthington Street
Oconoowoc, WI 53066

TACTAID I AND II

Audiological Engineering Corp.
9 Preston Road
Sommerville, MA 92143

TACTICON

Tacticon Corp.
4295 Oakwood Court
Concord, CA 94521

G E R A L D   E.   L O E B

NEURAL PROSTHETIC STRATEGIES FOR YOUNG CHILDREN

Neural prosthetic devices employ electronics to replace damaged or missing parts of the nervous system. One of the most complex and successful applications to date of this general notion is the cochlear implant. As encouraging experience accumulates with various designs in adults, there is increasing interest in applying this new technology to children. The transfer of therapeutic techniques from adults to children always requires special attention to those features of their bodies and lives that are not simply scaled-down versions of adults. This is particularly true when dealing with the nervous system which, unlike most organ systems, undergoes most of its functional development throughout childhood.

This chapter presents some of the physical and functional features of the immature, developing nervous system that suggest both special hope and special caution for neural prosthetics in children. Many of these features apply to clinical problems other than deafness, and much of the data must be extrapolated from neurophysiological inquiries in areas other than audition, one of the less well understood senses. However, these considerations provide what little objective direction is now available to help develop promising strategies for cochlear implantation. Given the shortage of unambiguous answers to the questions raised here, it is always tempting to proceed by blind empiricism. In a field as complex as neural prosthetics, this default strategy is both unlikely to produce much progress and certain to leave us wanting for the very information that might provide a better sense of direction.

SPECIAL FACTORS FAVORING IMPLANTS IN CHILDREN

STIMULATION MIGHT PREVENT ATROPHY

In the past decade, the term *critical period* has assumed great importance and credibility in developmental psychology, largely as a result of neurophysiological research on the development of feature-detecting neurons in the visual cortex of young animals. Experiments in kittens have demonstrated that the selective sensitivity of these cells to visual features such as oriented lines is not present before the animal is exposed to such visual stimuli (Hubel & Wiesel, 1970). In fact, the acquisition of at least some of the neural sensitivity (and presumably the related perceptual resolution) occurs during relatively brief temporal windows of perhaps a few days in the postnatal animal. During these so-called critical periods, the distribution of neurons that become sensitive to different features of visual images depends on the frequency of occurrence of such features in the visual world. The absence of particular features may lead to a permanent shortage of neurons sensitive to those features and to permanent behavioral deficits (Von Noorden, 1973). In the absence of any organized sensory input during the critical period, there may be a significant reduction in the physical size of the deprived brain center, which cannot be reversed by stimulation later in life (see Freeman, 1978, for review).

One clinical consequence of these developmental windows was discovered with the advent of corneal transplants. Adults who developed corneal opacities in adulthood had almost perfect restoration of their visual acuity even if it had been lost many years previously. However, adults who had had corneal opacities from birth remained functionally blind even though the refractive properties of the eye and the function of the retina appeared to be normal following the surgery. Even with time and efforts at rehabilitation, the sensations evoked by visual stimuli continued to be uninterpretable and even distressing to these patients, leading at least one to commit suicide. Corneal opacities in neonates are now corrected by transplants soon after birth, with excellent functional results (Casey, 1984).

Although the existence of critical periods in audition is not nearly so clear, it seems likely that some such phenomena exist. Auditory deprivation has been shown to result in anatomical and metabolic changes in some brainstem auditory nuclei (Feng & Rogowski, 1981; Moore & Kitzes, 1984; Webster & Webster, 1977, 1979; Wong-Riley, Merzenich, & Leake, 1978). At higher cognitive levels, there is certainly a strong feeling among educators of the deaf that language acquisition, whether verbal or visual, is greatly compromised if training is not begun early; furthermore, once there is one effective communication channel, transfer of fluent linguistic capabilities to new forms of communication is much easier, even for the adult (Walley, Pisoni, & Aslin, 1981; also Chapter 14).

If critical periods exist in the development of auditory perceptual capabilities, then the absence of coherent neural activity in the sensory pathways of the child who is profoundly deaf may permanently limit the functional capabilities of the brain to respond to prosthetically introduced auditory information. This consideration would appear to introduce a certain urgency into the decision whether to implant devices that are now primitive but rapidly evolving. Unfortunately, so little is known about these hypothetical critical periods that there is little guidance available. On the one hand, the auditory system may retain throughout life enough developmental capability to handle the very crude information that can be provided by any auditory prosthesis now envisioned. At the least, electrical stimulation may prevent some atrophic changes resulting from disuse (Chouard et al., 1983; Wong-Riley et al., 1981). However, the critical period may occur entirely in utero, when the fetus can respond to acoustic stimuli transmitted through the amniotic fluid. The results of implanting auditory prostheses in children of various ages can provide better answers to such questions than any animal experimentation, but only if the questions are recognized and the devices and studies are properly designed to answer them.

CENTRAL NERVOUS SYSTEM PLASTICITY MIGHT OVERCOME DISTORTION

While there is a great range of information carrying capacity in the various single and multichannel prostheses now available, even the best designs are limited to extremely simplified and distorted reproduction of only a few of the salient aspects of acoustic information. Furthermore, there are clear theoretical indications that, at least for cochlear electrode placements, the limits of resolution are already being approached (Loeb, 1985; Loeb, White, & Jenkins, 1983; Shannon, 1983a, 1983b; White, 1978). Given such limitations, one obvious question has been the ability of the nervous system to learn to extract the information from the distortion and to translate unnatural sensations into "normal" percepts. Experience with adult patients who are postlingually deafened has suggested that many of the functional results of a given implant are realized soon after it has been properly tuned and the patient has become accustomed to its use. There is also some indication that, at least among those patients using multichannel devices, speech understanding has gradually improved as a result of increased duration of device use without formal rehabilitative intervention (Brown, Dowell, & Clark, 1987; Schindler &

Kessler, 1987; Youngblood & Robinson, in press). This improvement over time is particularly observable in the recognition of contextual (sentence) materials, although performance on open-set tests of monosyllabic word recognition and on closed-set tests of vowel, consonant, and prosodic discrimination has also shown improvement (Schindler & Kessler, 1987).

The more plastic nervous systems of young children might be able to learn to make much better use of the limited and distorted prosthetic input than can postlingually deafened adults, who presumably try to find similarities between the prosthetically induced sensations and fully formed memories of sound. That is, prelingually deaf children, lacking this phonologic reference system, might conceivably develop an entirely new representation of linguistic sounds in their nervous systems. Although statistical correlations are not available and there are many notable exceptions (Schindler et al., 1986a; Schindler et al., 1986b), it may be relevant that some of the best users of prostheses, the so-called "star patients" whose performance seems to defy the design limitations of their devices, appear to be those whose deafness came on gradually, perhaps starting before adulthood. These patients may have had considerable practice dealing with distortions and limitations at an age when their perceptual processes were still adaptive.

However, plasticity as a justification for implanting children carries two important implications for device design, implications that have so far been largely ignored. First, the brain cannot possibly make use of information that it has not received. If the sound processor or the biophysical relationships between the electrodes and the auditory nerve fibers simply do not permit certain aspects of the acoustic signal to be represented in the evoked neural activity, then that information is irrevocably lost. This simple fact suggests that greater attention must be focused on both the detailed processes of neuronal activation by electrical stimuli and the various acoustic cues that can be used to recognize speech sounds. Second, the strategies for preprocessing speech information to convey as much raw information to the patient as possible are different from those strategies used to extract and transmit specific, selected features of the speech signal. An adult trying to find similarities between prosthetically induced sensations and the remembrance of natural sounds may well benefit from sophisticated preprocessing to present certain formants unambiguously to the auditory system. However, such a strategy must necessarily throw away information whose importance to and interpretability by the young nervous system is completely unknown. Preprocessing for children who are prelingually deaf should probably be limited to simple filtering and compression that compensates only for the transmission properties between electrodes and neurons, rather than attempting to emulate any guesses about normal speech recognition algorithms derived from the psychophysics of normal hearing research subjects.

SPECIAL PROBLEMS WITH IMPLANTS IN CHILDREN

HEAD GROWTH

In all of the currently proposed or available cochlear prostheses, an electrical cable traversing the external canal and middle ear cavity conveys the stimulus to the cochlea either from an implanted, superficially located, receiver, or from a percutaneous connector. If such a prosthesis has been implanted before the cranium reaches full development, something must give, eroding the tissue, breaking the lead, or dislodging the electrode. Luxford and House (1985; 1987), using the 3M/House single-channel implant, reported that this electrode's length is sufficient to accommodate increases in the height and width of the skull. Provided that the electrode is firmly anchored at the round window and the temporal squama, gradual straightening of the excess electrode lead occurs in the air-containing mastoid cavity. One possibility being explored is the use of coiled leads that can stretch to accommodate growth (O'Donoghue, Jackler, & Schindler, 1986). Although preliminary experiments have been encouraging, there are two fundamental properties of biological tissues that suggest long term problems. First, connective tissue tends to penetrate and encapsulate complex structures such as the interstices of a coil, eliminating compliance. This may be avoidable when crossing the air-filled middle ear space, but not all of the growth occurs exclusively across this space. Second, even tiny stresses that are continuously present tend to cause remodeling and erosion of connective tissue, which normally organizes itself in response to such stresses. The distended spiral, however elastic, will exert such forces at either end, perhaps eroding bone or loosening fixation, however secure initially. Such considerations seem to argue strongly for electrodes that are extracochlear and thus easily replaced, and perhaps for devices such as that developed at Guy's Hospital, London, which reach the promontory by surgically displacing the tympanic membrane to permit access via the external canal (Walliker et al., 1985).

The problem of head growth may be moot if it turns out to be impractical or unnecessary to implant children below the age of 2 to 3 years. O'Donoghue and colleagues (1986) have recently shown that most head growth is complete by 2 years of age. In initiating their Australian children's implant program with the Nucleus device, Clark and his associates (1987a) have begun with the 4-to-10-year-old age group in order to avoid, among other issues, the effect of skull growth on the electrode and lead wire assembly. In contrast, the American Nucleus children's program (Mecklenburg, 1987) considers 2 year olds as eligible for implantation, as does the 3M/House (Berliner, Eisenberg, & House, 1985) program.

INFECTION

Chronic and ascending middle ear infections constitute a major cause of sensorineural as well as conductive hearing loss in children, a fact of which otologists are all too aware. Inevitably, a certain percentage of auditory prostheses implanted in children will encounter infections. One of the best established truths of biomaterials science is the extreme difficulty, even impossibility, of completely eradicating an infection once it becomes entrenched around an avascular foreign body. Thus it seems inevitable that some of these devices will have to be completely removed to treat these infections. Even more ominous is the possibility that a cochlear implant may serve as a conduit for a middle-ear infection into the inner ear and central nervous system. If such infections can breach the normal, intact cochlear windows to give rise to sensorineural damage and meningitis, it seems likely that the presence of a foreign body, however well-sealed in place, will not prevent and may well exacerbate this problem. The tracking of middle ear infection into the implanted cochlea has been shown experimentally in cats by Leake, Rebscher, and Aird (1985), but House, Luxford, and Courtney (1985), in a questionnaire study, found no evidence of meningitis or inner-ear pathology in implanted children who developed middle ear infections. In more recent investigations in cats, results were mixed (Berkowitz et al., 1987; Cranswick et al., 1987; Franz, Clark, & Bloom, 1987). Depending upon the specific pathogen used to induce otitis media and the point in time following implantation at which the pathogen is introduced, the round window barrier may be ineffective, resulting in damage to cochlear structures.

The infection problem can only be viewed as a calculated risk in which some percentage of cochlear prostheses will eventually be associated with major and minor catastrophes, whether they caused them or not. At the very least, prudence would seem to dictate a very cautious approach to informed consent and a very aggressive approach to removing devices at the first signs of trouble. The risk of infection thus presents another consideration favoring minimally invasive, perhaps extracochlear, devices that can be easily removed without compromising surgical access for eventual replacement.

Device Life

The younger the patient, the longer the device has to survive or the more times it must be replaced over the life expectancy of the patient. Complex electromechanical devices interacting with living tissue have a great diversity of failure modes, many of which show no premonitory signs during early performance (see Loeb et al., 1982, for review). With a growing number of patients wearing devices for longer periods of time, a steadily increasing number and variety of device failures will inevitably be encountered. Luxford and House (1985) reported that 16 of 128 children required surgical revision or replacement, mostly for failures of the relatively simple 3M/House device in the first 2 to 3 years after implantation. Patients usually have two functional cochleas, so implants can be (and have been) inserted in the virgin ear; however, a patient with a failed device in one ear is then a patient being implanted with a device in his only good ear.

Replacing a failed implant in the same ear may be problematic. In the case of small, minimally invasive cochlear electrodes and certainly for extracochlear electrodes, replacement appears to be possible. However, the best functional results are likely to come from the relatively bulky and deeply inserted multichannel electrodes. When such devices are encapsulated by the usual scar tissue, they may be difficult to remove without damaging the basilar membrane or osseous spiral lamina, and they may leave cavities into which the insertion of a similar or larger, more complex electrode is not feasible. If the cavity must be left vacant for some time (e.g., to permit an infection to be eradicated), scar tissue is likely to obliterate the cavity, preventing replacement with a comparable electrode. In a few instances, single-channel electrodes have been replaced by longer multiwire electrode arrays without apparent trauma or impact on patient performance (Lindeman, Mangham, & Kuprenas, 1987; Luxford & House, 1987). Clark and his associates (1987c) have reported that, in 3 patients, a long prototype multielectrode array was replaced with its clinical counterpart, without difficulties and, again, without effecting performance. In all these instances, an electrode was explanted and immediately replaced with another; cases in which reimplantation was attempted following a lapse of time during which scar tissue might develop have not been reported in the literature.

One approach (Loeb, White, & Jenkins, 1983; Loeb et al., 1983; Simmons et al., 1979) was based on the assumption that the relatively simple, passive electrode assembly should be the least likely to fail or need upgrading. Accordingly, surgical disconnects are incorporated to allow the electrode to be left in place while the electronics package containing the receiver and stimulator circuits is replaced. However, this solves only part of the problem while adding substantially to the number and complexity of components then subject to failure (e.g., the connector itself). Clark and his colleagues (1987a) reported that, because failures in the connector may be as likely to occur as in the receiver, the disconnect system of the Nucleus system was recently eliminated in the course of producing a smaller device suitable for children. The irony of this situation is obvious: the design feature permitting easy access for upgrading or replacement of the receiver without disturbing the intracochlear electrode, and thus avoiding potential damage to cochlear structures, has been eliminated for the very population most likely to need this feature.

The thorny problem of device failure, coupled with the still uncertain advantages of multichannel devices (particularly for subjects who are prelingually deaf), seems to argue again in favor of simple, single-channel, minimally invasive prostheses that are easily removed and replaced in toto.

ASSESSMENT

There is probably no greater stumbling block to the comparison of auditory prosthesis designs in adults than the absence of effective and efficient assessment tests of every sort. Much of the variability in patient performance, particularly with multichannel devices, undoubtedly comes from enormous differences in the condition of the spiral ganglion cells. However, only a suggestion for a preoperative screening test (Smith & Simmons, 1982) and only the rudiments of parametric tests that can be used postoperatively to assess this most basic consideration are available (Shannon, 1983b; White, 1984; White, Merzenich, & Gardi, 1984). As the numbers of channels and parameters in the sound processing units increase to improve performance, the number of simultaneous variables to be explored in the postoperative tuning of the devices rises at least geometrically, requiring lengthy fitting sessions and the communication of many objective and subjective impressions from the patient to the practitioner. Clearly, fitting procedures applied to adults may be beyond the capabilities and patience of young patients with little or no previous auditory experience. Although there has been a laudable, if frequently ignored, attempt to standardize speech related tests in adults, namely, the Minimal Auditory Capabilities Battery (Owens et al., 1985), the testing of children who may have no preexisting vocabulary and who are acquiring verbal communication exclusively through their prosthetic devices poses much more formidable problems (Clark et al., 1987b; Nienhuys et al., 1987; Thielemeir et al., 1985; also see Chapters 11 and 12).

As multichannel devices become more complex, offering options both in speech coding strategies (Schindler et al., in press; Wilson, in press-a; in press-b) and in increased numbers of channels, questions concerning the selection of an appropriate processing scheme for the very young, nonverbal child become critical. Methods for objectively mapping both the magnitude and location of surviving auditory nerve fibers must be developed. Once such techniques are developed, the data collected on the choice of a processing scheme for adults who demonstrate similar patterns of nerve survival can be applied (albeit tentatively) to infants, just as conventional pediatric hearing aid fittings depend on a pool of accumulated adult data. Having selected the appropriate processor and channels for stimulation through objective assessment techniques, the clinician must then employ behavioral methods to fine-tune the device, extending to the utmost the capability and patience of both the clinician and child and bringing to bear the techniques of audiologic pediatric testing. Noninteractive functional tests, such as the acoustic brainstem response (ABR), have been under investigation in the fitting of hearing aids to young children (Mahoney, 1985). Currently, work is in progress on the use of electrically evoked brainstem responses (EABR), both preoperatively and for postoperative device adjustment (Brightwell, Rothera, Conway, & Graham, 1985; Chouard, Meyer, & Danadieu, 1979; Dobie & Kimm, 1980; Gardi, 1985; Starr & Brackmann, 1981; Stypulkowski, van den Honert, & Kvistad, 1986; Waring, Don, & Brimacombe, 1985). However, until such technically sophisticated tests are feasible and interpretable, yet another argument is found in favor of simple, single channel prostheses that can be easily upgraded as the patient gets old enough and experienced enough to provide the necessary feedback.

SPECIAL RESEARCH TOPICS IN CHILDREN

GRADUAL ONSET OF STIMULUS AWARENESS

A generally familiar phenomenon among clinicians experienced in fitting hearing aids to young deaf children is the gradual onset of stimulus awareness. Eisenberg and House (1982) have commented anecdotally on an observation in one of their youngest implant patients, a child aged 3 years 6 months. When tested shortly after implantation, the child responded only inconsistently to sound. The stimulator was gradually set at its maximum voltage. The child then showed a complete lack of awareness to stimulation, suggesting a possible device malfunction. Lacking any electronic or biological assay of a failure mode, the clinicians were fortunate to note that involuntary responses (eye blinks, body reflexes, and arousal) could be obtained to sounds presented via the prosthesis during sleep. They then observed sound awareness during waking in the form of the child lowering her voice, which developed slowly over several weeks. Gradually, as the child became more sensitized to sound, device loudness was adjusted over time according to the way in which the child modulated her voice at different settings. These observations constitute a salient demonstration of both the complete inappropriateness of procedures and expectations based on experience with adult patients and the largely unknown plasticity of the immature nervous system. Cochlear implants in young children offer a gold mine of opportunities to learn about cognitive development through carefully designed observations and psychophysical experiments.

EXTRACTION OF TEMPOROSPATIAL CUES

One of the remarkable findings for all prosthesis designs and all adult subjects tested is the almost complete absence of stimulus frequency discrimination above 300 Hz (Eddington, 1980; Shannon, 1983a). At the same time, there is considerable evidence suggesting that electrical stimulation causes phase-locking of auditory nerve discharge at frequencies up to at least 3000 Hz (Loeb, White, & Merzenich, 1983) and that phase-locked information contributes to pitch perception in hearing individuals (Sachs & Young, 1980). Although individual neurons cannot fire action potentials faster than about 300 pps, they tend to respond specifically during one phase of a much higher frequency acoustic or electrical stimulus; the combined activity of an ensemble of such neurons thus encodes this higher frequency. The absence of pitch sensations above 300 Hz in prosthesis patients suggests that the way in which the nervous system normally interprets phase-locked information is incompatible with some aspects of the temporospatial pattern of auditory nerve activity induced by the electrical stimulation strategies employed to date (Loeb, White, & Merzenich, 1983). However, the more adaptable nervous systems of children might possibly learn to extract pitch information from electrical stimulus frequencies over the entire speech recognition range, thus augmenting the highly limited place information possible with intracochlear electrodes. The potential of the developing nervous system argues for avoiding complex preprocessing algorithms developed for adults that tend to eliminate high frequency information. Again, careful psychophysical experiments could produce a wealth of information about normal hearing, as well as providing objective data to guide the improvement of prostheses intended specifically for children.

General Strategies

The development of a complex implantable device such as a cochlear prosthesis requires a major investment of time, personnel, and money. Thus, despite the above arguments, it is most likely that children will continue to receive devices designed for adults for some time to come. The decision facing the regulatory agencies will be whether to permit any general marketing of existing devices for implantation in children. The decision facing the individual clinician and the patient's family will be which device to choose.

There is little doubt that even poorly designed devices intended for adults will be attractive to the parents and teachers who must cope with a child who is profoundly deaf. Furthermore, once implanted, there will be ringing testimonials from those parties who are not directly aware of the device's design limitations and who are not in a position to weigh the technical merits of alternatives. It is tempting to suggest that a prohibition on implanting children would motivate the researchers and the industry to develop devices specifically geared to the needs of children. However, the regulatory system requires only devices that are "safe and efficacious," not theoretically or technically "optimal." Efficacy has been fairly easy to demonstrate and safety is a relative judgement that affects implants of any design. An artificially imposed prohibition would delay the availability of any prosthesis to many children during their formative childhood years and would foreclose the most important source of data needed to answer the very difficult theoretical and technical questions posed earlier.

Given that relatively large numbers of children are likely to receive auditory prostheses over the next several years, the following considerations may help maximize the research benefits while minimizing the individual patient risks:

CONSIDER MINIMALLY INVASIVE DEVICES. For a single-channel device, there is no functional or physiological disadvantage to an extracochlear electrode placement. Minor technical problems regarding fixation, power consumption, and current spread to pain and vestibular fibers have been noted, but these are easily corrected with much less design effort than has gone into intracochlear electrodes.

USE PREPROCESSING AND TRANSMISSION SCHEMES THAT DISTORT ONLY MINIMALLY THE ACOUSTIC SIGNAL. The plasticity and capacity of the brain cannot be evaluated as long as the information capacity of the prosthesis insults the brain's supposed capacity. Well-developed biophysical principles underlying neural responses to electrical stimuli must be drawn upon in ascertaining that the psychophysically important features of the acoustic signal are in some way reflected in the evoked neural activity. The lack of such considerations is an important failing of the 3M/House design, which employs an over-modulated, unrectified 16kHz stimulus waveform simply because it is easily transmitted across the skin.

DEVELOP AND APPLY OBJECTIVE SCREENING TESTS FOR THE CONDITION OF THE AUDITORY CENTRAL NERVOUS SYSTEM. Given the tremendous variability in pathology, intelligence, and device function that will be encountered in patients, it will take a large data base to learn to interpret and to use predictively such tests as the EABR. However, the longer we postpone gathering these data, the longer we will be forced to make individual therapeutic choices in the dark.

DEVELOP AND APPLY PSYCHOPHYSICAL AND FUNCTIONAL TESTS THAT MIGHT REVEAL THE PLASTICITY AND ADAPTATION THAT ARE ANTICIPATED IN RESPONSE TO AN IMPLANTED DEVICE. If there were nothing special about children's nervous systems, then implantation might be postponed until patients reach maturity when they can give informed consent, by which time devices might be vastly improved. If plasticity is going to be used to justify an invasive, experimental procedure on children who may not even be aware of their disability, then some special obligations are imposed upon those recommending such a procedure. Not the least of these is the promotion of the rapid advancement of cochlear implant science, so that the number of patients who must inevitably be subjected to the tentative first applications of a newly emerging therapy is minimized.

REFERENCES

Berkowitz, R., Franz, B., Shepherd, R., Clark, G., & Bloom, D. (1987). Pneumococcal middle ear infection and cochlear implantation. *Annals of Otology, Rhinology and Laryngology, 96* (Suppl. 128), 55–56.

Berliner, K. I., Eisenberg, L. S., & House, W. F. (Eds.) (1985). The cochlear implant: An auditory prosthesis for the profoundly deaf child. *Ear and Hearing, 6* (Suppl.), 1S–69S.

Brightwell, A., Rothera, M., Conway, M., & Graham, J. (1985). Evaluation of the status of the auditory nerve: Psychophysical tests and ABR. In R. Schindler & M. Merzenich (Eds.), *Cochlear implants* (pp. 343–349). New York: Raven Press.

Brown, A., Dowell, R., & Clark, G. (1987). Clinical results for postlingually deaf patients implanted with multichannel cochlear prostheses. *Annals of Otology,*

Rhinology and Laryngology, 96 (Suppl. 128), 127–128.

Casey, T. (1984). *Corneal grafting: Principles and practice.* Philadelphia: W. B. Saunders.

Chouard, C., Meyer, B., & Danadieu, F. (1979). Auditory brainstem potentials in man evoked by electrical stimulation of the round window. *Acta Otolaryngologica, 87,* 287–293.

Chouard, C., Meyer, B., Josset, P., & Buche, J. (1983). The effect of the acoustic nerve chronic electric stimulation upon the guinea pig cochlear nucleus development. *Acta Otolaryngologica, 95,* 639–645.

Clark, G., Blamey, P., Busby, P, Dowell, R., Franz, B., Musgrave, G., Nienhuys, T., Pyman, B., Roberts, S., Tong, Y., Webb. R., Kuzma, J., Money, D., Patrick, J., & Seligman, P. (1987a). A multiple-electrode intracochlear implant for children. *Archives of Otolaryngology, 113,* 825–828.

Clark, G., Busby, P., Roberts, S., Dowell, R., Tong, Y., Blamey, P., Nienhuys, T., Mecklenburg, D., Webb, R., Pyman, B., & Franz, B. (1987b). Preliminary results for the Cochlear Corporation multielectrode intracochlear implant in six prelingually deaf patients. *American Journal of Otology, 8,* 234–239.

Clark, G., Pyman, B., Webb, R., Franz, B., Redhead, T., & Shepherd, R. (1987c). Surgery for the safe insertion and reinsertion of the banded electrode array. *Annals of Otology, Rhinology and Laryngology, 96* (Suppl. 128), 10–12.

Cranswick, N., Franz, B., Clark, G., Shepherd, R., & Bloom, D. (1987). Middle ear infection postimplantation: Response of the round window membrane to *Streptococcus Pyogenes. Annals of Otology, Rhinology and Laryngology, 96* (Suppl. 128), 53–54.

Dobie, R., & Kimm, J. (1980). Brainstem responses to electrical stimulation of the cochlea. *Archives of Otolaryngology, 106,* 573–577.

Eddington, D. (1980). Speech discrimination in deaf subjects with cochlear implants. *Journal of the Acoustical Society of America, 68,* 885–891.

Eisenberg, L., & House, W. (1982). Initial experience with the cochlear implant in children. *Annals of Otology, Rhinology and Laryngology, 91* (Suppl. 91), 67–73.

Feng, A., & Rogowski, B. (1981). Effects of monaural and binaural occlusion on the morphology of neurons in the medial superior olivary nucleus of the rat. *Brain Research, 189,* 530–534.

Franz, B., Clark, G., & Bloom, D. (1987). Effect of experimentally induced otitis media on cochlear implants. *Annals of Otology, Rhinology and Laryngology, 96,* 174–177.

Freeman, R. (1978). *Developmental neurobiology of vision.* New York: Plenum Press.

Gardi, J. (1985). Human brain stem and middle latency responses to electrical stimulation: Preliminary observations. In R. Schindler & M. Merzenich (Eds.), *Cochlear implants* (pp. 351–363). New York: Raven Press.

House, W., Luxford, W., & Courtney, B. (1985). Otitis media in children following the cochlear implant. *Ear and Hearing, 6* (Suppl.), 24S–26S.

Hubel, D., & Wiesel, T. (1970). The period of susceptibility to the physiological effects of unilateral eye closure in kittens. *Journal of Physiology* (London), *206,* 419–436.

Leake, P., Rebscher, S., & Aird, D. (1985). Histopathology of cochlear implants. In R. Schindler & M. Merzenich (Eds.), *Cochlear implants* (pp. 55–64). New York: Raven Press.

Lindeman, R. C., Mangham, C. A., & Kuprenas, S. V. (1987). Single-channel and multichannel performance for a reimplanted cochlear prosthesis patient. *Annals of Otology, Rhinology and Laryngology, 96* (Suppl. 128), 150–151.

Loeb, G. (1985). Single and multichannel cochlear prostheses: Rationale, strategies, and potential. In R. Schindler & M. Merzenich (Eds.), *Cochlear implants* (pp. 17–28). New York: Raven Press.

Loeb, G., Byers, C., Rebscher, S., Casey, D., Fong, M., Schindler, R., Gray, R., & Merzenich, M. (1983). Design and fabrication of an experimental cochlear prosthesis. *Medical and Biological Engineering and Computing, 21,* 241–254.

Loeb, G., McHardy, J., Kelliher, E., & Brummer, S. (1982). Neural prosthetics. In D. William (Ed.), *Biocompatibility in clinical practice* (Vol. 2, pp. 123–149). Boca Raton: CRC Press.

Loeb, G., White, M., & Jenkins, W. (1983). Biophysical considerations in the electrical stimulation of the auditory nervous system. *Annals of the New York Academy of Sciences, 405,* 123–136.

Loeb, G., White, M., & Merzenich, M. (1983). Spatial cross-correlation: A proposed mechanism for acoustic pitch perception. *Biological Cybernetics, 47,* 149–163.

Luxford, W., & House, W. (1985). Cochlear implants in children: Medical and surgical considerations. *Ear and Hearing, 6* (Suppl.), 20S–23S.

Luxford, W. & House, W. (1987). House 3M cochlear implant: Surgical considerations. *Annals of Otology, Rhinology and Laryngology, 96* (Suppl. 128), 12–14.

Mahoney, T. (1985). Auditory brainstem response hearing aid applications. In J. T. Jacobson (Ed.), *The auditory brainstem response* (pp. 349–370). San Diego, CA: College-Hill Press.

Mecklenburg, D. J. (1987). The Nucleus children's program. *American Journal of Otology, 8,* 436–442.

Moore, D., & Kitzes, L. (1984). Projections from cochlear nucleus to inferior colliculus in normal and unilateral neonatal cochlear ablated gerbils. *Abstracts of the Society for Neurosciences, 10* (Abstract No. 333.2), 1147 .

Nienhuys, T., Musgrave, G., Busby, P., Blamey, P., Nott, P., Tong, Y., Dowell, R., Brown, L., & Clark, G. (1987). Educational assessment and management of children with multichannel cochlear implants. *Annals of Otology, Rhinology and Laryngology, 96* (Suppl. 128), 80–82.

O'Donoghue, G., Jackler, R., Jenkins, W., & Schindler, R. (1986). Cochlear implantation in children: The problem of head growth. *Otolaryngology-Head and Neck Surgery, 94,* 78–81.

O'Donoghue, G., Jackler, R., & Schindler, R. (1986). Observations on an experimental expansile electrode for use in cochlear implantation. *Acta Otolaryngologica, 102,* 1–6.

Owens, E., Kessler, D., Raggio, M., & Schubert, E. (1985). Analysis and revision of the Minimal Auditory Capabilities (MAC) battery. *Ear and Hearing, 6,* 280–290.

Sachs, M., & Young, E. (1980). Effects of non-linearities on speech encoding in the auditory nerve. *Journal of the Acoustical Society of America, 68,* 858–875.

Schindler, R., & Kessler, D. (1987). The UCSF/Storz cochlear implant: Patient performance. *American Journal of Otology, 8,* 247–255.

Schindler, R., Kessler, D., Jackler, R., & Merzenich, M. (in press). Multichannel cochlear implants: Current status and future directions. In J. Johnson (Ed.), *American Academy of Otolaryngology-Head and Neck Surgery: Instruction course* (Vol. 1). St. Louis, MO: C. V. Mosby.

Schindler, R., Kessler, D., Rebscher, S.J., & Yanda, J. (1986a). The University of California, San Francisco/Storz cochlear implant program. *Otolaryngologic Clinics of North America, 19,* 287–305.

Schindler, R. A., Kessler, D. K., Rebscher, S. J., Yanda, J., and Jackler, R. K. (1986b). The UCSF/Storz multichannel cochlear implant: Patient results. *Laryngoscope, 96,* 597–603.

Shannon, R. (1983a). Multichannel electrical stimulation of the auditory nerve in man. I. Basic psychophysics. *Hearing Research, 11,* 157–189.

Shannon, R. (1983b). Multichannel electrical stimulation of the auditory nerve in man. II. Channel interaction. *Hearing Research, 12,* 1–16.

Simmons, F., Mathews, R., Walker, M., & White, R. (1979). A functioning multi-channel auditory nerve stimulator. *Acta Otolaryngologica, 87,* 170–175.

Smith, L., & Simmons, F. (1982). Estimating eighth nerve survival by electrical stimulation. *Annals of Otology, Rhinology and Laryngology, 92,* 19–23.

Starr, A., & Brackmann, D. (1981). Brain stem potentials evoked by electrical stimulation of the cochlea in human subjects. *Annals of Otology, Rhinology and Laryngology, 88,* 550–556.

Stypulkowski, P., van den Honert, C., & Kvistad, S. (1986). Electrophysiologic evaluation of the cochlear implant patient. *Otolaryngologic Clinics of North America, 19,* 249–257.

Thielemeir, M., Tonokawa, L, Peterson, B., & Eisenberg, L. (1985). Audiological results in children with a cochlear implant. *Ear and Hearing, 6* (Suppl.), 27S–35S.

Von Noorden, G. (1973). Experimental amblyopia in monkeys. Further behavioral observations and clinical correlations. *Investigative Ophthalmology, 12,* 721.

Walliker, J., Douek, E., Frampton, S., Abberton, E., Fourcin, A., Howard, D., Nevard, S., Rosen, S., & Moore, B. (1985). Physical and surgical aspects of external single channel electrical stimulation of the totally deaf. In R. Schindler and M. Merzenich (Eds.), *Cochlear implants* (pp. 143–155). New York: Raven Press.

Walley, A., Pisoni, D., & Aslin, R. (1981). The role of early experience in the development of speech perception. In J. Alberts & M. Petersen (Eds.), *The development of perception: Vol. I. Audition, somatic perception and the chemical senses* (pp. 219–255). New York: Academic Press.

Waring, M., Don, M., & Brimacombe, J. (1985). ABR assessment of stimulation in induction coil implant patients. In R. Schindler & M. Merzenich (Eds.), *Cochlear implants* (pp. 375–378). New York: Raven Press.

Webster, D., & Webster, M. (1977). Neonatal sound deprivation affects brainstem auditory nuclei. *Archives of Otolaryngology, 103,* 392–396.

Webster, D., & Webster, M. (1979). Effects of neonatal conductive hearing loss on brainstem auditory nuclei. *Annals of Otology, Rhinology and Laryngology, 88,* 684–688.

White, M. (1978). *Design considerations of a prosthesis for the profoundly deaf.* Unpublished doctoral dissertation, University of California, Berkeley.

White, M. (1984). The multichannel cochlear prosthesis: Channel interactions. In *Proceedings of the 6th Annual Conference of IEEE Engineering for Medicine and Biology Society* (pp. 396–400).

White, M., Merzenich, M., & Gardi, J. (1984). Multichannel cochlear implants: Channel interactions and processor design. *Archives of Otolaryngology, 110,* 493–591.

Wilson, B. S., Finley, C. C., Farmer, J. C., Lawson, D. T., Weber, B. A., Wolford, R. D., Kenan, P. D., White, M. W., Merzenich, M. M., & Schindler, R. A. (in press-a). Comparative studies for speech processing strategies for cochlear implants. *Laryngoscope.*

Wilson, B. S., Schindler, R. A., Finley, C. C., Kessler, D. K., Lawson, D. T., & Wolford, R. D. (in press-b). Present status and future enhancements of the UCSF cochlear prostheses. In P. Banfai (Ed.), *Cochlear implants 1987.* New York: Springer-Verlag.

Wong-Riley, M., Leake-Jones, P., Walsh, S., & Merzenich, M. (1981). Maintenance of neuronal activity by electrical stimulation of unilaterally deafened cats demonstrable with cytochrome oxidase technique. *Annals of Otology, Rhinology and Laryngology, 90* (Suppl. 82), 30–32.

Wong-Riley, M., Merzenich, M., & Leake, P. (1978). Changes in endogenous enzymatic reactivity to DAB induced by neuronal inactivity. *Brain Research, 141,* 185–192.

Youngblood, J., & Robinson, S. (1988). Ineraid (Utah) multichannel cochlear implants. *Laryngoscope, 98,* 5–10.

C H A P T E R 9

ROBERT K. JACKLER
GRANT J. BATES

MEDICAL AND SURGICAL CONSIDERATIONS OF COCHLEAR IMPLANTATION IN CHILDREN

Cochlear implantation during early childhood presents medical, surgical, and technical complexities not encountered in adults. Merely arriving at the diagnosis of profound deafness requires sophisticated audiologic methodology and may require prolonged therapeutic trials with hearing aids and educational programs. In addition, the causes of deafness among children differ considerably from those encountered in the adult population. In congenital losses, co-existing neural deficits may limit the potential benefit from electrical stimulation of the auditory end organ. In early acquired losses, in which meningitis predominates, cochlear patency is frequently compromised and may render insertion of long intracochlear devices difficult or impossible.

To achieve implantation in children, surgical techniques must be modified due to the thinness of the skull and incomplete development of the ear canal and mastoid. An accommodation must be made for the eventual growth of the temporal bone and skull. Redundancy of the electrode lead wire is needed to prevent dislodgement of its intracochlear portion. As children frequently suffer from middle-ear infection, a barrier must be constructed to protect the inner ear from intracochlear spread of infection. Suppurative labyrinthitis in the implanted ear may damage the surviving neural population.

Additional device modifications, especially further miniaturization and enhanced long-term component stability, must be achieved before widespread application of cochlear implant technology in children who are deaf is undertaken. Because long term device failures are probable and because future technological breakthroughs may provide a compelling need to upgrade existing hardware, the eventual necessity of replacing an indwelling device in the pediatric population is very likely. The potential detrimental effects of explantation followed by reimplantation of a new device on cochlear patency and eighth nerve survival are currently unknown.

THE ETIOLOGIES OF PROFOUND SENSORINEURAL HEARING LOSS IN CHILDREN

Profound sensorineural hearing loss (SNHL) in childhood may be classified according to the age of onset, whether it is genetic or nongenetic in origin, and by specific etiology. A congenital hearing loss is defined as one that is present at birth. Although it is usually genetic (Beighton & Sellars, 1982), nongenetic causes occur when the auditory system of the fetus is damaged in utero. A postnatal hearing loss is defined as one that occurs after birth. This type of hearing loss is usually acquired, but may be due to genetic factors that manifest on a delayed basis.

The distinction between congenital and postnatal SNHL is important because it affects the management of the child. The acquisition of language skills is widely believed to be most easily achieved during a "critical period" that exists early in childhood (see Chapter 14). Although the presence of profound deafness can usually be ascertained audiometrically at a very early age (see Chapter 4), possible difficulties in establishing a diagnosis and necessary delays in evaluating other rehabilitative measures means that cochlear implantation will seldom be feasible before the age of 2 years. Delays in undertaking cochlear implantation in congenitally deafened individuals may limit the potential utility of the device because of possible limitations in central auditory development. Establishing the exact etiology of the deafness may permit earlier intervention based upon knowledge of the natural history of the disease. Many children with profound SNHL are clearly pre- or postlingual. However, a disconcerting number of these young deaf children are *perilingual,* having had initial exposure to sound that may have permitted limited speech and language acquisition followed by the early onset of deafness. In this group, identification of the underlying disease process and ascertaining its prognosis are critical if clinicians are to make informed decisions concerning appropriate intervention.

CONGENITAL PROFOUND CHILDHOOD SNHL

GENETIC CAUSES

Genetic causes account for approximately 50 percent of cases of congenital deafness. Of these, 30 percent are due to autosomal dominant traits, 68 percent to recessive traits, and 2 percent to X-linked inheritance (Beighton & Sellars, 1982). The majority of congenital SNHL is neither part of a recognizable syndrome nor is it associated with abnormalities of other parts of the body. However, there are about 70 recognized genetic syndromes in which SNHL does accompany other malformations. It is convenient to consider these syndromes according to the region of the body that is affected. The more common syndromes are those of Waardenburg, Jervell and Lange–Nielsen, Pendred, Usher, and Alport.

DERMATOLOGICAL SYNDROMES. Waardenburg syndrome accounts for approximately 2 percent of congenital deafness (Beighton & Sellars, 1982). It is inherited by an autosomal dominant gene, the expression of which is extremely variable. Major characteristics that can occur in any combination include laterally displaced medial canthi making the eyes appear widely spaced (83 percent), a broad nasal root (68 percent), hyperplasia of the eyebrows (57 percent), heterochromia of one or both irides (51 percent), and a white forelock (48 percent). Congenital hearing loss occurs in about 50 percent of affected individuals and may be unilateral or bilateral. In the majority of affected individuals, the hearing loss is profound (Ruben, 1983).

OPHTHALMOLOGICAL SYNDROMES. The three syndromes in which retinitis pigmentosa accompanies SNHL are Usher's, Refsum's, and Alstrom's. Usher's is the most frequent of the three and occurs in between 3 percent and 10 percent of children who are profoundly deaf. It can be distinguished from the other two syndromes because the deafness affects both ears equally. Usher's syndrome is transmitted as an autosomal recessive gene. The characteristic retinal changes are granular accumulations of pigment that begin at the optic macula and extend to the periphery. To identify this disease entity, every child with profound congenital SNHL should have a fundoscopic examination. An early diagnosis and rehabilitation is particularly important to an individual who will eventually experience combined visual and auditory impairments (Kumar, Fishman, & Torok, 1984).

CARDIOVASCULAR SYNDROMES. The Jervell and Lange–Nielsen syndrome consists of profound SNHL and cardiac abnormalites which result in syncopal episodes. It has an autosomal recessive inheritance and has an incidence of 1 percent in children who are severely deaf (Jervell, 1985). It is important to identify this syndrome early because treatment with beta blockers may reduce the incidence of sudden death that is associated with the cardiac abnormalities (Olley & Fowler, 1979). The characteristic electrocardiographic (EKG) changes are enlarged T-waves and a prolonged QT interval. All children with idiopathic SNHL should have an EKG recording. There is also the possibility of identifying heterozygote family members by EKG recordings.

ENDOCRINE SYNDROMES. Pendred's syndrome is characterized by severe SNHL and thyroid goiter. It has an autosomal recessive form of inheritance and accounts for between 1 percent and 2 percent of children who are profoundly deaf (Thould & Scowen, 1964). In this study, 13 out of 23 individuals had a profound hearing loss with the remainder partially impaired. A thyroid goiter may be present at birth and is usually apparent by the age of 8. The patients are euthyroid and the goiter usually responds to treatment with exogenous thyroid hormone (Das, 1987).

RENAL SYNDROMES. Alport's syndrome accounts for 1 percent of genetic deafness. It consists of chronic nephritis with intermittant hematuria which leads to progressive renal failure. The SNHL is progressive and usually does not become apparent until after the age of 10. Typically the hearing loss is of the order of 50 dB, so the majority of these children can be helped with hearing aids. The syndrome is more common in boys, who are also more severely handicapped, and have a life expectancy of 30 years (Konigsmark & Gorlin, 1976).

NONGENETIC CAUSES

There are a variety of intrauterine insults that may cause SNHL in the fetus. The earlier in the pregnancy the insult occurs the more severe the consequences. This is because embryological differentiation of the inner ear takes place during the first trimester of pregnancy. An interruption to development at this stage results in severe malformations.

INFECTIONS DURING PREGNANCY. A variety of maternal infections may cause SNHL in the fetus (Pappas & Mundy, 1982). Viruses are the most common infectious agents and often occur with minimal signs and symptoms in the mother. Viruses that are known to affect the developing auditory system include rubella, influenza, cytomegalovirus, and herpes.

Other microrganisms, notably syphilis and toxoplasmosis, may also have a teratogenic effect on the inner ear.

Despite widespread vaccination programs, maternal rubella remains an important cause of SNHL. The severity of SNHL varies and it may be progressive. In patients with cogenital rubella, SNHL is often the only manifestation and this may cause diagnostic difficulty. The diagnosis is made by physical examination and immunological techniques. During physical examination the stigmata of cogenital rubella should be sought. These include "salt and pepper" retinitis, congenital heart disease, lesions of the long bones, microcephaly, and jaundice. The presence of rubella-specific IgM antibodies at birth in the umbilical cord, or during the first 6 months of life in the mother's or infant's serum, is diagnostic. Maternal infections are often subclinical and only in about one third of cases is the fetus affected (Parving et al., 1980).

It is estimated that between 0.7 percent and 6 percent of women develop a primary cytomegaloviral (CMV) infection during pregnancy (Strauss, 1985). Most of these infections pass unrecognized. CMV is the most common cause of congenital viral infection with an incidence of between 0.4 percent and 2.3 percent of live births. Of these neonates only a small proportion are symptomatic and therefore have true cytomegaloviral disease (CID). Among children with CID the quoted range of SNHL is between 20 percent and 65 percent. The SNHL may be unilateral or bilateral and the degree of severity varies considerably (Strauss, 1985).

MEDICATIONS TAKEN DURING PREGNANCY. Drugs, both medical and illicit, may have an adverse affect on the fetus. Those that are definitely known to cause hearing impairment include the aminoglycosides, quinine, chloroquine phosphate, and thalidomide. Among the aminoglycosides, streptomycin in particular has been linked with severe human fetal hearing loss. However, virtually all the other members of the aminoglycoside group are known to cause fetal hearing loss in pregnant animals (Siegel & McCracken, 1981). Thalidomide caused severe middle and external ear abnormalities as well as deformities of the bony and membranous labyrinths. Chemical teratogens are particularly dangerous in the first trimester of pregnancy. Because inner ear organogenesis has often initiated before the mother is aware of her pregnancy, it is prudent for all women at risk of pregnancy to avoid such agents.

MISCELLANEOUS CAUSES. Fetal hypoxia is associated with SNHL due to damage to the cochlear nuclei (Bergstrom, 1980). Infantile hyperbilirubinemia with an unconjugated bilirubin level exceeding 20 mg per 100 ml of blood has potential for similar deleterious effect on the brainstem nuclei. This condition occurs in from 0.5 percent to 1.5 percent of children with SNHL. A long term study of children with severe hyperbilirubinemia (kernicterus) found that 22 percent had profound SNHL (Ruben & Rozycki, 1970).

There are various other factors that can cause fetal hearing loss many of which are not fully understood. Maternal nutrition affects the weight and general condition of the fetus without producing specific anatomical deformities. Prematurity carries an increased risk of fetal hypoxia. Because premature infants are also generally of low birth weight, any neonate weighing under 1500 grams at birth is considered to be at risk for congenital hearing loss. The role of fetal autoimmune disease and other factors such as maternal endocrine disease are yet to be established.

POSTNATAL CHILDHOOD PROFOUND SNHL

GENETIC CAUSES

Many genetic abnormalities that cause SNHL may not become manifest until after birth. This is particuarly true of autosomal dominant conditions in which there is a tendency for the SNHL to be progressive. An example of a genetic syndrome that may not manifest until after birth is Alport's syndrome in which hearing loss does not usually make its appearance until late childhood.

NONGENETIC CAUSES

INFECTIONS. Meningitis accounts for 7 to 8 percent of severe childhood SNHL and is the most common form of acquired postnatal SNHL (Dahnsjo et al., 1976). It occurs throughout the pediatric age range, but is most common during the first 3 years of life. Approximately 6 percent of patients suffering acute bacterial meningitis will develop SNHL (Keane et al., 1979). The incidence of hearing loss was found to vary with the type of organism (Dodge et al., 1984). In a study of 185 children the incidence of hearing loss was 31 percent with *Streptococcus pneumoniae,* 10.5 percent with *Neisseria meningitidis,* and 6 percent with *Hemophilus influenzae.*

Postnatal viral infections may also cause profound SNHL. Examples include mumps, measles, Epstein-Barr, CMV, herpes zoster, influenzae, cocksackie, and adenoviruses (Pappas & Mundy, 1982). Many of these infections cause a transient hearing loss and the impairment may be confined to one ear.

OTOTOXIC MEDICATIONS. The aminoglycoside antibiotics are the most frequent group of drugs implicated in ototoxicity. Children at greatest risk are those with impaired renal function and pre-existing SNHL of other causation. Those simultaneously receiving multiple ototoxic agents (e.g., an aminoglycoside and a loop diuretic) are at particular risk for auditory injury. Care should be taken in monitoring drug dosage with peak and trough blood levels and maintaining an adequate state of hydration. Frequent audiologic monitoring during therapy is advisable.

TRAUMA. Head injury seldom fractures both bony labyrinths, but when this occurs anacusis may result. Head trauma without fracture may, in rare instances, result in labyrinthine hemorrhage with profound SNHL. Severe acoustical trauma (e.g., a bomb blast) may also result in permanent deafness.

PATHOLOGICAL FEATURES OF PROFOUND CHILDHOOD SNHL

IMPLICATIONS FOR COCHLEAR IMPLANTATION

Most types of SNHL are caused by loss of cochlear hair cells, accompanied to a greater or lesser extent by degeneration of the neural elements of the cochlea (Bergstrom, 1980). The amount an individual can be helped by a cochlear implant may be largely determined by the proportion of ganglion cells that survive. Below a certain number of neurons, the cochlear implant may be of extremely limited use. At the present time, there is no reliable preoperative test for determining the proportion of surviving neurons.

NEURAL SURVIVAL RATES BY ETIOLOGY. Normal individuals in the first decade of life have approximately 36,000 spiral ganglion cells in each cochlea and subsequently lose these at a rate of about 2000 per decade. Ten thousand spiral ganglion cells appear necessary in order to achieve some degree of speech discrimination, with at least 3000 of these located in the apical 10 mm of the cochlea. This region of the cochlea serves frequencies up to 900 Hz and these low frequencies are thought to be important for speech reception in cochlear implants (Otte, Schuknecht, & Kerr, 1978).

Congenital Profound SNHL

WAARDENBURG SYNDROME. The inner ear pathology of a 3-year-old girl with profound deafness was described by Fisch (1959). The organ of corti was absent in all turns and there was poor spiral ganglion survival.

USHER'S SYNDROME. On histologic examination, this syndrome shows degeneration of the organ of corti and spiral ganglion cells in the basal turn, but apical structures were well preserved (Belal, 1975). Schmidt (1985) reported a patient with a profound SNHL above 1000 Hz in which 18,171 spiral ganglion cells remained in the right cochlea and 21,870 in the left, with 6000 cells in each apex.

JERVELL AND LANGE–NIELSEN SYNDROME. The histopathology of the inner ear showed a normal bony labyrinth with degeneration of the organ of corti and spiral ganglion in all turns (Friedmann, Fraser, & Froggat, 1966).

PENDRED'S SYNDROME. The temporal bones of one patient were reported to show only two turns and complete absence of the neuro-epithelium and ganglion cells (Hvidberg-Hansen & Jorgensen, 1968).

ALPORT'S SYNDROME. One patient with Alport's syndrome with moderate hearing loss had 22,914 spiral ganglion cells in the right cochlea and 22,347 in the left, with over 5000 cells in the apical segment (Schmidt, 1985).

VIRAL INFECTIONS. Most available information applies to patients with congenital rubella (Bordley & Alford, 1970). Usually there is a normal bony labyrinth, with varying degrees of membranous degeneration. Schmidt (1985) reported on the spiral ganglion counts in one ear of a Rubella patient with a profound SNHL; there were 13,311 remaining neurons in the ear, with less than 3000 in the apex.

INNER EAR MALFORMATIONS. Kerr and Schuknecht (1968) examined four temporal bones from patients with profound congenital SNHL. Two out of three ears had deformities limited to the membraneous labyrinth (cochleosaccular dysplasia) in which there was a normal number of spiral ganglion cells. The one ear with Mondini's dysplasia that was studied also had a good population of spiral ganglion cells in the existing turns. However, Schmidt (1985) examined the cochlear neuronal populations of eight patients with Mondini's dysplasia (a partially developed cochlea of 1-and-one-half turns and an incomplete scalar septum) and found that the spiral ganglion cell counts ranged from 7,677 to 16,110 with an average of 11,478.

POSTNATAL PROFOUND SNHL

Kerr and Schuknecht (1968) evaluated the spiral ganglion count in 37 temporal bones from postnatal patients who were profoundly deafened. Bacterial labyrinthitis accounted for 17 ears in which severe destruction of the membranous labyrinth was found. This was usually accompanied by an extensive loss of spiral ganglion cells. In cases of viral labyrinthitis in 9 ears, variable amounts of degeneration of membranous and neural structures were encountered.

The spiral ganglion survival rate has been examined in other conditions. Fractures of the temporal bone and ototoxically damaged ears are accompanied by good neural survival (Otte, Schuknecht, & Kerr, 1978). In patients deafened by hypoxia and kernicterus, the brainstem nuclei are mainly affected so that normal cochleas have been found in most instances (Ruben, 1983). When the brainstem nuclei are affected, it is doubtful whether peripheral stimulation with a cochlear implant would be of benefit. A possible exception might occur if stimulation was commenced very early while central plasticity remains.

CONGENITAL MALFORMATIONS OF THE INNER EAR. Eighty percent of children with congenital SNHL have lesions limited to the membranous labyrinth. The most common histopathologic finding is cochleosaccular dysplasia, also know as Schiebe's dysplasia. In 20 percent of deaf children the otic capsule is malformed. A broad spectrum of anomalies may be seen, most of which can be explained by an arrest of inner ear development at some stage in its embryogenesis. The malformed cochlea may consist of only a small bud (cochlear hypoplasia), a partially developed coiled structure of 1-and-one-half turns (incomplete partition), or a cystic structure lacking in internal architecture (common cavity). Deaf children with these congenital cochlear anomalies may present unique technical challenges to those designing cochlear implants. Foremost is the need for an electrode that adapts to the altered cochlear lumen in a fashion that permits selective control of cochlear nerve populations. These children are known to be at increased risk of developing CSF leaks with the possible consequence of meningitis (Monsell, Jackler, & Motta, 1987), and there is also an increased incidence of a dehiscent facial nerve. In one study of four children implanted with a single-channel device, all of whom had malformations of the bony labyrinth, two were nonusers because of cross stimulation of the facial nerve (Jackler, Luxford, & House, 1987). With a multichannel system, facial nerve stimulation might be isolated to one or two channels that could be disconnected without depriving the child of sound from the remaining channels.

COCHLEAR PATENCY PROBLEMS. The pathological processes that damage the inner ear often lead to osteoneogenesis within the cochlea. This is particuarly true of meningitis, in which granulation and fibrous tissue that result from the labyrinthitis are followed by new bone growth. The extent of osteoneogenesis within the cochlea can be assessed radiographically, as discussed in a later section of this chapter devoted to the issue of cochlear patency.

PREOPERATIVE MEDICAL EVALUATION OF PEDIATRIC COCHLEAR IMPLANT CANDIDATES

In the child with profound SNHL a history, physical examination, and certain diagnostic investigations are indicated to identify potentially reversible otologic conditions and associated systemic disorders. Genetic aspects need to be explored to facilitate reproductive counseling and to identify relatives at risk of developing hearing loss.

POTENTIALLY REVERSIBLE OTOLOGIC CONDITIONS

Profound SNHL is seldom reversible, but there are some exceptions. One of these is endolymphatic hydrops, which may occur in childhood, although it is rare (Hausler et al., 1987). This diagnosis may be suspected from a history of fluctuating hearing loss accompanied by episodic vertigo and tinnitus. Reduction of endolymphatic pressures by medical or surgical means may help to stabilize hearing. Treatable infections, especially syphilis, should be identified because appropriate antibiotic treatment may avoid further cochlear damage (Kerr, Smyth, & Cinnamond, 1973). Serologic testing for syphilis is obtained for all children with SNHL (Hughes & Rutherford, 1986). In otosyphilis, prolonged high dose intravenous antibiotics, at times accompanied by anti-inflammatory corticosteroids, is required. Immune-related inner-ear dysfunction is another treatable cause of SNHL. This may result from either cellular or humoral immune system dysfunction. Cogan's syndrome, autoimmune SNHL accompanied by interstitial keratitis, has been reported in childhood (Kundell & Ochs, 1980). Often auditory dysfunction is part of a systemic immunological disorder, such as systemic lupus erythrematosis, polyarteritis nodosa, or sarcoidosis (Schatz & Zeiger, 1987). SNHL may also be the sole manifestation of the patient's immune dysfunction (Veldman, 1987). Treatment is with corticosteroids and immunosuppressive agents; occasional dramatic improvements in hearing thresholds have been reported. Perilymphatic fistula may occur in children and should be suspected in patients with post-traumatic, sudden, or fluctuant SNHL (Supance & Bluestone, 1983). They are also associated with congenital malformations of the inner ear. Surgical intervention may prevent further deterioration of hearing, but significant improvement is unlikely.

It is common for a conductive hearing loss (CHL) to accompany SNHL in young children. The most common cause is middle-ear effusion, which occurs frequently in this age group. It may be detected by pneumatic otoscopy and tympanometry. Congenital middle-ear or ear-canal anomalies may also be associated with profound SNHL. Common signs include low-set or deformed pinnae, meatal atresia, and pre-auricular sinuses. Identification of CHL is important, as this is often medically or surgically reversible and may make the difference between success or failure with hearing aids. Also, hearing evaluation in the child with profound SNHL is complicated by the presence of a co-existing conductive deficit. Auditory Brainstem Responses (ABR) are frequently absent in such patients even when residual cochlear and central auditory function is present. In children who present with both profound SNHL and middle ear effusion, ventilating tubes should be inserted and then the hearing level re-evaluated.

IDENTIFICATION OF ASSOCIATED SYSTEMIC DISEASES

Although it is not usually the case, a child with profound SNHL may be harboring a serious underlying systemic disorder. Most common among these are renal dysfunction, syphilis, viral infection (e.g., CMV), cardiac rhythm disturbance, and hypothyroidism. The history should include a thorough systems inquiry. The general physical examination should be conducted by a pediatrician because the signs of systemic disease can be diverse and subtle. Routine laboratory investigations provide a screen for systemic disorders. A summary of recommended routine laboratory tests is provided at the end of this section.

GENETIC ASPECTS OF PROFOUND CHILDHOOD SNHL

Approximately 30 percent of all deafness can be demonstrated to be genetic (Beighton & Sellars, 1982). The mechanism of inheritance in systemic syndromes is generally known and counseling can be given accordingly. Classically, autosomal dominant inheritance involves 50 percent of offspring; however, due to variability in penetrance, in reality this is seldom the case. In recessive syndromes with a well established family pattern, the risk to offspring is as much as 25 percent. In the most common clinical situation, namely, sporadic deafness with no familial history, an uncommon recessive allele is often responsible. Because a fraction of these patients have nongenetic causes that are beyond clinical detection, the recurrence risk for siblings of such patients is far less than the postulated 25 percent expected for recessive inheritance. In sporadic congenital deafness, the probability of sibling inheritance is approximately 5 percent (Beighton & Sellars, 1982). Also, the offspring of such patients are seldom deaf, although they may become carriers of the recessive gene. A history of consanguinity in the family increases the chances of genetic disease (Costeff & Dar, 1980).

It is best to carefully trace the origins of both sides of the family for three or four generations. Attention should be given to any history of premature hearing impairment in siblings and other family members. Once a genetic disease has been diagnosed, referral to a professional genetic counselor is advisable.

SUMMARY OF EVALUATION PROCEDURES

The following medical evaluations are considered routine in all children who are newly diagnosed as profoundly deaf. Audiological investigations required to establish the diagnosis of deafness are not included.

PREGNANCY HISTORY. Maternal infections (rubella, CMV, toxoplasmosis), potential ototoxic drugs, radiation exposure. Stress events in the first trimester. Birth history (hypoxia, kernicterus, trauma, toxemia, prematurity).

POSTNATAL HISTORY. Head trauma, meningitis, systemic infections (measles, mumps, syphilis), ototoxic exposure, detailed otologic history.

FAMILY HISTORY. Premature hearing loss in blood relations through at least two generations. Identify consanguinity if present. All siblings should undergo audiologic evaluation.

PHYSICAL EXAMINATION. Otologic examination to identify malformations, infection, cholesteatoma, or signs of trauma. General examination by pediatrician to evaluate for systemic disease. Ophthalmologic examination to exclude keratitis (syphilis, Cogan's), retinitis pigmentosa (Usher's), viral inclusions (CMV, toxoplasmas).

LABORATORY TESTING. Renal function: (1) blood urea nitrogen and creatinine; (2) urinalysis for hematuria and proteinuria (Alport's, polycystic kidney disease).

Metabolic function: (1) thyroid function tests (Pendred's, cretinism); (2) blood and urine glucose (diabetes).

Complete blood count (anemia, infections).

Luetic serology.

Immune function: (1) erythrocyte sedimentation rate, anti-nuclear antibodies (Cogan's, autoimmune disease); (2) Specific immunological tests if viral disease is suspected as in rubella and CMV.

ELECTROCARDIOGRAM (EKG). Prolonged QT interval of Jervell and Lange–Nielsen syndrome or other abnormalities.

COMPUTED TOMOGRAPHY OF THE TEMPORAL BONES. To investigate for malformation (cochlea, semicircular canals, vestibular and cochlear aqueducts, internal auditory canal, middle ear), cholesteatoma, fracture, or osteodystrophy.

If any of the above tests are abnormal the next line of investigation is instituted. For example, in an individual with profound SNHL and proteinuria, an ultrasonic examination of the kidneys would be appropriate.

SURGICAL TECHNIQUE FOR COCHLEAR IMPLANTATION IN CHILDREN

Cochlear implantation in childhood requires a general anesthetic, usually lasting between 1.5 and 3 hours. The retroauricular incision must be placed sufficiently posterior to allow the device to lie entirely under the skin flap and not in proximity to the incision. Implanted hardware that underlies an incision is at risk of extrusion. The receiving (internal) coil should not be positioned beneath the auricle as it may interfere with placement of the external coil and also cause patients discomfort when lying on their side. In children, the thinness of the skull permits little countersinking of the receiver into bone in an effort to reduce its thickness. Devices appropriate for use in young children must be very thin (preferably less than 1 cm thick) to avoid excessive tension on the skin flap. While thinning of the flap to reduce the amount of tissue interposed between the internal and external coils is routine in adults, this should not be performed in children. Anchoring the implant to the cranium is also more difficult in a child. This may be achieved with acrylic cement or a suture placed through a superficial tunnel created in the outer table of the skull.

Two surgical approaches to the round window region are in widespread use by cochlear implant surgeons: the posterior canal wall groove and the transmastoid-facial recess routes. In the posterior canal wall groove method, a trough is drilled in the posterior aspect of the external auditory canal to accommodate the electrode lead wire (Schindler et al., 1987). After reflecting the tympanic membrane, the surgeon works through the ear canal to obtain wide exposure of the round window and basal scala tympani. This approach provides access to the cochlea at an angle favorable for atraumatic electrode insertion. Its main disadvantage is the proximity of the lead wire to the epithelial surface of the ear canal. This risks infection and possible extrusion. In adults this problem has been largely overcome through the use of a deep bony channel segregated from the lumen by bone paté and pieces of cortical bone. For several reasons, however, this technique is not suitable for young children. The primary difficulty lies in the narrowness of the developing external auditory canal. This provides only limited surgical exposure and prohibits creation of a bony groove of sufficient depth to prevent electrode extrusion. An additional problem with this approach is that it places the extracochlear portion of the electrode almost entirely within subcutaneous soft tissue. This location is less favorable than placing the electrode within a pneumatized space when it is intended to undergo gradual elongation during head growth.

The transmastoid-facial recess approach is preferred in young children (Clark et al., 1987b; House, 1982). In preparation for opening the facial recess, an intact canal wall mastoidectomy must be performed. In infancy and early childhood the mastoid is smaller and less well pneumatized than in adults. At birth, only the mastoid antrum is pneumatized and the mastoid tip is completely undeveloped. This places the stylomastoid foramen on the lateral aspect of the temporal bone. Thus, in infants the location of the facial nerve may restrict the available mastoid exposure and make cochlear implantation quite difficult. By the age of two, progressive pneumatization and mastoid tip growth have enlarged the exposure sufficiently to permit fairly reliable exposure of the facial recess via this route. Access to the middle ear is via the facial recess, a narrow opening into the posterior tympanum between the facial and chorda tympani nerves. Fortuitously, the facial recess is nearly adult size at birth. This technique provides adequate exposure to the round window region to permit insertion of either single- or multichannel implants. It is essential that placement of an intracochlear electrode be atraumatic. Efforts at deeper insertion should be abandoned when significant resistance is encountered. The primary disadvantages of the facial recess approach are a somewhat less direct access to the scala tympani and the remote possibility of facial nerve injury while opening the facial recess or manipulating the electrode during insertion. The advantages of this technique are that it widely separates the electrode from epithelial surfaces and it creates an air containing space into which redundant loops of electrode may be placed to allow for future head growth.

STRATEGIES FOR THE ACCOMMODATION OF HEAD GROWTH

A problem unique to cochlear implantation in childhood is the effect of head growth. Because the cochlea is adult sized at birth, the intracochlear portion of the electrode need not be expansile. However, because the squamous, petrous, and mastoid portions of the temporal bone are destined to enlarge, the lead wire between the antenna and receiver package and the round window must be capable of gradual elongation. Furthermore, it must be engineered to retain this property for as long as 18 years, until the child reaches full growth. Should it not have this feature, tension would develop along the axis of the lead wire. As the receiver package is firmly fixed to the cranium, the most likely consequence of these forces is extraction of the active electrode from the cochlea.

The magnitude of postnatal temporal bone growth has been estimated in two recent studies. In a study of 103 computed tomographic scans in children from birth to age 18, over 50 percent of postnatal temporal bone growth was found to occur during the first 2 years of life (O'Donoghue et al., 1986). Thereafter, growth continued at a more gradual pace until the late teen-age years. A second study of 253 plain skull radiographs in children yielded similar findings (Eby & Nadol, 1986). In addition, it revealed a second, but lesser phase of accelerated growth during adolescence. These investigations suggest that a cochlear implant placed at the age of 2 years must be capable of accommodating approximately two to three centimeters of growth if it remains in place until maturity.

One possible solution to the problem of growth would be to periodically explant the ear and reinsert a larger device. However, this would subject a growing child to numerous surgical procedures, and the repeated explantations and reimplantations may cause damage to the cochlea and surviving neurons. Clearly, the preferable strategy is to utilize an expandable device. A number of bioengineering obstacles must be overcome to achieve a reliable expansile cochlear implant system. The materials, especially the electrode wire and its insulating sheath, must remain pliable for many years despite constant contact with physiologic fluids. Many prosthetic materials gradually gain rigidity under such conditions. Also, the external surface of the cable must not adhere to its surrounding fibrous tissue envelope. A recent study indicates that merely placing excess lengths of lead wire is not sufficient to ensure expandability (O'Donoghue, Jackler, & Schindler, 1986). When in subcutaneous tissue, redundant electrode coils become bound down by dense fibrous tissue and do not extend. Enclosing the redundant electrode in a sheath designed to prevent the ingrowth of fibrous tissue may overcome this problem. Such a solution has not yet been demonstrated in the temporal bone, although it has shown some promise in other pediatric prosthetic applications (Hooper, 1969; Sato & Glenn, 1970). O'Donoghue, Jackler, and Schindler (1986) also demonstrated that coiled wire placed within an air-containing space, such as the middle ear or mastoid, will successfully elongate during head growth. Therefore, it has been suggested that the optimal surgical technique for children should maximize the amount of air containing space and mininize the amount of soft tissue traversed by the electrode lead wire. This is one factor favoring the transmastoid-facial recess surgical approach, as this technique places the majority of the lead wire in pneumatized space.

An additional strategy to discourage dislodgement of the intra-cochlear electrode as a consequence of head growth is to solidly fix it at its entry into the scala tympani. This may be achieved by adding a cuff of bioactive material (such as hydroxyapatite ceramic) to the electrode at the round window level. By adhering to surrounding bone and soft tissue, the electrode may then be stabilized against extracting forces.

COCHLEAR PATENCY PROBLEMS: DIAGNOSIS AND MANAGEMENT

In most forms of sensory deafness the hair cell population is depleted while the macroscopic cochlear architecture remains unaltered. Examples of such etiologies include ototoxicity, viral infection, metabolic dysfunction, and most forms of familial losses. Other causes of deafness, however, may be associated with varying degrees of distortion or obliteration of the cochlear scalae. The most prominent examples are deafness resulting from meningitis, otitis, otosclerosis, and temporal bone fracture. By far the most common histopathologic finding in these ears is osteoneogenesis within the cochlear scalae as a consequence of either suppurative labyrinthitis or intralabyrinthine hemorrhage. In these cases, insertion of a conventional multichannel scala tympani electrode may be difficult or impossible. The incidence of cochlear patency problems is higher in children who are deaf than in adults, largely because of the frequency of meningitis and otitis in this age group.

In many cases, compromised cochlear patency may be identified by preoperative radiographic studies (Balkany, Dreisbach, & Seibert, 1986;

Jackler et al., 1987). The investigation of choice is high-resolution computed tomography (CT). To adequately image the minute inner ear structures, scans must be taken in thin sections (1.0 or 1.5 mm) and enhanced for osseous detail with a bone review program. An abnormal preimplant CT scan is a reliable predictor of compromised cochlear patency at operation. Endocochlear ossification may be partial or complete and may be localized to one or more cochlear turns (Becker et al., 1984; Swartz et al., 1985). Unfortunately, a normal preimplant CT scan does not exclude the possibility of encountering impaired cochlear patency during insertion. Because CT has limited spatial resolution, it may fail to detect subtle degrees of endocochlear ossification. Also, CT does not reliably image abnormal endocochlear soft tissue, and most fibrous scalar obliteration will pass undetected until surgery. Magnetic resonance imaging, which provides excellent visualization of the eighth nerve and central auditory system, has not proven useful in the evaluation of cochlear patency.

Narrowing or obliteration of the cochlear lumen has not been a critical problem for short, single-channel intracochlear devices, such as the 3M/House design. These electrodes have been inserted, with some success, into completely ossified cochleas following creation of a bony channel with a drill (Eisenberg et al., 1984). However, such ears do tend to require more power to achieve audiometric thresholds comparable to those obtained by nonossified cochleas. Compromises of cochlear patency are much more problematic for long multichannel electrodes that are designed to be inserted well into the second cochlear turn. Implant teams using such devices must be prepared with backup electrodes appropriate for whatever existing or surgically created lumen may be available. The suggestion of a cochlear patency problem on preoperative CT scan does not preclude an attempt at insertion of a sophisticated multichannel device. Often, by widely fenestrating an obliterated base turn, the surgeon will encounter an adequate scalar lumen further anteriorly. Failing this, a shorter, narrower intracochlear device or extracochlear strategy may be successful.

Congenital malformations of the inner ear where cochlear anatomy is distorted present unique cochlear patency problems. A fundamental assumption of multichannel scala tympani devices is the selective control of discrete auditory nerve segments utilizing the neural organization in the osseous spiral lamina and spiral ganglion. In anomalous cochleas, where the scalae are often confluent, an electrode inserted via the round window may have no predictable relationship to neural structures. While limited success with single channel devices has been obtained in such ears (Jackler, Luxford, & House, 1987; Miyamato et al., 1986), multichannel electrodes may need to be of custom design to achieve optimal stimulation.

OTITIS MEDIA IN THE IMPLANTED EAR

The design of a cochlear implant intended for use in deaf children must take into account the frequency of otitis media in this age group. By the age of 6, approximately 84 percent of otherwise healthy children have suffered at least one episode of acute otitis media (Brownlee et al., 1969). Scala tympani electrodes, which traverse the middle ear before entering the cochlea, may serve as conduits by which middle ear infection can enter the inner ear and, from there, potentially the central nervous system. Investigations in the cat have revealed that the implanted round window membrane shows increased permeability to horseradish peroxidase for at least 2 weeks following implantation (Franz, Clark, & Bloom, 1984), indicating that the implanted cochlea is particularly vulnerable to early postoperative middle-ear infection. After this initial period, a membrane forms around the lead wire as it traverses the round window. This tenuous neomembrane may not be sufficient to resist the destructive enzymes and toxins secreted by bacteria during middle ear infection. The devastating effects of bacterial infection on the cochlea and its neural elements have been well described (Paparella & Sugiura, 1967). In implanted animals with experimentally induced *Staphylococcus aureus* otitis media, extensive cochlear damage including osteoneogenesis, destruction of the Organ of Corti, and profound neural degeneration have been seen (Leake, Rebscher, & Aird, 1985). Although less severe, similar damage has been demonstrated in implanted ears infected with *Streptococcus pneumoniae* (Berkowitz et al., 1987) and *Pseudomonas aeruginosa* (Berkowitz et al., 1985). *Streptococcus pyogenes* middle ear infection in the implanted cat did not traverse the round window neomembrane, unless it was mechanically disrupted at the time of innoculation (Cranswick et al., 1987). It should be noted that marked differences exist in the virulence of organisms among species, and care must be taken in generalizing from studies in the cat to the human condition.

Middle ear infection in the implanted ear may have an impact on implant performance. In the worst case, the implant may become a nidus for infection that ultimately necessitates its removal. This is a common result when implanted prosthetics, such as heart valves or hip prostheses, become infected. However, in an epithelium lined body cavity, such as the middle ear, infection may resolve following treatment with appropriate antibiotics. But even after infection has been controlled, long term deleterious effects on implant performance may ensue. The most important consequence is loss of neurons, as this may impair speech discrimination. An additional factor is the slow process of post-labyrinthitis osteoneogenesis, which insulates the active electrodes from neural elements and may increase the electrical threshold for auditory stimulation.

Two strategies designed to protect the implanted ear from middle ear infection have been evaluated. The technique most studied involves reestablishing the separation between the inner ear and the middle ear by means of a seal around the electrode at the level of the round window. Both autogenous and alloplastic material have been studied. Two studies evaluated autogenous fascia wrapped around the electrode as a round window seal with mixed results. In four cats infected with *S. aureus,* fascia did not prevent intracochlear infection (Jackler, O'Donoghue, & Schindler, 1986). In three cats infected with *S. pyogenes,* intracochlear infection did not occur (Clark et al., 1984). However, subsequent studies have indicated a lack of virulence for this organism in the cat (Cranswick et al., 1987). The difficulty in obtaining a biologically effective seal against infection with autogenous tissue lies in the fact that the outer surface of the electrode is either silastic or a noble metal, neither of which adhere to living tissue. Thus, a potential space at the electrode-tissue interface exists which is vulnerable to penetration by bacterial enzymes. Three prosthetic materials, which can be hermetically adhered to the electrode, have been evaluated. Dacron® has been abandoned because it causes a strong intracochlear inflammatory reaction (Clark et al., 1984). A Teflon® felt disc glued to the electrode shows some promise as a round window sealant (Clark et al., 1984), as does the bioactive ceramic Ceravital® (Jackler, O'Donoghue, & Schindler, 1986). An ideal material for round window sealing is one that can be hermetically glued to the inert electrode surface and provide a broad flange of bioactive material that will strongly adhere to living tissue. Hydroxyapatite ceramic surrounded by a bone paté of high osteoblastic potential is currently under evaluation as a round window seal.

A second strategy for protecting the implanted cochlea from middle ear infection involves separating the entire electrode lead wire from the mucosal envelope of the middle ear and mastoid (Bates et al., 1987). In this technique, the electrode is buried in bone throughout its course. In the mastoid and ear canal the electrode is laid in the bottom of a surgically created bony trough and covered by bone paté and cortical bone plates. The hypotympanum, including the round window area, is then filled with bone paté. In preliminary animal experiments this technique has shown much promise as a means of separating the entire implanted device from infections which involve the mucosally lined cavities of the temporal bone.

In the only clinical study of otitis media in implanted children reported to date, neither the severity nor the incidence of this illness was increased (House, Luxford, & Courtney, 1985). However, all of these children were implanted with the 3M/House device, which has a short single channel electrode. With short implants the peri-implant fibrous sheath is usually continuous with the round window neomembrane. In this situation the entire electrode is often externalized, essentially forming a diverticulum of the middle ear space. This may limit infection to the basal region of the cochlea thereby reducing neural damage and the risk of intracranial spread of infection. It is reassuring that no case of meningitis or other intracranial infection has been reported in implanted children.

COMPLICATIONS OF COCHLEAR IMPLANTATION IN CHILDREN

SURGICAL COMPLICATIONS

Complications of cochlear implantation in children may occur as an immediate consequence of the implant surgical procedure or, more commonly, arise on a delayed basis due to some biological or technical failure (Cohen, Rosenberg, & Goldstein, 1987; Gray & Schindler, 1985). Surgical complications have fortunately been rare. The most common operative mishap is damage to the device during its placement. Breaks in the insulating sheath of the electrode lead wire or antenna coils may result in seepage of physiologic fluids and short out the device. Also, manipulation may work-harden wires and cause their fracture. This is especially likely to occur where the wire exits the cannister containing the implanted electronics.

Mis-insertion of the intracochlear electrode has occurred where the electrode has been advanced into a hypotympanic air cell tract rather than into the cochlear lumen. This may be identified by postoperative CT scan (Ball, Miller, & Hepfner, 1986). Traumatic insertion of a scala tympani electrode may damage the cochlea, possibly causing neural damage or leading to intracochlear ossification that impairs stimulability. It may also result in kinking of the electrode or even its folding and doubling back on itself within the scala tympani.

Injury to the facial nerve during implant surgery is unlikely because otologic surgeons are experienced with the identification and preservation of this structure. However, the facial nerve may be at risk when a surgeon not experienced with the facial recess approach attempts this route. This is especially true in young children whose incomplete mastoid development affords limited exposure. Even in the hands of experienced surgeons, the facial nerve may be in jeopardy when it follows a congenitally anomalous course. This situation may be anticipated, to some degree, by preoperative radiographic studies.

Mistakes in the design of the post-auricular skin flap can also occur. Should the antenna or receiver cannisters lie beneath the skin incision, device extrusion might take place (Luxford & House, 1985). Over-thinning of the skin flap could have similar consequences. Conversely, inadequate thinning of the skin flap may substantially increase the power requirements of transcutaneous transmission, although this is unlikely to be a factor in young children in whom thinning is usually unnecessary.

Cerebrospinal fluid (CSF) leak is a rare complication of cochlear implantation. In some individuals the perilymphatic and CSF spaces are confluent via the internal auditory canal or a widely patent cochlear aqueduct. This results in profuse CSF drainage upon surgically entering the scala tympani (Miyamoto et al., 1986). Congenitally malformed inner ears are especially prone to develop CSF fistulae (Phelps, 1986), which may be managed by packing a tissue seal of muscle or fat around the electrode. Meningitis is a potential complication of cochlear implantation, but has yet to be reported.

POSTOPERATIVE COMPLICATIONS

Infection following cochlear implantation may result from contamination during insertion, exposure of the device through an epithelial surface, or via otitis media or mastoiditis. Early infections following implant surgery have not been common due to the maintenance of strict aseptic technique and the use of prophylactic antibiotics (Clark, Pyman, & Pavillard, 1980). Most clinically significant infections derive from extrusion of the device. This has been particularly a problem with devices routed via the ear canal, a technique that affords little separation between the electrode and the ear canal skin.

Cross-stimulation of adjacent nerves may be problematic, especially when high levels of current are required to achieve auditory stimulation. Facial twitching (facial nerve) and pain (Jacobson's nerve) are the two most common clinical manifestations of cross-stimulation. The facial nerve, at its closest approach, lies several millimeters from the round window. Facial stimulation at this level is most common with extracochlear devices. Intracochlear monopolar devices, which have current paths between the active electrode and a distant ground (usually in the eustachian tube or under the temporalis muscle), may also activate the facial nerve on the medial wall of the middle ear. The closest approach between an active intra-cochlear electrode and the facial nerve is at the start of the second cochlear turn where it lies less than one millimeter from the cochlear endosteum. Cross-stimulation at this location is more likely to occur when the otic capsule is deficient, as it may be in otospongiosis. Con-genitally malformed ears also have a high incidence of facial cross-stimulation (Jackler, Luxford, & House, 1987). As with facial stimulation, pain associated with electrical stimulation may limit use of certain elec-trode channels or even render the implant unusable. Pain most probably arises from Jacboson's nerve, a component of the ninth cranial nerve, which courses across the cochlear promontory (Banfai et al., 1986). Its hypotympanic branch is in close proximity to the round window. It is uncertain whether resection of this nerve during implant surgery (there are no adverse consequences) will obviate this problem.

Significant vertigo following cochlear implantation is suprisingly uncommon, probably because most patients have pre-existing vestibular hypofunction. In those patients with residual vestibular function, vertigo may result from direct electrical stimulation of the vestibular end organ. In such cases, the symptom resolves when the device is inactivated (Burien, Hochmair-Desoyer, & Eisenwort, 1986). Persistent vertigo with the device turned off may indicate a perilymphatic fistula or labyrinthine trauma. Vertigo that is not controlled with routine medical therapy may, theoretically, be managed with labyrinthectomy or by the administration of drugs toxic to vestibular hair cells (e.g., streptomycin). Preoperative electronystagmography may detect residual vestibular function, thereby predicting the risk of postoperative vertigo.

The most frequent cause of failure in cochlear implantation is inadequate electrical stimulation of the cochlea due to lack of sufficient neural population. This failure of candidate selection is currently un-avoidable and will remain so until a reliable method of predicting nerve survival has been developed. All implant teams are faced with the pro-bability that some implanted patients will derive little or no benefit from their devices.

Generally, there are few postoperative restrictions placed on implanted children. They are able to participate in most physical activi-ties. Obviously, they must use caution in those sports in which a blow to the head is highly likely. The single precaution that children must take is to avoid very powerful magnetic fields, such as a Magnetic Resonance Imaging (MRI) scan, and strong radiofrequency energy that have the potential to cause electrical or electro-mechanical interactions with the implant.

COCHLEAR IMPLANT REVISION:
THE EFFECTS OF EXPLANTATION FOLLOWED BY REIMPLANTATION

In the future, the need for removal of an indwelling cochlear implant electrode followed by reimplantation with a new device is likely to increase substantially for several reasons: (1) over 1000 early generation devices have been implanted worldwide that lack internal disconnect systems to allow replacement of failed antenna or receiver components without removal of the intracochlear electrode; (2) the intracochlear electrode arrays themselves, although designed to be long lasting, will probably fail after decades long periods of use; and (3) the future development of highly superior multichannel electrode arrays will undoubtedly raise the issue of risk versus benefit concerning the extraction of existing devices for upgrading. These considerations are especially germane to the implantation of deaf children because device failures and compelling upgrades are a virtual certainty over a 70-year-plus lifespan.

The removal of an indwelling cochlear implant electrode followed by reinsertion of a new device is a maneuver of uncertain consequences to the cochlea and its surviving neural population. A scala tympani electrode rapidly becomes encased in a dense fibrous envelope. From histologic studies, it is known that this peri-implant fibrous sheath usually remains in situ following extraction of the electrode (Leake-Jones & Rebscher, 1983). Osteoneogenesis is also frequently found in the scala tympani, which may further stiffen the cuff surrounding the implant. Due to these restrictions in the cochlear lumen, it is probable that a replacement electrode that is longer or wider than the explanted one will not pass atraumatically into the cochlea. Attempts at forceful insertion may damage the delicate electrode contact surfaces or cause cochlear injury that may further deplete neural elements. Reimplantation with an electrode that is either identical to the explanted one, or shorter and narrower, is likely to proceed easily and atraumatically (Hochmair-Desoyer & Burian, 1985). Such a reinsertion may, in fact, be safer than primary implantation, as the peri-implant fibrous sheath provides a channel that guides the electrode and mimimizes the chance of cochlear damage.

As future intracochlear electrodes are likely to be longer and more complex than current ones, it is probable that their insertion will be difficult or impossible in most previously implanted ears. The exception to this general rule is the replacement of a very short, single-channel device with a long multichannel one. Successful replacements of single-channel 3M/House implants (a bare 6 mm wire) with multichannel Nucleus devices have been reported (Lindeman, Mangham, & Kuprenas, 1987).

Such transitions probably succeed because the peri-implant reaction is limited to the most basal region of the scala tympani, and an adequate lumen remains apical to this location. However, the great majority of future implant revisions will involve replacement of long intracochlear devices that have failed or become obsolete. Because such procedures may have deleterious effects, it is prudent at this time to perform only unilateral cochlear implantation in the pediatric age group. This allows for the placement of future upgrades in the virginal cochlea.

CONCLUSION

Although current generation multichannel implant systems are not yet "ideal" for young deaf children, technological advances in the near future promise to provide such devices. An ideal system must be miniaturized until its receiver package is as thin as possible, preferably less than 1 cm thick. The new Nucleus "mini" 22-channel implant for children has achieved a thickness of 6 mm (Clark et al., 1987a), but it lacks the other characteristics essential for implantation of the very young. The ideal implant also requires expansile properties to accommodate for head growth, modifications to prevent the medial spread of middle ear infection into the cochlea, and a capability for replacing and upgrading the existing electrode without further damage to the cochlea or its neural population. Although the ideal implant is not yet available, the authors do support the unilateral placement of sophisticated, multichannel intracochlear devices in young children at the present time. Less capable devices, such as extra- or intracochlear single-channel systems, may have limited potential for auditory rehabilitation.

ACKNOWLEDGMENT

Supported in part by the National Institutes of Health, Contract numbers NS-7-2391 and NS-3-2353.

REFERENCES

Balkany, T. J., Dreisbach, J. N., & Seibert, C. E. (1986). Radiographic imaging of the cochlear implant candidate: Preliminary results. *Otolaryngology-Head and Neck Surgery, 95,* 592–597.
Ball, J. B., Miller, G. W., & Hepfner, S. T. (1986). Computed tomography of single channel cochlear implants. *American Journal of Neuroradiology, 7,* 41–47.

Banfai, P., Karczag, A., Kubik, S., Luers, P., & Surth, W. (1986). Extracochlear sixteen channel electrode system. *Otolaryngologic Clinics of North America, 19,* 371–408.

Bates, G. J., Marks, D., Jackler, R. K., Leake, P. A., Snyder, R., Greenberg, S., & Merzenich, M. M. (1987). *Studies on pediatric auditory prosthesis implants.* National Institutes of Health, 1st Quarterly Progress Report, Contract No. NS 7-2391.

Becker, T. S., Eisenberg, L. S., Luxford, W. M., & House, W. F. (1984). Labyrinthine ossification secondary to childhood bacterial meningitis: Implications for cochlear implant surgery. *American Journal of Neuroradiology, 5,* 739–741.

Beighton, P., & Sellars, S. (1982). *Genetics and otology.* New York: Churchill-Livingstone.

Belal, A. (1975). Usher's syndrome (retinitis pigmentosa and deafness). *Journal of Laryngology and Otology, 89,* 175–181.

Bergstrom, L. (1980). Pathology of congenital deafness: Present status and future priorites. *Annals of Otology, Rhinology and Laryngology, 89* (Suppl. 74), 31–42.

Berkowitz, R. G., Franz, B. K., Shepard, R. K., Clark, G. M., & Bloom, D. M. (1985). Cochlear implant and otitis media: A pilot study to assess the feasibility of *Pseudomonas Aeruginosa* and *Streptococcus Pneumoniae* infection in the cat. *Journal of the Otolaryngology Society of Australia, 5,* 297–299.

Berkowitz, R. G., Franz, B. K., Shepard, R .K., Clark, G. M., & Bloom, D. M. (1987). Pneumococcal middle ear infection and cochlear implantation. *Annals of Otology, Rhinology and Laryngology, 96* (Suppl. 128), 55–57.

Bordley, J. E., & Alford, B. R. (1970). The pathology of rubella deafness. *International Audiology, 9,* 58–76.

Brownlee, R. C., DeLoache, W. R., Cowan, C. C., & Jackson, H.P. (1969). Otitis media in children: Incidence, treatment, and prognosis in pediatric patients. *Journal of Pediatrics, 75,* 636–642.

Burian, K., Hochmair-Desoyer, I. J., & Eisenwort, B. (1986). The Vienna cochlear implant program. *Otolaryngologic Clinics of North America, 19,* 313–328.

Clark, G. M., Pyman, B. C., & Pavillard, R. E. (1980). A protocol for the prevention of infection in cochlear implant surgery. *Journal of Laryngology and Otology, 94,* 1377–1386.

Clark, G. M., Shepard, R. K., Franz, B., & Bloom, D. M. (1984). Cochlear implant round window sealing procedures in the cat. *Acta Otolaryngologica, Suppl. 410,* 5–15.

Clark, G. M., Blamey, P. J., Busby, P. A., Dowell, R. C., Burkhard, K. H., Musgrave, G. N., Nienhuys, T. G., Pyman, B. C., Roberts, S. A., Tong, Y. C., Webb, R. L., Kuzma, J. A., Money, D. K., Patrick, J. F, & Seligman, P. M. (1987a). A multiple-electrode intracochlear implant for children. *Archives of Otolaryngology, 113,* 825–828.

Clark, G., Pyman, B., Webb, R., Franz, B., Redhead, T., & Shepherd, R. (1987b). Surgery for the safe insertion and reinsertion of the banded electrode array. *Annals of Otology, Rhinology and Laryngology, 96* (Suppl. 128), 10–12.

Cohen, N. L., Rosenberg, R., & Goldstein, S. (1987). Problems and complications of cochlear implant surgery. *Annals of Otology, Rhinology and Laryngology, 96* (Suppl. 128), 14–15.

Costeff, H., & Dar, H. (1980). Consanguinity analysis of congenital deafness in northern Israel. *American Journal of Human Genetics, 32,* 64–68.

Cranswick, N. E., Franz, B. K., Clark, G. M., Shepard, R. K., & Bloom, D. M. (1987). Middle ear infection postimplantation: Response of the round window membrane to Streptococcus Pyogenes. *Annals of Otology, Rhinology and Laryngology, 96* (Suppl. 128), 53–54.

Dahnsjo, J., Andersson, H., Hallander, H. O., & Rudberg, R. D. (1976). Tone audiometry control of children treated for meningitis with large intravenous doses of ampicillin. *Acta Paediatrica Scandinavica, 65,* 733–737.

Das, V. K. (1987). Pendred's syndrome with episodic vertigo, tinnitus, and vomiting and normal bithermic caloric responses. *Journal of Laryngology and Otology, 101,* 721–722.

Dodge, P. R., Davis, H., Feigin, R. D., Holmes, S. J., Kaplan, S. L., Jubelirer, S. P., Stechenberg, B. W., & Hirsh, S.K. (1984). Prospective evaluation of hearing impairment as a sequel of acute bacterial meningitis. *New England Journal of Medicine, 311,* 869–874.

Eby, T. L., & Nadol, J. B. (1986). Postnatal growth of the human temporal bone. Implications for cochlear implants in children. *Annals of Otology, Rhinology and Laryngology, 95,* 356–364.

Eisenberg, L. S., Luxford, W. M., Becker, T. S., & House, W. F. (1984). Electrical stimulation of the auditory system in children deafened by meningitis. *Otolaryngology-Head and Neck Surgery, 92,* 700–705.

Fisch, L. (1959). Deafness as part of an hereditary syndrome. *Journal of Laryngology and Otology, 73,* 355–383.

Franz, B., Clark, G. M., & Bloom, D. M. (1984). Permeability of the implanted round window membrane in the cat. *Acta Otolaryngologica, Suppl. 410,* 17–23.

Friedmann, I., Fraser, G. R., & Froggat, P. (1966). Pathology of the ear in the cardio-auditory syndrome of Jervell and Lange–Nielsen (recessive deafness with electrocardiographic abnormalities). *Journal of Laryngology and Otology, 80,* 451–470.

Gray, R. F. & Schindler, R. A. (1985). Complications and failures of cochlear impants. In R. F. Gray (Ed.), *Cochlear implants* (pp. 152–162). San Diego, CA: College-Hill Press.

Hausler, R., Toupet, M., Guidetti, G., Basseres, F., & Montandon, P. (1987). Meniere's disease in children. *American Journal of Otolaryngology, 8,* 187–193.

Hochmair-Desoyer, I. J., & Burian, K. (1985). Reimplantation of a molded scala tympani electrode: Impact on psychophysical and speech discrimination abilities. *Annals of Otology, Rhinology and Laryngology, 94,* 65–70.

Hooper, R. (1969). A lengthening procedure for ventriculo-atrial shunts. *Journal of Neurosurgery, 30,* 93–96.

House, W. (1982). Surgical considerations in cochlear implantation. *Annals of Otology, Rhinology and Laryngology, 91* (Suppl. 91), 15–20.

House, W. F., Luxford, W. M., & Courtney, B. (1985). Otitis media in children following the cochlear implant. *Ear and Hearing, 6* (Suppl.), 24S–26S.

Hughes, G. B., & Rutherford, I. (1986). Predictive value for serologic tests for syphilis in otology. *Annals of Otology, Rhinology and Laryngology, 95,* 250–259.

Hvidberg-Hansen, J., & Jorgensen, M.B. (1968). The inner ear in Pendred's syndrome. *Acta Otolaryngologica, 66,* 129–135.

Jackler, R. K., Luxford, W. M., & House, W. F. (1987). Sound detection with the cochlear implant in five ears of four children with congenital malformations of the cochlea. *Laryngoscope, 97* (Suppl. 40), 15–17.

Jackler, R. K., Luxford, W. M., Schindler, R. A., & McKerrow, W. S. (1987). Cochlear patency problems in cochlear implantation. *Laryngoscope, 97,* 801–805.

Jackler, R. K., O'Donoghue, G. M., & Schindler, R. A. (1986). Cochlear implantation: Strategies to protect the implanted cochlea from middle ear infection. *Annals of Otology, Rhinology and Laryngology, 95,* 66–70.

Jervell, A. (1985). The surdo-cardiac syndrome. *European Heart Journal, 6* (Suppl. D), 97–102.

Keane, W. M., Postic, W. P., Rowe, L. D., & Konkoe, D. F. (1979). Meningitis and hearing loss in children. *Archives of Otolarygology, 105,* 39–44.

Kerr, A., & Schuknecht, H. F. (1968). The spiral ganglion in profound deafness. *Acta Otolaryngologica, 65,* 586–598.

Kerr, A. G., Symth, G. D., & Cinnamond, M. J. (1973). Congenital syphilitic deafness. *Journal of Laryngology and Otology, 87,* 1–12.

Konigsmark, B. W., & Gorlin, R. J. (1976). *Genetic and metabolic deafness.* Philadelphia, PA: W. B. Saunders Co.

Kumar, A., Fishman, G., & Torok, N. (1984). Vestibular and auditory function in Usher's syndrome. *Annals of Otology, Rhinology and Laryngology, 93,* 600–608.

Kundell, S. P., & Ochs, H.D. (1980). Cogan syndrome in childhood. *Journal of Pediatrics, 97,* 96–98.

Leake, P. A., Rebscher, S. J., & Aird, D. W. (1985). Histopathology of cochlear implants: Safety considerations. In R. A. Schindler & M. M. Merzenich (Eds.), *Cochlear implants* (pp. 55–64). New York: Raven Press.

Leake-Jones, P. A., & Rebscher, S. J. (1983). Cochlear pathology with chronically implanted scala tympani electrodes. In C. W. Parkins & S. W. Anderson (Eds.), Cochlear prostheses: An international symposium. *Annals of the New York Academy of Sciences, 405,* 203–223.

Lindeman, R. C., Mangham, C. A., & Kuprenas, M. A. (1987). Single-channel and multichannel performance for reimplanted cochlear prosthesis patient. *Annals of Otology, Rhinology and Laryngology, 96* (Suppl. 128), 150–151.

Luxford, W. M., & House, W. F. (1985). Cochlear implants in children: Medical and surgical considerations. *Ear and Hearing, 6* (Suppl.), 20S–23S.

Miyamoto, R. T., Robbins, A. M., Myres, W. A., Pope, M. L. (1986). Cochlear implantation in the Mondini inner ear malformation. *American Journal of Otology, 7,* 258–261.

Monsell, E. M., Jackler, R. K., & Motta, G. (1987). Congenital malformations of the inner ear: Histologic findings in five temporal bones. *Laryngoscope, 97* (Suppl. 40), 18–24.

O'Donoghue, G. M., Jackler, R. K., Jenkins, W. M., & Schindler, R. A. (1986). Cochlear implantation in children: The problem of head growth. *Otolaryngology-Head and Neck Surgery, 94,* 78–81.

O'Donoghue, G., Jackler, R., & Schindler, R. (1986). Observations on an experimental expansile electrode for use in cochlear implantation. *Acta Otolaryngologica, 102,* 1–6.

Olley, P. M., & Fowler, R. S. (1979). The surdo-cardiac syndrome and therapeutic observations. *British Heart Journal, 32,* 467–471.

Otte, J., Schuknecht, H. F., & Kerr, A. G. (1978). Ganglion cell populations in normal and pathological cochleae: Implications for cochlear implantation. *Laryngoscope, 88,* 1231–1246.

Paparella, M. M., & Sugiura, S. (1967). The pathology of suppurative labyrinthitis. *Annals of Otology, Rhinology and Laryngology, 76,* 554–586.

Pappas, D. G. & Mundy, M. R. (1982). Sensorineural hearing loss: Infectious agents. *Laryngoscope, 92,* 752–754.

Parving, A., Vejtorp, M., Moller, K., & Moller, J. K. (1980). Congenital hearing loss and rubella infection. *Acta Otolaryngologica, 90,* 262–266.

Phelps, P. D. (1986). Congenital cerebrospinal fluid fistulae of the petrous temporal bone. *Clinical Otolaryngology, 11,* 79–92.

Ruben, R. J. (1983). Diseases of the inner ear and sensorineural deafness. In C. D. Bluestone & S. E. Stool (Eds.), *Pediatric otolaryngology* (Vol. 1, pp. 577–604). Philadelphia: W. B. Saunders.

Ruben, R. J., & Rozycki D. (1970). Diagnostic screening for the deaf child. *Archives of Otolaryngology, 91,* 429–432.

Sato, G., & Glenn, W. W. L. (1970). Teflon envelope protection for cardiac electrodes in the growing swine. *Journal of Thoracic and Cardiovascular Surgery, 59,* 830–836.

Schatz, M., & Zeiger, R. S. (1987). Otologic manifestations of systemic immunologic diseases. In J. M. Bernstein & P. L. Ogra (Eds.), *Immunology of the ear* (pp. 481–487). New York: Raven Press.

Schindler, R. A., Kessler, D. K., Rebscher, S. J., Jackler, R. K., & Merzenich, M. M. (1987). Surgical considerations and hearing results with the UCSF/Storz cochlear implant. *Laryngoscope, 97,* 50–56.

Schmidt, J. M. (1985). Cochlear neuronal populations in developmental defects of the inner ear: Implications for cochlear implantation. *Acta Otolaryngologica, 99,* 14–20.

Siegel, J. D., & McCracken, G. H. (1981). Aminoglycoside ototoxicity in children. In S. Lerner, G. Matz, & J. Hawkins (Eds.), *Aminoglycoside ototoxicity* (pp. 341–353). Boston: Little Brown.

Strauss, M. (1985). A clinical pathologic study of hearing loss in congenital cytomegalovirus infection. *Laryngoscope, 95,* 951–962.

Supance, J. S., & Bluestone, C. D. (1983). Perilymph fistulas in infants and children. *Otolaryngology-Head and Neck Surgery, 91,* 663–671.

Swartz, J. D., Mandell, D. M., Faerber, E. N., Popky, G. L., Ardito, J. M., Steinberg, S. B., & Rojer, C. L. (1985). Labyrinthine ossification: Etiologies and CT findings. *Radiology, 157,* 395–398.

Thould, A. K., & Scowen, E. F. (1964). The syndrome of congenital deafness and simple goiter. *Journal of Endocrinology, 30,* 69–77.

Veldman, J. E. (1987). Immune mediated inner ear disorders. New syndromes and their etiopathogenesis. In J. E. Veldman & B. F. McCabe (Eds.), *Otoimmunology* (pp. 125–138). Amsterdam: Kugler Publications.

DORCAS K. KESSLER

PRESENT STATUS OF COCHLEAR IMPLANTS IN CHILDREN

As documentation on the benefits provided by cochlear implants has accumulated and as implantation has gradually gained wider clinical acceptance, interest in applying these devices for the rehabilitation of young profoundly deaf children has grown. Since the House Ear Institute (HEI) of Los Angeles initiated a children's implant program in 1980 (Berliner & Eisenberg, 1985), the number of children receiving cochlear implants has rapidly increased.

In the United States, only two devices have been applied to children: the 3M/House single-channel implant and the Nucleus 22-electrode system. Presently, both of these programs retain investigational status, having received Food and Drug Administration (FDA) Investigational Device Exemptions (IDEs) permitting clinical trials of implantation in children. As investigational programs monitored by the FDA, careful documentation of both pre- and postoperative status is required to establish the safety and efficacy of the devices and to prove their viability for "premarket approval" (Berliner & Eisenberg, 1985; Yin & Segerson, 1986).

Children are also implanted in at least two European programs. In France, a 12-channel intracochlear system, called Chorimac, is implanted in children aged 7 years and older (Chouard, Fugain, & Meyer, 1985; Chouard et al., 1986). In Germany, children are implanted beginning at 6 years of age with a 16-channel extracochlear system (Banfai et al., 1986). However, reports on patient performance with these devices do not consider children independently from adults; rather, data are presented for the total patient samples. In this chapter, consideration is thus restricted to the 3M/House and Nucleus implants. Several reports on the performance of children with the 3M/House device have appeared since the early 1980s. Data on the performance of children with the Nucleus system are sparse because the program has only recently begun. The literature on children with these two cochlear implants is reviewed and summarized, and some of the more prominent issues concerning these data are discussed.

SINGLE-CHANNEL STIMULATION

THE 3M/HOUSE COCHLEAR IMPLANT

The first House single-channel device with a wearable, external processor was implanted in 1972 by William F. House. This implant served as the model for all subsequent House single-channel systems. In 1981, following an agreement with the 3M Company, the House device underwent slight modifications (Fretz & Fravel, 1985), including replacement of the 15-mm electrode with a 6-mm electrode in order to reduce the chances of traumatic insertion and the use of magnets for holding the wearable transmitter in place. It is this modified device that has been implanted in the majority of children.

The internal components of the 3M/House single-channel implant, shown in Figure 10–1(A), consist of the receiver and a single platinum ball electrode. The system uses monopolar stimulation, with the titanium receiver can acting as the ground (Luxford & House, 1987) and the short active (uninsulated) electrode portion inserted a distance of 6 mm into the scala tympani. The electrode lead was designed to be of sufficient length (64 mm) to accommodate head growth in young children. According to Luxford and House (1985; 1987), the excess electrode length gradually straightens in the air-containing mastoid cavity provided that the electrode is firmly attached at its two ends, the round window and the temporal squama. The external components of the 3M/House system, consisting of the processor, the microphone, and the transmitter, are shown in Figure 10–1(B).

In the House speech processing strategy, an amplified signal is bandpass filtered between 340 and 2700 Hz. This filtered signal is used to amplitude modulate a 16 kHz sinusoidal carrier, which is set just below audibility. After amplitude modulation, no further processing occurs. Processor controls allow the clinician to adjust the carrier level and limit the maximum output (peak clipping) for each individual patient. The constant 16 kHz carrier was selected, according to Fretz and Fravel

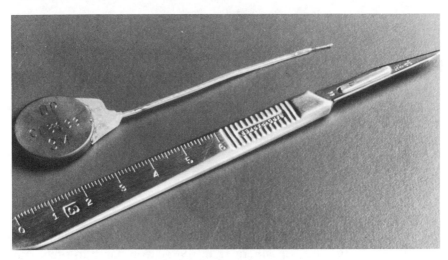

A

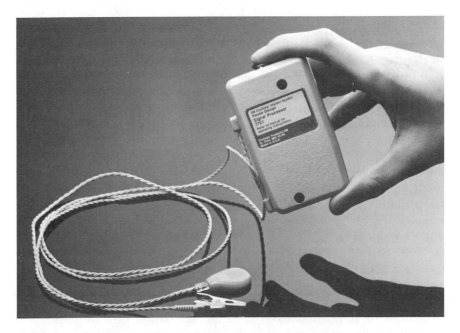

B

FIGURE 10–1. A. The internal components of the 3M/House implant, consisting of the receiver and the electrode. B. The external components of the 3M/House implant, consisting of the speech processor, the microphone, and the transmitter. Courtesy of the 3M Company.

(1985), because frequencies near 16 kHz are easily and efficiently transmitted across the skin. They also assert that use of this signal makes device fitting easier than with more complex systems, because lengthy loudness and frequency equalization procedures are avoided. Both Pfingst (1986) and Moore (1985) have referred to this form of single-channel processing as the modulated-carrier, analog approach, defining it as a strategy in which the waveform itself is used to drive the electrode and in which an attempt is made to squeeze the entire speech signal into a single channel.

BACKGROUND

The decision to proceed with a children's program was based on results obtained with adults using the House single-channel system (Berliner & Eisenberg, 1985; Eisenberg et al., 1983). Compared to preoperative performance with hearing aids, adult implant users showed improvement in auditory thresholds and in the ability to make prosodic discriminations. Implant use reportedly enhanced communication skills and encouraged feelings of confidence. Almost no adverse effects were reported among adults and it was determined that the benefits of implantation far outweighed the risks (Berliner, 1982).

Three categories of medical and surgical risks were considered (Berliner, 1982; Berliner & Eisenberg, 1985; Eisenberg et al., 1983): those involved with mastoid surgery, those involved with implantation and the ongoing presence of a foreign body in the ear, and those concerned with electrical stimulation of the auditory nervous system. Although the effects of long-term electrical stimulation on the developing nervous system remain unknown, the risks entailed in the surgical procedure itself and in the insertion and presence of a device were deemed minimal based on adult experience. Despite the high incidence of otitis media in the pediatric population, the potential for tracking infection into the inner ear was also considered minimal based on the successful treatment of adult implant recipients with otitis media using conventional antibiotics. The possibility for dislodgement of the intracochlear electrode portion as a result of head growth was considered resolved by allowing sufficient electrode length for straightening and by anchoring the electrode in place. (For detailed discussions of the medical and surgical considerations of implantation in children, see Chapters 8 and 9.)

Among the risks considered for children were the impact of deafness on the social, emotional, and educational development of the child (Berliner, 1982; Berliner & Eisenberg, 1985; Eisenberg et al., 1983). Eisenberg and colleagues (1983) noted that "Even minimal auditory input can have a significant impact on language acquisition and educational success" (p. 42). Citing research on early deprivation studies indicating the atrophy of cells in the central auditory pathways, the authors stated that "Early auditory experience may be important in developing basic concepts about sound and its meaningfulness, and may be an important determinant in whether a child can later in life make effective use of auditory input" (p. 49). In response to the question whether implantation in children should be postponed until better devices are available, the House group argued that there is no evidence to support the contention that a child implanted now may not be able to benefit in the future from an improved device. They also stated that "In addition, only one ear is implanted [the poorer ear], leaving the better ear for future use" (p. 49). In summary, Eisenberg and colleagues (1983) reasoned as follows:

> Given that some children do not have the hair cell population to benefit from [hearing] aids, that deprivation of sound causes further degeneration, and that early auditory experience is so influential in the child's development and for future use of sound, it would appear that the cochlear implant is an appropriate alternative." (p. 49)

According to Eisenberg (1982), a study of implantation in 12 adults who were prelingually deaf was undertaken as a preliminary to the implantation of children. Eight of the 12 subjects were considered successful implant users, wearing their devices on a daily basis. Of these 8, 6 were congenitally deaf. Audiologic findings for these subjects were similar to those for postlingually deafened adults. On the one hand, although implant stimulation did not alter the life style of these subjects, and although 4 of the 12 patients rejected device use, it was concluded that these prelingual subjects accepted and enjoyed sound (Eisenberg, 1982). On the other hand, experience with prelingually deaf adults suggested that there may be a point in time beyond which sound did not provide meaningful information (House, Berliner, & Eisenberg, 1983). These findings further encouraged the House group to proceed with the implantation of children.

PREOPERATIVE AND POSTOPERATIVE EVALUATION PROCEDURES

PATIENT SELECTION

The patient selection procedures for children for the 3M/House implant have been described in a number of publications (Berliner & Eisenberg, 1985; Eisenberg et al., 1983). Children must be at least 2 years of age, with 17 years as the upper-age limit. The selection process includes medical, audiological, and psychological evaluations. The primary criterion is the confirmation of profound hearing loss, although a specific definition of "profound" is not supplied. The child's ability to make use of a hearing aid is the second primary area of consideration. The child's aided performance on specific tests of auditory discrimination in the ear selected for implantation must be poorer than or equal to the average test results from children using a cochlear implant. The ear demonstrating the poorest aided results is selected for surgery (Thielemeir et al., 1985). The reason for accepting children whose aided results are equal to average implant performance is not explained; evidence indicating that such children, once implanted, always exceed that average is not provided.

Psychologically, children who demonstrate signs of psychosis, mental retardation, organic brain damage or severe behavioral problems are eliminated from consideration. Additionally, the family's expectations regarding the implant and their ability to follow-through with a postimplant rehabilitation program are considered (Tiber, 1985). Those children selected for implantation are also administered a battery of speech and language evaluations. According to Eisenberg and associates (1983), the speech and language ability of a child is not a criterion in the selection process; rather, this information is used as baseline information with which to compare postoperative results.

POSTOPERATIVE EVALUATION

Berliner and Eisenberg (1985) have identified several methodological difficulties in attempting to study deaf children. Among these are the inability to separate the effects of intervention from the effects of maturation, and the heterogeneity of the population. Such factors as age, duration of deafness, age at onset of deafness, and educational training and communicative environment (i.e., aural/oral, manual, total) present an array of confounding variables. They concluded that the number of variables that must be considered in creating a matched control group for experimental study was nearly impossible. Rather, a single-group repeated measures design is employed in which each child serves as his or her own control. As with adult implant evaluation protocols, preoperative measures are repeated postoperatively, with preoperative results considered the baseline data against which postoperative performance is compared.

In the 3M/House protocol, followed by each of eight coinvestigational facilities, children return home after surgery for a 1- to 2-month healing period. They then return to the clinic for device fitting and for training, called *Basic Guidance.* After optimum device settings have been established and some basic audiometric measures obtained, the children again return home and to their regular educational settings. A full evaluation is first administered 6 months after the initial device fitting and Basic Guidance (Thielemeir et al., 1985). Medical, audiological, psychological, and speech and language re-evaluations are then performed at 6-month intervals for children under 8 years of age, and annually for children 8 years and older.

Of necessity, the evaluation of a cochlear implant for children is much more complex than for postlingual adults. Speech and language abilities are generally intact in adults who are postlingually deafened, and evaluation procedures concentrate on measuring aspects of auditory speech reception. In contrast, profound hearing impairment in children may have an effect on auditory speech reception, language acquisiton, speech production, educational achievement, and psychological status. Consequently, in order to determine benefit and the effects of intervention with a sensory aid, each of these areas must be assessed. The manner of assessment and the materials used will vary depending on the age and linguistic abilities of the child. The 3M/House evaluation protocol consists of batteries of tests for each of the areas potentially effected by implant use. These have been described by Berliner, Eisenberg, and House (1985), and will be summarized as results are reviewed.

SUBJECTS

Accounts of patient data encompass patients from each of the eight investigational centers participating in the 3M/House children's program. According to the most recent report (Berliner et al., 1987), as of mid-1987, a total of 282 children had been implanted with the 3M/House device. One of these patients was designated as *in process* and three patients are deceased, leaving a total of 278. Of these 278 patients, 32 either were not using or were unable to use their devices. These 32 patients were assigned to various categories: 14 *nonusers;* 5 *awaiting revision;* 8 *nonstimulable;* and 5 *devices removed.* This leaves a total of 246 *users;* conversely, 12 percent of the patient sample were not using their devices at that time. Explanations for these categories are not provided; for example, reasons for device removal are not discussed and *user* is not defined. In previous accounts, the definition of *user* has varied, including from 5 to 13 hours a day (Eisenberg & House, 1982), from 8- to 10-hours a day (Eisenberg et al., 1983), and device use on a "regular basis," usually "all day, everyday" (Berliner & Eisenberg, 1985). The manner in which the average hours of daily usage are derived (e.g., clinician observation, questionnaire, teacher report, parent report) is not supplied.

Since the inception of the children's program, the total number of surgical revisions performed either because of internal device failure or in order to upgrade the system cannot be calculated from published reports. For example, Eisenberg and associates (1983) referred to one patient who underwent a successful surgical revision, and Berliner and Eisenberg (1985) referred to 13. In all of these 13 cases, no decrements in performance were observed following revision. Because the most recent count of *awaiting revision* is 5, it can be assumed that, once successfully accomplished, patients with surgical revisions return to the overall data pool. Surgical revisions have been described as relatively easy procedures, usually involving only replacement of the receiver rather than the full electrode and receiver assembly (Luxford & House, 1985; 1987). Luxford and House (1987) reported that all patients who have undergone a revision now have functioning devices. This suggests that *device removal* is an option for patients confronting a second surgical procedure because of an internal failure. Indeed, Luxford and House (1985) reported that the parents of three children, in whom revision could not be accomplished immediately because of infection and subsequent device rejection, decided to have the other ear implanted rather than wait for the infection to heal and revision to occur. Implantation on the opposite ear was successfully performed, and, presumably, these three patients are now also part of the total patient sample. On the other hand, in one case discussed by Eisenberg and colleagues (1986a), device removal was the option selected by the parents of a young child when the internal coil failed.

In the recent patient tally by Berliner and associates (1987), patients were placed in three age categories. Subtracting the one *in process,* the three deceased, and the 32 various nonusers, the distribution of patients by age was as follows: 112 were from ages 2 through 5, 107 were from ages 6 through 12, and 27 were teenagers, from 13 to 17 years. The teenage category claimed the largest number of nonusers. From 43 patients placed in this age category (the total actually sums to 44, with one apparently unaccounted), 7 were either awaiting revision, nonstimulable, or had their devices removed, while 10 were labeled *nonusers.* Thus, 40 percent of the adolescent population were not using their devices at that time, and 30 percent (10 *nonusers* and 3 *devices removed*) had apparently elected this alternative. The reluctance of teens to use their implants has been acknowledged in several reports and has recently become the focus of a clinical study (Chute et al., 1987). Generally, adolescent device rejection has been attributed (Berliner & Eisenberg, 1985; Luxford et al., 1987) to self-consciousness concerning the cosmetic aspects of the implant and peer pressure (see Chapter 15 for a discussion of this issue).

In a report on 164 children, Berliner and Eisenberg (1985) provided detailed information on patient demographics. The majority of these children (N = 98) were implanted at the House Ear Institute, while the remaining 66 children were implanted at the seven co-investigating facilities. Of these 164 children, 91 were males and 73 were females; 106 of the children had an acquired hearing loss, 55 were congenitally deaf, and in 3 cases the onset of deafness was unknown. The etiology in the majority of cases was bacterial meningitis, being the cause of deafness in 98 of the 164 children. The age range of the children at time of implant was 2 years 5 months to 17 years 11 months, with a mean of 8 years 4 months. The majority of children were implanted in the preschool and elementary school ages. For the acquired loss group, the mean age at onset of deafness was 2 years 5 months. With the congenital and acquired loss groups combined, the mean age of onset was 1 year 7 months. The majority of implanted children were prelingually deaf. The duration of deafness prior to implantation ranged from 5 months to 17 years 6 months, with a mean of 6 years 7 months.

As the number of implanted children has grown, these statistics appear to remain fairly stable. In a report on 189 children, for example, Luxford and colleagues (1987) stated that one-third of the children were congenitally deaf and two-thirds had an acquired hearing loss. Bacterial meningitis remained the primary etiology for the majority of children. Although the incidence of cochlear ossification in cases of meningitis is high, for the most part the House group has reported successful implantation of these children (Eisenberg et al., 1984). In a study comparing 25 meningitis children with 10 congenitally deaf children, some degree of ossification was found in 20 of the meningitis children and in only one of the congenitals. The meningitis group demonstrated electrical and auditory thresholds comparable to those of the congenital group, although significantly greater power was needed to achieve a response. From this study it was concluded that auditory neural elements are present in cases of both partial and complete cochlear obliteration resulting from meningitis and that neither of these conditions were contraindications to implant surgery.

RESULTS

The pilot study and first account (Eisenberg & House, 1982) of House cochlear implants in children concerned 12 subjects who had been implanted as of December, 1981. These 12 children ranged in age from 3 years 5 months to 17 years, with a mean age of 10 years 3 months. Six of the children were congenitally deaf; 6 had an acquired loss, with meningitis as the etiology for 5 of the acquired loss group. Eight of the children were using hearing aids at the time of implantation. Results for these 12 children were consistent with those of adult House implant users. Mean warble tone thresholds with the implant, ranging from 59 to 64 dB SPL over 250 to 3000 Hz, were considerably improved relative to preoperative aided thresholds. The children were also able to make timing and intensity differentiations (e.g., loud versus soft, long versus short, and continuous versus interrupted) that could not be done preoperatively, although test data to support these results were not reported. Eisenberg and House (1982) stated that among these 12 children, no adverse reactions were noted. However, one subject developed an infection over the incision and two children experienced otitis media; all three cases were treated and resolved without incident.

Tyler, Davis and Lansing (1987) suggested that this small study is of particular interest because, rather than simply presenting group means as in reports on larger numbers of subjects, individual preimplant and postimplant data are shown. For the 11 children for whom preoperative hearing aid information was available, they noted that 8 subjects demonstrated a clear improvement in thresholds with their implants, 2 showed equivocal results, and 1 child displayed a decrement of hearing at 500 and 1000 Hz.

In the most complete report to date (Berliner, Eisenberg, & House, 1985), the status of 164 children, who had received the 3M/House implant as of December, 1984, was reviewed. In this monograph, each area of assessment was considered and the evaluation instruments used were described. Subsequent publications (Berliner & Eisenberg, 1987; Berliner et al., 1987; Eisenberg et al., 1986b; Luxford et al., 1987) have added to the patient data, analyzed particular aspects of the data in detail, or presented recent results using new evaluation tools.

AUDIOLOGIC PERFORMANCE

Preoperatively, implant candidates are given an audiologic and hearing aid evaluation, including impedance audiometry and, for those under 6 years of age, Auditory Brainstem Response testing (Thielemeir et al., 1985). In addition to warble tone thresholds, a speech detection threshold (SDT) and a speech uncomfortable loudness level (ULL) are obtained in the unaided condition. Thresholds, SDTs, and ULLs are also measured with hearing aids for each ear separately. The ear providing the best aided response is selected for speech discrimination testing.

TEST MATERIALS. The primary materials used for the evaluation of speech perception are the Discrimination After Training Test (DAT) and the Test of Auditory Comprehension (TAC). The same battery of tests is administered postoperatively. The DAT (Thielemeir et al., 1985) is intended for use with children and adults who are prelingually deaf. The stimuli for the test items are taken from the Monosyllable, Trochee, Spondee (MTS) test (Erber & Alencewiecz, 1976), designed to assess the perception of the durational and stress patterns of speech. The test proceeds through 12 levels that progress in difficulty. Level 1 is a lipreading task to ensure that the child understands the task; level 2 tests auditory-only speech detection; levels 3 through 5 test discriminations of gross durational and timing cues; and levels 6 through 12 evaluate discriminations of speech pattern (stress) perception. The test is administered live voice, and the child responds by pointing to a picture or by saying or signing the correct item. The test score is the highest level passed.

Using a closed-set format and recorded voice, the TAC (Los Angeles County, 1980) evaluates the comprehension of environmental sounds and speech. The test contains 10 subtests, ranging in difficulty from subtest 1, in which a discrimination between a linguistic and nonlinguistic sound is required, to subtest 10, in which the subject is required to recall five details of a story presented in the presence of a competing message. The ten subtests are presented in sequence, with the child responding by pointing to a picture. As with the DAT, the test score is the highest level passed.

AUDIOMETRIC DATA. Thielemeir and colleagues (1985) analyzed data for 126 children. Preoperatively, mean aided warble-tone thresholds for 124 of these children ranged from 82 to 100 dB SPL over 250 to 4000 Hz. An aided mean SDT of 82 dB SPL was obtained. Postoperatively, at the first audiometric testing, mean thresholds ranged from 50 to 64 dB SPL across 250 to 4000 Hz for 114 children, with an average SDT of 57 dB SPL. Thresholds are similar at the 6-month evaluation (N = 62) and at the 12-month evaluation (N = 35). However, because the number of subjects at both pre- and postoperative intervals is not held constant, the same children are not being consistently compared and results are difficult to interpret.

CLOSED-SET SPEECH PERCEPTION. According to Thielemeir and colleagues (1985), the majority of 106 children tested preoperatively with hearing aids on the DAT could not detect the tester's voice (level 2) at a distance of 1 to 2 feet. The preoperative aided DAT mean score was 2.16, but the median was only 1.0. A mean test score of 6.7 (level 6 = monosyllable versus spondee) was obtained for 39 of these 106 children at their 6-month postimplant evaluations. Although the mean DAT test scores show some slight improvement at each 6-month postoperative interval, the number of subjects reported progressively decreases from 30 at the

12-month evaluation to 3 at the 36-month evaluation, making a comparison over time of questionable validity.

A second analysis of pre- and postimplant performance on the DAT for HEI children who had completed at least their 6-month followup evaluations was provided (Thielemeir et al., 1985). The mean duration of implant use at test time was 13 months. Preoperatively (N = 41), only 40 percent of the subjects could pass level 2 with their hearing aids, whereas all of the children could pass level 2 postimplant (N = 45). Less than 30 percent of the children could pass levels higher than 2 with hearing aids, but postimplant 80 percent could pass level 6 and over 60 percent could pass level 8 (monosyllable versus trochee).

In a 3-year followup study, Allsman and Tonokawa (1987) demonstrated improvement over time with the implant for 21 subjects on the DAT. At the 6-month assessment their mean DAT score was 6.7, and at the 3-year evaluation, the mean was 9.2 (level 9 = two-choice spondee). Improvement over time was confirmed in a recent study of DAT results (Johnson, 1987a), in which a statistical analysis of covariance was undertaken to determine factors associated with high performance. The following variables were evaluated: months of cochlear implant use, preoperative baseline scores, age at onset of deafness, age at time of implantation, duration or years of profound deafness, age at time of postoperative evaluation, and mode of communication. This statistical investigation found that duration of implant use, or months of stimulation, showed significant consistent association with increasing DAT scores. That is, experience with the implant was the predominant factor in predicting DAT performance.

Berliner and Eisenberg (1987) showed raw DAT scores for 73 children who were tested preoperatively with hearing aids and then postoperatively with the implant. The best implant score for each child was used. For 66 of the 73 subjects, better scores were achieved with the implant than with the hearing aid. Viewing the DAT results from a new perspective, Berliner and Eisenberg (1987) grouped the twelve DAT levels according to the categories of speech perception skills developed by Geers and Moog (1987; 1988; Chapter 11). However, they have added a fifth category, designated category 0, in which to place children who have no auditory detection. DAT levels 1 and 2, auditory detection only, fit perceptual category 1; DAT levels 3 through 8 fit category 2, or pattern perception; DAT levels 9 through 11 (two- and three-choice spondees) fit category 3, or partial word identification; and DAT level 12 (four-choice spondee) fits category 4, or consistent word identification. An analysis of the DAT data according to this scheme placed 7 percent of the 73 subjects in either category 0 or 1, 53 percent in category 2, 32 percent in category 3, and 8 percent in category 4. Geers and Moog (1988; Chapter 11) reported identical results for this sample of 73 children. They also analyzed the earlier DAT results reported by Thielemeir and colleagues (1985) for 54 children and noted that the majority (70 percent) were in perceptual category 2. Whereas 20 percent of the children were in categories 3 and 4 in the early sample, 40 percent attained these categories in the later sample. Geers and Moog concluded that the success rate doubled as a result of 2 additional years of experience with the implant. However, both a discrepancy in sample size and the fact that the later report (Berliner & Eisenberg, 1987) stated that the children's best scores were used regardless of the point in time at which they were attained, makes this conclusion somewhat tenuous.

The TAC appears to be a much more difficult test for these children. Thielemeir and associates (1985) reported that of the 39 children tested with hearing aids preoperatively, 63 percent were unable to take the test because they could not detect the test stimuli at the required standardized level (76 dB SPL). Presumably, they were assigned a score of 0, because the mean TAC score reported for these 39 preimplant subjects was well below 1 (0.13). At the 6-month postimplant assessment (N = 39), the mean remained below 1 (0.90), and at the 12-month postimplant interval (N = 32), a mean of 1 was finally achieved, indicating that the children were able to discriminate between a linguistic and a nonlinguistic stimulus.

In a separate analysis, 14 percent of 21 subjects who were able to take the test preoperatively with a hearing aid in the implant ear could pass subtest 1, but none could pass subtest 2. Postimplant, 71 percent of 49 children could pass subtest 1, 22 percent passed subtest 2 (linguistic versus human nonlinguistic versus environmental sounds), and a few could pass levels 3 through 5.

In their 3-year followup study, Allsman and Tonokawa (1987) found only very slight improvement over time for 23 implanted children on the TAC, with a mean of 1.0 at the 6-month test interval and a mean of 1.4 at the 3-year evaluation. These children had not yet achieved subtest 2, the ability to discriminate among a linguistic, a human nonlinguistic, and an environmental sound.

OPEN-SET SPEECH RECOGNITION. In their 1985 report, Thielemeir and associates discerned the emergence of certain trends among the 126 implanted children whose audiological results were presented. They noted that children who were deafened at age 2 years or older and who used some form of oral communication (auditory/verbal, oral/aural, cued speech) performed above average with the implant. They speculated that both age at time of onset and duration of profound loss at time of implant may affect performance. They further observed that the best performers were either those deafened at a later age or those postlingually deafened preschool aged children who were implanted shortly after the onset of deafness. Results were described for three children cited as their "best performers." Two of these 3 children, or 1.5 percent of the total sample of 126 subjects, obtained some sentence and word recognition in a live-voice auditory-only open-set format, using stimuli from the Glendonald Auditory Screening Procedure (GASP) (Erber, 1982).

The GASP, originally intended as a closed-set test of words and simple phrases using a picture pointing response format, consists of 12 words and 10 sentences. The 12 words, rich in duration/timing cues, include 3 monosyllables (e.g., shoe), 3 trochees (e.g., pencil), 3 spondees (e.g., airplane), and 3 polysyllabics (e.g., elephant). The 10 sentences consist of familiar, everyday questions, such as "What is your name?", "How old are you?", and "What color are your shoes?" Berliner and Eisenberg (1987) reported that these stimuli are being used in a live-voice, open-set auditory-only format to evaluate 3M/House children who are demonstrating open-set speech recognition. They provided results for 10 children tested on the GASP word items, 9 of whom obtained some word recognition, and for 19 children tested on the questions, 10 of whom showed some sentence comprehension. It is not stated whether these were independent subject groups or whether the 10 children tested on words were among the 19 tested on question comprehension. In addition, Berliner and Eisenberg (1987) presented results for one postlingually deafened adolescent whose 3-year postimplant scores on open-set tests of the Minimal Auditory Capabilities (MAC) Battery (Owens et al. 1985) and on tracking (DeFilippo & Scott, 1978) were similar to those of postlingually deafened adults with multichannel implants (see Chapter 3).

Berliner and Eisenberg (1987) have also identified characteristics among those children achieving auditory-only speech recognition. Comparing patient data for the 10 children who attained some comprehension of the GASP questions with the 9 that did not, they noted that age at onset of deafness and duration of implant use may be variables that affect performance. The 10 children who achieved some sentence recognition had a mean age at onset of 3 years 11 months and a mean duration of implant use of 2 years 5 months. In contrast, the 9 children unable to achieve sentence recognition had a mean age at onset of deafness of 2 years 2 months, with a mean duration of implant use of 1 year 7 months. All the children who achieved some open-set recognition had acquired deafness as the result of meningitis.

Results for 3M/House children on the GASP recognition tasks have been recently updated by Tonokawa and Dye (1987). Of 49 children tested on word items, 24 achieved some open-set recognition with a mean of 30.5 percent and a range of 8.3 to 75 percent. Of 41 children tested on the GASP questions, 15 obtained some open-set understanding, with a mean of 29.3 percent and a range of 10 to 100 percent. In contrast to conventional practice, the means for the total group tested were not reported. Twenty-five children failed to achieve open-set understanding of words, resulting in a mean for the total patient sample of approximately 15 percent; 26 children were unable to recognize the GASP questions, yielding a mean for the total patient sample of about 11 percent. Again, information concerning the total number of children tested and the total number obtaining some open-set speech recognition was not provided; that is, whether the 15 children achieving question comprehension were among the 24 demonstrating word understanding was not specified.

Tonokawa and Dye (1987) reported that most of the children showing some open-set speech understanding have acquired deafness and are in educational settings that emphasize auditory training. In contrast to a previous suggestion of Berliner and Eisenberg (1987), data analyses for these children indicated that age at onset of deafness does not appear to be a factor in high performance. Rather, the length of auditory deprivation prior to implantation, as previously suggested by Thielemeir and colleagues (1985), and the length of time of device use, also suggested by Berliner and Eisenberg (1987), do appear to affect performance. Johnson (1987a) asserts that duration of deprivation, mode of communication, and age at onset of deafness are all factors in high performance. She noted that those children obtaining open-set speech recognition have been deaf for shorter periods of time, are oral rather than manual, and were deafened later in life.

SPEECH/LANGUAGE PERFORMANCE

The following three areas of speech and language performance are evaluated in 3M/House children (Kirk & Hill–Brown, 1985): speech production, language reception, and language expression. A battery of tests is applied in each of these areas, using the communication mode (manual, spoken, total) that the child customarily uses at home and at school.

SPEECH PRODUCTION. Speech production is evaluated using the Ling Phonetic and Phonologic Speech Evaluations (Ling, 1976). The Phonetic Level tests the child's imitative responses and the Phonologic Level analyzes spontaneous production. Each Level is concerned with both the nonsegmental (prosodic) and the segmental (phonemes) aspects of speech. At the Phonetic Level, the nonsegmental and segmental features are tested in increasingly complex phonetic environments. At the Phonologic Level, a spontaneous speech sample is analyzed. For purposes of the implant evaluation, responses are quantified by assigning a numerical value to each type of response depending upon the phonetic environment (Kirk & Hill–Brown, 1985). Apparently, no measures of overall speech intelligibility are administered.

Kirk and Hill–Brown (1985) reported that, as of July 1984, pre- and postimplant data had been collected on 78 children. Paired comparisons of the children's performance preoperatively and postoperatively showed significant improvements in both imitative and spontaneous speech production abilities. Relative to the preoperative imitative performance for 78 children, improvement was observed in the ability of 42 children to produce the nonsegmentals, vowels, diphthongs, and simple consonants at the 6-month postoperative evaluations. These improvements were maintained at the 1-year evaluation for 24 children. The imitative skills of the children were analyzed according to the following age categories: 2 to 5 years, 6 to 12 years, and 13 to 18 years. It was found that the greatest number of improvements at the 6-month postimplant interval were made by the children in the youngest age group, 2 to 5 years. Children in the 13- to 18-year old category, on the other hand, displayed some decrements in performance. Additional analysis revealed that children trained orally had better imitative production skills than those in total communication programs. This was attributed to a later mean age at onset of deafness for the orally trained children. Generally, children in total communication programs made a greater number of improvements than did orally trained children, although the oral children began at a higher level and retained higher absolute scores.

Kirk and Hill–Brown (1985) found similar postimplant improvements at the Phonologic (spontaneous) Level. Compared to preimplant results (N = 69), improvement was observed for the nonsegmentals and the segmental production of vowels, diphthongs and simple consonants at the 6-month test interval (N = 40). Improvements continued in these areas at the 1-year evaluation (N = 24). An analysis by age category again revealed that the youngest children showed the greatest number of gains.

In a recent report on speech production using paired comparisons of the Ling Evaluation Levels, Johnson (1987b) focused on children who had received their 30-month postoperative evaluation. The data indicated that for each area of phonetic and phonologic production postimplant scores were considerably improved over preimplant results. Recalling the order of normal speech acquisition, Johnson asserted that the implanted children were progressing and mastering specific articulations in the same order of development as would normal hearing children. As with speech reception, an analysis of covariance was performed to investigate the contributions of factors to changes in speech production for children who had used the implant for at least 30 months. This study indicated that duration of implant use has the highest association with gains in speech production scores, showing greater influence than such variables as age of onset of deafness, duration of deafness, and communication mode.

Because improvements in the production of speech sounds were observed so rapidly following implantation (i.e., at the 6-month test interval), Kirk and Hill–Brown (1985) suggested that improvements were most likely due to the implant. However, they acknowledged that it is impossible to determine definitively whether such changes are a direct result of the implant as opposed to maturation or rehabilitative intervention. In an effort to control for maturation, they developed an experimental control group among prospective implant candidates whose preimplant scores were age-matched and compared to results for implanted children. The abilities of this control group, who meet audiological and other criteria for implantation, are assumed to represent the skill levels that would have been attained by the implanted children. Both the control and implanted groups were divided into three age categories, and the implanted children were further divided according to duration of implant use. Six postimplant groups emerged who were compared to the control groups in four areas of speech production (both the phonetic and phonologic nonsegmentals and segmentals) for a total of 24 contrasts. The implanted children scored higher than their age-matched nonimplanted peers in all but one of these contrasts.

Using the same experimental design for comparing age-matched unimplanted and implanted children, Hill–Brown (1987) has more recently divided children into four age categories (four-, five-, six- and seven-year-olds) and three categories of implant use (zero or the unimplanted controls, less than 2 years of stimulation, and more than 2 years of stimulation). The means for the implanted children were higher than those of the age-matched controls for all phonetic and phonologic speech scores. Statistical analysis revealed a significant effect for length of device use. It was also demonstrated that, among implanted 5- to 6-year-olds on the spontaneous (phonologic) nonsegmentals, scores were better for children with more than 2 years of stimulation than for their age-matched peers with less than 2 years of implant use.

LANGUAGE RECEPTION/EXPRESSION. For the measurement of language reception of children wearing the 3M/House implant, the following instruments are used (Kirk & Hill–Brown, 1985): the Peabody Picture Vocabulary Test (PPVT) (Dunn, 1965), which measures vocabulary recognition age; the Test for Auditory Comprehension of Language (Carrow, 1973), which measures morphological constructions, grammatical categories, and syntactic structures; the SKI*HI Language Development Scale (Tonelson & Watkins, 1979), which assesses both receptive and expressive language skills of children from birth to 5 years, according to parental ratings of the child's skill level; and, the Grammatical Analysis of Elicited Language — Pre-Sentence Level (GAEL-P) (Moog & Geers, 1983), which evaluates both reception and expression for children who are neither understanding nor producing sentences. Expressive language is evaluated with both the SKI*HI and the GAEL-P as well as either the Grammatical Analysis of Elicited Language — Simple Sentence Level (GAEL-S) (Moog & Geers, 1979) or the Grammatical Analysis of Elicited Language — Complex Sentence Level (GAEL-C) (Moog & Geers, 1980), which each elicit specific language structures that may not occur in a spontaneous language sample.

Unfortunately, the postimplant data available on language expression and reception is very limited. Kirk and Hill–Brown (1985) reported that marked delays, as a result of profound hearing impairment, were seen in both receptive and expressive language skills at each test interval. On three of the four receptive measures, improvements were observed relative to preoperative results, although sample size was very small. The mean 6-month postimplant scores for the SKI*HI (N = 8) and the PPVT (N = 11) indicated a growth in receptive language equal to or greater than the chronological time period; the same observations on the SKI*HI (N = 3) and the PPVT (N = 6) were made at the 1-year postimplant test interval. However, relative to preimplant results, a statistically significant decrease in performance was noted on the Test for Auditory Comprehension of Language at the 1-year evaluation (N = 7). On expressive language measures, Kirk and Hill–Brown (1985) reported that only one test, the parent rating scale or the SKI*HI, showed significant improvement (N = 9) at the 6-month postimplant test date.

A pre- and postimplant comparison of language results for six children was recently reported by Robbins and Miyamoto (1987). Dividing the children into two groups of three each, those implanted before the age of 10 and those implanted after 10 years, they observed that the younger age group achieved higher language quotients on all tests and seem to be rapidly approaching their chronological age in terms of language acquisition. They concluded that age at onset of deafness and duration of hearing loss are important factors in attaining age-appropriate language skills, while communication mode in and of itself is not a predictor of success.

PSYCHOLOGICAL STATUS

According to Tiber (1985), a preoperative family interview is conducted in which parent–child interactions are observed. Parents are required to complete both a Cochlear Implant Questionnaire, which explores their expectations and understanding of the implant, and a Child Behavior Rating Scale (Cassel, 1962), in which the parent rates the child's adjustment at home, school, and socially. Children are administered the nonverbal performance scale from one of several standardized intelligence tests. The choice of test is dependent on the age of the child. In addition to intelligence, neuropsychological function is assessed with the Halstead–Reitan Test of Lateral Dominance (Reitan & Davison, 1974) and the Bender–Gestalt (Bender, 1938), and academic achievement is evaluated using the Wide Range Achievement Test (WRAT) (Jastak & Jastak, 1978). These same tests are administered postoperatively in order to monitor the psychological effects of implantation.

According to Tiber (1985), the cochlear implant had no negative effects on the children and, based on 6-month followup data, they continued to function well. Preoperatively, 86 children were tested. The mean age of the children was 8 years and they were evenly distributed by sex. As a group, intelligence testing placed them at the upper end of the average range with a mean performance IQ of 109. The majority of the children (52) were tested on the Wechsler Intelligence Scale for Children-Revised, geared for ages 6½ to 16½. Of these 52 children, pre-and postoperative comparisons were reported for 19 subjects. The mean preoperative IQ for these 19 children was 106, whereas the mean 6-month postimplant IQ was 115. Tiber asserted that improvement is not the result of test practice effect because of the selective nature of the subtests on which the children improved; rather, he attributed this improvement to increased attention span and a reduction in distractibility observed in many of the implanted children.

Pre- and postimplant Bender data were reported for 22 children (Tiber, 1985). Preoperatively, these 22 children showed a lag of 2 years 2 months; postoperatively, no lag in perceptual motor function was seen. According to Tiber, this growth is much greater than can be expected from a 6-month period of maturation, and, again, he attributed this change to longer attention spans and decreased distractibility. Behaviorally, based on the Child Behavior Rating Scale, pre- and postimplant comparisons indicated that there were no significant changes in the parents' ratings of their children's general adjustment following implantation.

EDUCATION AND REHABILITATION

As previously noted, children return to their regular educational settings following implantation. The majority of children implanted at HEI are enrolled in self-contained classes that use total communication (Selmi, 1985). Preoperatively, as part of the selection process, the child's educational records, and history of hearing aid use and auditory training are reviewed. An educator for the deaf meets with parents and discusses educational needs and goals. Six weeks prior to each followup evaluation, classroom teachers are sent the Teacher Evaluation Form, in which they are asked to rate the child's auditory responses in the classroom. A rating scale of *always/almost always* (assigned 3 points), *sometimes* (2 points), and *seldom/never* (1 point) is used. Mean ratings for a sample of 41 to 50 children revealed that on 12 "awareness to sound" tasks ratings ranged from 1.2 to 2.7, and on seven tasks labeled "discriminates between suprasegmental features," ratings ranged from 1.4 to 2.3. The majority of teachers rated the implanted children as *seldom/never* on the comprehension of single words or short phrases and on the comprehension of details in sentences. Unfortunately, preoperative data on the same rating scale is not provided. Furthermore, the conditions under which ratings are taken is not specified; that is, it is unknown whether teachers make judgements based on responses in auditory-only situations or on responses in auditory plus vision conditions.

Citing research that indicates a direct correlation between hearing loss and educational options, Selmi (1985) states that the severity of the loss often determines the child's communication mode and that those with profound loss are usually limited to total communication programs at schools for the deaf. She reported that use of the cochlear implant in a program offering good auditory rehabilitation may affect educational placement. Over a period of 4 years, 14 children implanted with the 3M/House device (presumably from a total of 98 seen at HEI) changed educational settings. Generally, these children shifted from total programs to oral/aural classrooms; some changed from self-contained classrooms to mainstreamed programs.

Controlled studies on the effects of rehabilitation with 3M/House implant children and investigations comparing the efficacy of specific methodologies and training strategies are not available. As described by Eisenberg (1985), Basic Guidance is "analogous to an extended hearing aid fitting program," rather than an intensive program of auditory/verbal therapy. In discussing treatment, Tyler, Davis, and Lansing (1987) reported that there is a complete absence of information on the efficacy of rehabilitative attempts with implanted children. They noted that one of two approaches is possible: to view the implant as simply another form of amplification and to continue with procedures used in the past with deaf children; or, to consider the elecrical signal as unique and to develop programs based on the particular signal being transmitted to the child. They prefer the latter approach, stating that training activities must consider the speech processing characteristics of the particular implant used by the individual child.

It has been consistently reiterated by 3M/House associates (Eisenberg, 1985; Eisenberg et al., 1986b; Johnson, 1987a; Selmi, 1985; Thielemeir et al., 1985) that those children involved in auditory/verbal training and educational programs emphasizing the development of oral/aural skills appear to achieve higher levels of performance with the implant. Furthermore, Eisenberg (1985) asserts that the 3M/House children are not meeting their potential: "It is felt that as a group they could do better than they are presently doing, and that [auditory] training is the critical factor toward optimized implant performance" (p. 61S). As a result of these observations, Eisenberg (1985) advocates specific rehabilitation strategies for incorporation into an extended training program. Despite encouraging strong auditory/verbal training, she states that methods for providing acoustic information to the child must be adapted to the child's educational setting and mode of communication. Regardless of modality, the goal of training is always "the enhancement of aural/verbal communication skills by effectively increasing reliance on auditory cues" (p. 68S). Followup reports on the implementation of such an extended 3M/House training program and its efficacy are not available.

INTERPRETATION OF 3M/HOUSE DATA

As indicated throughout the discussion of patient results, difficulty in interpreting the 3M/House implant data occurs because the means reported for preoperative and postoperative comparisons of both auditory reception and speech and language tasks differ in sample size. This problem is noted by Tyler, Davis, and Lansing (1987) and discussed at some length by Geers and Moog (1986). In addition, Geers and Moog (1986) pointed out that tests for statistical significance were conducted by paired comparisons of still different numbers of subjects than those for whom performance means are provided.

In response to the 1985 House Ear Institute monograph (Berliner, Eisenberg, & House), problems that prevent a clear-cut determination of the degree of benefit provided by the implant were itemized by Geers and Moog (1986). Among the most prominent of these is the failure to report results of the child's overall binaural auditory functioning. This concern was also expressed by Owens (1986), who, in addition, had reservations about the restrictions on gain and MPO placed by HEI on the hearing aids used for preoperative evaluation. Although it was reported (Thielemeir et al., 1985) that the majority of children (87 percent at the

House Ear Institute) use an aid in their unimplanted ear and that the ear with the poorest aided performance is selected for implantation, 3M/House results are presented for the implanted ear alone. Geers and Moog recall a basic fact of auditory functioning: the handicap associated with auditory deficits is largely dependent on the auditory capabilities of the better ear. This fundamental tenet of auditory behavior is the basis for a single case study conducted by Popelka and Gittelman (1984). Their subject was an 8-year-old boy who had acquired hearing loss at 3 years 7 months as a result of meningitis. He had been fit with a hearing aid shortly after his illness and was wearing binaural aids by the age of 5 years. Tests of auditory perception were conducted prior to and 1 month and 6 months after he received a 3M/House implant. Results for nine tests indicated that, relative to preoperative aided performance on the implanted ear, cochlear implant performance was poorer for four tests, better for three tests, and showed no change on two tests; monaural aided tests on the better (unimplanted) ear showed that six of seven tests were superior with conventional amplification in this ear than with the implanted ear; of six tests administered binaurally, three showed an increase in performance and three showed a decrease in performance relative to the aided better ear. Popelka and Gittelman (1984) concluded that performance of the implanted ear was inferior to performance of the aided opposite ear. Further, because binaural scores increased on some tasks and decreased on others, binaural results were equivocal as whether the implant enhanced or interfered with functioning of the unimplanted aided ear.

Geers and Moog (1986) noted that, generally, results would have greater validity if binaural comparisons were made both preoperatively and postoperatively and if preimplant results were compared with postimplant results in both the device on and device off conditions (with an aid in the unimplanted ear). In response, Berliner, Eisenberg, and House (1986) asserted that there is a misunderstanding regarding the amount of residual hearing in the contralateral ear. Losses in the opposite ear, they stated, are very profound and receive only minimal, if any, benefit with even the most powerful aids.

More recently, a study (Bell & Tonokawa, 1987) of 31 subjects comparing implant and aided performance indicated that, for the implant ear, there was a statistically significant improvement from aided preimplant results to postimplant scores on all auditory measures. On the DAT, all 31 children showed improvement with the implant relative to aided preimplant results; with the nonimplant (aided) ear, only 11 showed improvement and 7 decreased in scores. On the TAC, 24 of 31 subjects showed improvement with the implant over aided results in the implant ear, while only two improved relative to performance with their hearing aid in the opposite ear. Because training and maturation was the same for both ears, Bell and Tonokawa (1987) concluded that the implant provides benefit greater than what might have been anticipated with a hearing aid. This study, as with Berliner and Eisenberg's (1987) examination of DAT aided performance on the unimplanted ear, failed to evaluate binaural function.

In regard to speech production, Geers and Moog (1986) noted that the effects of training were not effectively separated from the effects of the implant itself. They state that Kirk and Hill–Brown's (1985) study was marred because the implant children had received Basic Guidance whereas the control group had not. Tyler, Davis, and Lansing (1987) pointed out that the control group was matched for age only. Furthermore, Geers and Moog remarked that statistically significant gains in speech production were observed only for the 2- to 5-year old group where progress in response to training is most likely to occur in any event. In contrast, significant improvement was not observed in the nonsegmental skills of the oral group who had presumably already acquired these skills. Berliner, Eisenberg, and House (1986), dismissing Basic Guidance, responded that training was not controlled because it was not considered influential; the implant children were provided with no special training and returned to their prior educational settings.

Considering language growth, Geers and Moog believe that measurements of benefit provided by the implant do not separate changes in sign language proficiency from an increase in spoken language acquisition as a result of the implant. Because tests are administered in the communication mode customarily used by the child, most children are tested with total communication. Significant improvements on the PPVT (Kirk & Hill–Brown, 1985), for example, may be measuring increases in sign acquisition rather than increased comprehension of spoken language. Berliner, Eisenberg, and House (1986) responded that the PPVT is always administered with speech rather than sign, thus contradicting the report of Kirk and Hill–Brown (1985).

In summary, Geers and Moog (1986) suggested that the House Ear Institute studies would be strengthened by reporting results for the same subjects both pre- and postoperatively. Because most children continue to wear a hearing aid in the unimplanted ear, auditory speech perception should be evaluated and compared in several conditions: with the hearing aid alone in the unimplanted ear, with the implant alone, and, finally, in the binaural condition with both implant and hearing aid (see also Chapter 11). In regard to the development of speech production and oral language acquisiton, Tyler, Davis, and Lansing (1987) and Geers and Moog (1986) reached the same conclusion: namely, because many of the implanted children had well-developed skills before losing their hearing, because some use sign and others do not, and because some continued to use hearing aids in conjunction with the implant, the contribution of the implant to development in these areas cannot be determined without the use of matched control groups.

MULTICHANNEL STIMULATION

THE NUCLEUS 22-ELECTRODE IMPLANT

The Nucleus device was developed in Australia at the University of Melbourne under the direction of Graeme M. Clark (Clark, 1986; Clark et al., 1983; Tong et al., 1982; 1983) and is distributed in the U.S. by Cochlear Corporation of Nucleus. The electrode, which may be inserted 25 mm into the scala tympani, consists of 22 platinum–iridium circumferential bands around a tapered Silastic® carrier. Bipolar stimulation occurs between adjacent bands or between alternating bands. The receiver, housed in a hermetically sealed titanium capsule, is built around a custom microprocessor chip which digitally selects the level and rate of stimulation and the electrode pair to which the signal is passed. Stimulation occurs in biphasic charge-balanced pulses and is nonsimultaneous, sequentially exciting different electrode pairs with differently processed signals.

The speech processing strategy of the Nucleus system is designed to transmit specific speech features: fundamental frequency is coded by the rate of stimulation pulses, first and second formant by electrode position, and signal intensity by the amplitude of the pulses. This information is then referred to the digital memory of the speech processor where the appropriate electrode, current amplitude, and stimulus rates are assigned. These assignments, based on psychophysical data concerning thresholds, comfort and discomfort levels, and pitch scaling, are obtained during the early stages of device fitting with a computer programming unit. Until recently, the processor was limited to the transmission of the fundamental frequency and second formant information (the $f0/f2$ device). Currently, the Nucleus system has added the first formant to its coding scheme (the $f0/f1/f2$ processor) (Dowell et al., 1987; Millar et al., 1987).

Both Moore (1985) and Pfingst (1986) have referred to this form of speech processing as the feature extraction approach. In this strategy, only those patterns or features of speech considered most salient for normal adult speech perception are transmitted, the rest of the acoustic signal being discarded. This method of coding assumes that certain linguistic aspects of the acoustic signal are sufficient for identification of the whole signal and that, when presented in isolation, identification is easier than if the entire signal were transmitted.

The decision to proceed with the implantation of children was, as with the 3M/House device, based on favorable results obtained with adult postlingual patients (Mecklenburg, 1987). In developing a children's program, certain physical aspects of the device were modified to accommodate the special characteristics of children (Clark et al., 1987a; Mecklenburg, 1987). In order to create a smaller device, the height of the internal receiver capsule was reduced from 10 mm to 6 mm, although the length of the total implant was thereby slightly increased. In addition, as with the 3M/House device, magnets were incorporated into the receiver and the external transmitter, providing an easy mechanism by which to hold and align the external transmitter in place (Clark et al., 1987a). Finally, in developing a smaller system, the connector or surgical disconnect was discarded (Clark et al., 1987a; see Chapter 8 for a discussion of this issue). Clark and associates explained that this decision was based on three factors: (1) although unlikely, failures could occur in the connector and electrode array as well as in the receiver; (2) animal studies have demonstrated that the Nucleus electrode could be explanted and reimplanted without trauma; and (3) clinical studies have demonstrated that explantation and reimplantation did not result in decrements in performance. For these reasons and for purposes of creating a smaller system, the need for retaining ready access to the receiver/stimulator without disturbing the intracochlear electrode did not seem justified. The processing strategy and the 22-banded electrode array used in the *mini-unit* are identical to those of the larger adult version. Figure 10–2 shows both the internal and external components of the *mini* Nucleus 22-electrode device.

PREOPERATIVE AND POSTOPERATIVE EVALUATION PROCEDURES

PATIENT SELECTION

A Nucleus children's program has been initiated both in Australia and the United States. From published accounts, it is not possible to discern whether a single protocol exists that applies to all children implanted with the Nucleus device regardless of their geographic location. It is known, however, that the same regulatory control exerted in the United States is not applicable in Australia. For purposes of discussion, except where specifically noted, it will be assumed that a single pre- and postoperative protocol is used.

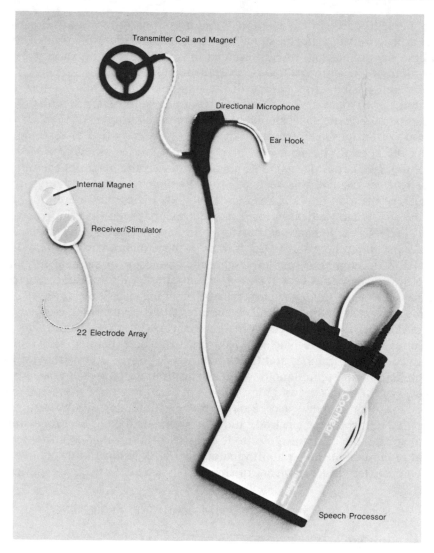

FIGURE 10–2. Both the internal and external components of the Nucleus *mini* 22-electrode implant. Courtesy of Cochlear Corporation.

In the United States, two childrens' programs, each administered under a separate IDE, are in progress with the Nucleus implant (Mecklenburg, 1987). One concerns children aged 10 through 17 years, and the other involves children from 2 to 10 years. According to published accounts (Clark et al., 1987a), the youngest age at which the Australian program considered children was 4 years. Specific factors pertinent to children younger than 4 were thus avoided. For example, in children 4 years and older, hearing thresholds can be accurately assessed using conventional methods, increases in the skull are less than at a younger age, and middle ear infection is less frequent. More recently, however, after a consideration of recent evidence on the age and rate of head growth, the Australian group has successfully implanted a child of 2 years 5 months (D. Mecklenburg, personal communication, June 1988). In contrast, the American program has always considered children from ages 2 to 4 "under special consideration" (Mecklenburg, 1987), although these considerations are not specified.

Until recently, the selection criteria for each of these age groups differed in some regards (Mecklenburg, 1987). The protocol for the younger children did not distinguish between pre- and postlingual deafness. This is consistent with a current awareness of the difficulty in classifying young deaf children on the basis of pre- or postlingual loss (Mecklenburg, 1987). Although 2 years of age is the conventional cut-off in defining pre- and postlingual (Northern et al., 1986), some children deafened in the later preschool years might be considered functionally prelingual, particularly if they have experienced a long period of auditory deprivation following the onset of deafness. HEI had made a similar observation and is in agreement with this point (Eisenberg et al., 1986b). Mecklenburg (1987) has suggested the term *perilingual* to define children who have had hearing and some level of spoken language, but at the time of implant exhibit spoken language skills consisting of utterances of less than three words. In contrast, for the 10- to 17-year olds, only postlingually deafened youngsters were considered eligible for implantation. Alternatively, children in this age range who had exposure to auditory stimulation for at least 1 year in conjunction with an oral education program and auditory training are considered eligible. This option allowed children with a single-channel implant to be converted to a multichannel system (Mecklenburg, 1987). Since the formulation of the original protocol, however, the selection criteria for the older children have been expanded to include prelinguals as well (D. Mecklenburg, personal communication, June 1988).

The remaining selection criteria are similar to those for the 3M/ House device and implant programs generally. Children of both age groups must have profound or total bilateral sensorineural hearing loss. Evaluation consists of audiologic, medical, radiographic, and psychological assessments. For older children, preoperative electrical stimulation of the promontory, when possible to administer, should reveal consistent, positive results. Psychologically, older children are expected to be motivationally suitable; for younger children, families must demonstrate realistic expectations and a willingness to cooperate in pre- and postoperative training and assessment programs. Mecklenburg (1987) states that the goal of both sets of selection criteria is to provide a means of selecting children who will be optimal candidates. She outlines three factors considered important in predicting success with the implant: age at onset of profound deafness, duration of deafness, and type of educational program. The most promising candidates are considered to be those with deafness of short duration, those with a memory for spoken language, and those being educated in an oral/aural program.

Preoperatively, the primary consideration is the audiological assessment of the child and a determination of benefit provided by other sensory aids. Clark and colleagues (1987a) reported that children evaluated for the implant undergo a 6-month trial period with either a hearing aid or a tactile device. Busby and associates (1987) defined an extensive series of audiologic evaluations administered to prospective candidates, including both behavioral and objective measures of degree of hearing loss, speech perception studies, and psychophysical evaluation. If satisfactory progress with an aid or tactile device has not been made after the trial period, the child is accepted for the implant procedure (Clark et al., 1987b). Although speech production and communication skills are also assessed preoperatively, Mecklenburg (1987) reported that this is in order to gather baseline information. Changes in speech production and language competency are considered a "secondary benefit" of the implant (Mecklenburg, 1987; Mecklenburg et al., 1988); because the young child is constantly changing regardless of intervention, any changes that may occur in areas other than auditory perception cannot be attributed solely to the implant.

POSTOPERATIVE EVALUATION

As with the 3M/House program, investigations of the Nucleus device in children employ a "single-subject time-series" experimental design (Nienhuys et al., 1987; Mecklenburg et al., 1988). That is, the subject serves as his or her own control and test measures are repeated pre-and postoperatively. Nienhuys and associates (1987) asserted that previous studies with children have been unsatisfactory and have failed to provide evidence of benefit from implants because the children have lacked adequate preoperative assessments and educational evaluations. Postoperatively, long-term rehabilitation and training effects have not been taken into account. In contrast to Mecklenburg (1987), Nienhuys and colleagues apparently believe that these variables can be controlled. To establish a baseline of behavior, repeated behavioral observations are made in the preimplant period. Multiple observations are made postoperatively so that changes can be identified. In order to explore the full potential of the device, both analytic and global skills are evaluated. Following implantation, an ongoing diagnostic teaching approach is used by an educator or therapist who is part of the implant team. The first postoperative evaluation is administered 3 months after implantation and at 6-month intervals thereafter (Clark et al., 1987a).

The Nucleus protocol requires assessment in three areas: speech reception, speech production, and receptive and expressive language and communication (Mecklenburg, 1987; Nienhuys et al., 1987). Extensive test batteries (Clark et al.,1987a, 1987b; Nienhuys et al., 1987) are administered in each of these areas. The choice of test is dependent on the age and language abilities of the child. In the area of speech perception, each test is administered in the auditory-only, auditory-plus-vision, and vision-only conditions. The following aspects of speech perception are evaluated: segmental identification and speech feature analysis, suprasegmental discriminations, closed-set word identification, open-set word and sentence recognition. The evaluation of speech production includes both segmental and suprasegmental production, word production, speech intelligibility, and process analysis of a spontaneous speech sample. Language evaluation includes an assessment of the child's receptive and expressive skills and global communication ability, using formal tests of syntax and semantics, descriptive analyses of language samples, and analyses of interactional conversational samples.

SUBJECTS

As of May 1988, 83 children at 24 co-investigating centers in the United States had received the Nucleus 22-electrode system (Mecklenburg et al., 1988). The mean age for these children at time of implantation was 8 years 8 months. Fifty of these 83 children are included in the younger protocol, ranging in age from 2 years 5 months through 9 years 1 month, with a mean age of 6 years 3 months. The mean duration of deafness for the younger children was 4 years 4 months. Thirty-three of the 83 children are older, ranging in age from 10 through 16 years, with a mean of 13 years 9 months. The average duration of deafness experienced by the older children was 10 years 1 month. For the total group, the average length of deafness prior to implantation was 6 years 7 months. Most of the children are either congenitally deaf or were deafened under the age of 2 years, with 64 percent of the total population considered prelingual. The most common eitology among these children is meningitis, representing 51 percent of the total sample. According to Mecklenburg and associates (1988), cochlear ossification as a result of meningitis has not prevented the insertion of the long intracochlear Nucleus electrode. The mean distance of insertion into the scala tympani for the meningitis group is 20 mm, with only four of these children having less than 15 electrodes inserted.

There have been no internal device failures among these 83 children, and only a few medical or device complications have been reported (Mecklenburg et al., 1988). One child failed to stimulate as a result of inappropriate placement of the electrode during insertion. This device was subsequently removed and a new one was successfully reinserted. Two instances of incision (flap) complications occurred, requiring extended healing periods. Both problems were successfully resolved. In nine cases, children experienced transient loud sounds which were eliminated through processor reprogramming or replacement of external hardware. Incidents of otitis media, unassociated with the implant, did not result in complications.

According to Mecklenburg and colleagues (1988), all speech processors for these 83 children have been successfully programmed. Special techniques and materials, designed to teach the perceptual concepts of sound detection, loudness scaling, and loudness balancing, have been developed for purposes of device fitting, with initial device adjustment requiring from 3 to 7 days. Because of the complexity of the Nucleus system and its multichannel features, specific methods of device adjustment, especially for very young children, are of particular interest and concern. (See Chapter 8 for a discussion of this issue.) This device fitting process has been described in a recent presentation by Mecklenburg (1988). The two critical elements in device programming are the determination of the threshold and the maximum comfortable loudness level on each electrode. With these two measurements, an effective electrical dynamic range can be applied. In order to attain these measures, a pre-device fitting training program is provided in which the child is familiarized with the test situation and the tasks involved. Ideally, this training occurs after surgery but prior to the first fitting session. In addition, efforts are made to allow newly implanted children to observe another implant recipient in the device fitting process.

Training consists of establishing a clear response pattern to visual and tactile stimulation. Using a variety of materials, the concepts of *on-off, same-different, high-low,* and loudness scaling are taught. According to Mecklenburg (1988), threshold has been relatively easy to determine, but maximum comfortable loudness has proved more difficult. Using either a 10-point loudness scale or *progressive illustrations* of listening attitudes depicting appropriate gestures and facial expressions, this process is confounded by the small dynamic range and rapid growth in loudness that often characterizes electrical stimulation. In order to establish loudness balancing between electrodes, the concept of *same-different* is a prerequisite. Lacking this concept, the clinician must establish equalization based on extrapolations from previous experience. For pitch scaling, the child should be able to identify high-low differences. Without this ability, normal pitch order is simply assumed. Once all of the information has been obtained, the frequency boundaries for each of the electrodes are assigned. A quick check of the device is then performed through informal live-voice testing.

Although the functioning of each electrode is established during the initial fitting sessions by simply checking for the presence or absence of a sensation, the primary goal, according to Mecklenburg (1988), is to provide the child with a comfortable, working device as rapidly as possible. To this end, each of the electrodes need not be programmed during the early sessions. Gradually, over time, more electrodes are brought into use as appropriate psychophysical measurements are obtained. All but 3 children are reported to be full-time users of the device (Mecklenburg et al., 1988). Because 33 of these are teenagers, this report is in sharp contrast to the 3M/House experience. The device is said to be worn on an average of 10.5 hours per day, although methods for obtaining average daily usage are not given.

RESULTS

Since May 1988, only 4 percent of the children implanted with the Nucleus device had received evaluations beyond the 6-month time period. However, preliminary group data is reported for 36 children who have received their 6-month postoperative evaluations (Mecklenburg et al., 1988). Demographic characteristics of this group are considered representative of the total population. The average number of electrodes programmed and in use by these 36 children at 3 months postimplant is 17, with the younger children averaging 14. Because of differences in age and language abilities, not all children receive each test. Postoperative implant-only comparisions are made with the child's best preoperative aided performance, regardless of whether this condition was monaural, binaural, or tactile.

The test most frequently administered was the DAT. Of those children with preoperative comparative results, 58 percent attained postoperative improvement of 3 or more DAT levels. Among the 58 percent demonstrating improvement, 29 percent were congenitally deaf. Pre- and postoperative results for 26 children show that 4 had equivalent postoperative scores, 2 had poorer postimplant results, and 20 (77 percent) improved by one or more levels from their preoperative performance. Applying the perceptual categories developed by Geers and Moog (Chapter 11), 62 percent of these 26 children changed one or more categories, 35 percent achieved category 3, and 19 percent attained category 4. Four congenitally deaf children were among those who moved into categories 3 or 4.

A series of tape recorded tests is also administered to the children, although it is noted (Mecklenburg et al., 1988) that their performance is consistently poorer on recorded materials compared to live-voice presentations. Moreover, although several of the MAC (Owens et al., 1985) closed-set prosody and phoneme or word discrimination tests have been administered, these tests are considered inappropriate for young children and most of the reported results were obtained from teenagers. On the MAC Noise/Voice test, for example, 46 percent of those tested significantly improved relative to preoperative results. On prosodic tests, such as the MAC Spondee Same/Different, 40 percent demonstrated improvement. Taped tests of open-set speech recognition are also administered. As with adult implant patients, the most difficult items are the monosyllabic NU6 words, with only one child showing improvement. However, 45 percent showed significant changes with phoneme-scored NU6 words. On CID sentences, 29 percent of those tested improved significantly.

In summary, more than half of the children tested on both live-voice and taped closed-set materials demonstrated significant postoperative improvements. Among those showing such improvement, 22 percent were congenital. Thirty-five percent of the children who were administered open-set tests improved on one or more measures of auditory-only speech recognition. Congenitals are conspicuously absent from this group, and only children who were postlingually deafened are among the 35 percent who attained open-set speech understanding.

Individual case studies of children with the Nucleus implant have also been reported. Mecklenburg and colleagues (1987) presented four children who have experienced their device for 12 months or more. Two of these children were implanted in Australia and two in the United States. These four subjects have been the focus of several papers (Clark et al., 1987a, 1987b; Mecklenburg, 1987). One child, who became deaf at 3 years of age as a result of meningitis, received the new *mini* implant at age 5. Preoperatively, this child used binaural hearing aids, had a trial with a tactile device, and was enrolled in a cued speech program (Clark et al., 1987a, 1987b). In preparation for setting thresholds, comfort levels, and discomfort levels of the individual electrodes in the Nucleus electrode array, he was preoperatively conditioned in scaling the intensity of light and electrotactile stimulation using blocks of different sizes. Ac-

cording to Clark and colleagues (1987a, 1987b), this training proved successful in facilitating postoperative device adjustment. Preoperatively
(Mecklenburg et al., 1987), he received an age-equivalent score of 2 years
on the PPVT; at the 10-month postoperative test interval his receptive
language age-equivalent had increased to 4 years 3 months. On a closed-
set test of 12 words differing in syllable pattern and scored by both category of stress pattern and word identification, this child's categorization
skills were significantly above chance postoperatively and increased
from the initial postimplant test (3 months) to the 12-month test interval.

The second child considered by Mecklenburg and colleagues (1987)
received a *mini* device at 10 years of age. He had become deaf as a result
of meningitis at the age of 3½ years. According to Clark and colleagues
(1987a, 1987b), he used hearing aids after the onset of deafness and
entered a total communication program. Preoperatively, his speech intelligibility on the McGarr test (McGarr, 1983) was rated at 0 percent. With
speech training, his 6-month postimplant intelligibility score increased
to 47 percent. Clark and associates reported that he now attends a regular school. On the closed-set test of 12 words scored by category and
identification (Mecklenburg et al., 1987), his scores increased at all postimplant intervals on the identification task, improving from 17 percent
preimplant to 67 percent at 20 months postimplant. On a closed-set test
of vowel perception (11 vowels), his postoperative scores at the 7-month
test interval were 44 percent in the lipreading-alone condition and 65
percent for lipreading plus device. At 20 months postimplant, his lipreading-alone score had increased to 67 percent and the lipreading plus
device to 89 percent. Auditory-only results for vowel identification are
not reported. His ability to recognize keywords in sentences both visually and in the lipreading plus device condition is also reported to have
increased at all postimplant test periods.

Mecklenburg and associates (1987) next considered two adolescents
implanted in the United States. The first child received his Nucleus device at age 13 after experiencing progressive sensorineural loss since
early infancy. Mecklenburg (1987) reported that by 1 year of age his loss
was described as severe to profound and he was fit with binaural hearing
aids. The hearing loss continued to progress and, although he used an
aid in one ear for sound detection, he had experienced profound deafness for four years prior to implantation. Preoperatively, on seven closed-
set tests of the MAC battery, he received chance scores on each test.
Postoperatively, at the 12-month test interval, his scores were above
chance on all of the closed-set tests. On open-set tests of the MAC, he
uniformly scored 0 percent preoperatively; at 12-months postimplant, he
achieved some auditory-only understanding on tests of spondee recogni-

tion (about 50 percent), monosyllabic words (about 2 percent), and the CID Sentences (about 8 percent). A comparison of results at the 6- and 12-month test intervals demonstrates improvement over time.

The second teenager also experienced a progressive loss of hearing, initially noticed in one ear at 4 years of age (Mecklenburg, 1987). By age 10, he was fit with binaural aids. His loss continued to progress until 6½ months prior to implantation at which time he experienced total loss and was unable to use his hearing aids. He was implanted at age 15 and, according to Mecklenburg (1987), 3 days after being fit with his device, he was able to identify open-set words over the telephone when spoken by an unfamiliar speaker. On the MAC closed-set tests (Mecklenburg et al., 1987), his scores were well above chance at 12-months postimplant and were comparable to postlingual adult multichannel patients. On open-set tests of the MAC, he showed dramatic improvement relative to preimplant results, obtaining scores of 26 percent on monosyllabic words, 68 percent on spondee recognition, and approximately 60 percent on CID Sentences. A comparison of 6- and 12-month postimplant results shows improvement over time. This outstanding patient is also reported to achieve auditory-only tracking rates of 55 wpm.

Mecklenburg (1987) discussed the differences between these two teenagers at some length. While the second subject was very recently deafened prior to implantation, the first subject had sustained a severe or profound loss since early childhood and might more aptly be described as *perilingual*. According to Mecklenburg, this suggests that different learning rates might be observed relative to the duration of deafness and memory for speech. Moreover, children who are recently deafened appear to have the possibility of understanding ongoing speech without the aid of lipreading. Based on these two cases, Mecklenburg concludes that performance for the postlingual teenage population will not differ greatly from that of adult Nucleus patients.

In contrast to these adolescents, Clark and colleagues (1987b) present another teenager who obtained only minimal improvements with the implant. Deafened at 16 months of age from meningitis, this child had been fit with hearing aids and educated with cued speech. He received an implant at age 14 and had been using it regularly for 1-and-a-half years at the time of the report. With the implant, he was unable to obtain significant improvement on closed-set tests of vowel and consonant identification compared to the visual-only condition. On a prosodic speech perception task, a test of male and female discrimination, he was able to score well above chance, although preoperative data were not available for comparison. Accordingly, the implant appeared to offer him assistance in lipreading, with tracking rates improving from 25.4 wpm in the lipreading-only condition to 33 wpm in the lipreading plus device condition. This teenager, who had experienced prelingual deafness and long-standing auditory deprivation, appears to obtain benefits similar to those provided by a single-channel system.

Recently, Tonokawa, Berliner, and Dye (1987) have reported preliminary results for two children implanted at HEI with the Nucleus device. Both children were tested preoperatively with a tactile device and a hearing aid. Results for these children are particularly interesting because the subjects were tested with the same materials used to evaluate 3M/House patients. One child, who lost his hearing at 5 years 1 month of age as a result of meningitis, was implanted at 5 years 9 months. Nineteen of the 22 electrodes were inserted and 17 are in use. Results for only the initial evaluation at 3-months postimplant are available. On the DAT, preoperative scores with the tactile device were level 5 and with the hearing aid, level 1, whereas DAT level 12 was obtained with the implant. Word identification on the MTS with the tactile device was 1 of 24 words, with the hearing aid 2 of 24, and with the implant, 17 of 24. Categorization by stress pattern on the MTS was 10 of 24 for the tactile device, 12 of 24 with the hearing aid, and 21 of 24 with the implant. Postimplant open-set, auditory-only recognition was achieved using GASP stimuli, with a word recognition score of 5 out of 12 items and a sentence comprehension score of 1 out of 10. An auditory-only presentation of a PBK-50 (½) list resulted in 0 percent words correct and 18 percent phonemes correct. When presented in the device plus vision condition, results were 40 percent words correct and 71 percent phonemes correct.

The second child implanted at the HEI with the Nucleus device presents a very different history. She was a 9-year-old who became profoundly deaf at 8 months of age as a result of meningitis. She was fit with hearing aids at age 2 and received extensive training in an auditory program. Although all 22 electrodes were inserted, only 10 are in use. Tonokawa, Berliner, and Dye (1987) reported that initial stimulation and device setting were considerably more difficult with this prelingually deaf child who had experienced a long duration of deafness. Because she had not yet reached her 3-month postoperative evaluation period, only one pre- and postimplant comparison was available. Preoperatively, using a tactile device, she achieved level 6 on the DAT; with a hearing aid, she scored level 5; at 7 weeks postimplant, she obtained level 8 (although she was unable to pass levels 3 and 7).

SUMMARY AND CONCLUSION

The 3M/House single-channel implant appears to provide benefit to the majority of children who have received this device. For the most part, benefit is confined to the ability to make prosodic discriminations based on the timing and intensity information transmitted by the implant. That is, improvements are observed in the discrimination of speech patterns as determined on closed-set auditory-only tests, such as the DAT. Applying the categories of speech perception developed by Geers and Moog (Chapter 11), most 3M/House children achieve perceptual category 2, or speech pattern perception.

Among experts in the evaluation and training of auditory speech perception and production in deaf children, there appears to be some controversy regarding the contribution of speech perception abilities at this level to the development of spoken language (see Chapters 6, 11, and 12). Unfortunately, data on the contributions of the implant to the overall intelligibility of the child's speech are not provided, and the impact of reported improvements in the imitative and spontaneous production of suprasegmentals and segmentals is unknown. Lacking information on speech intelligibility, several questions remain unanswered: are vocalizations spontaneously increased; if so, are they intelligible to listeners inexperienced in listening to deaf speech; are they intelligible only to those familiar with the child? In short, the evidence regarding the acquisition or maintenance of intelligible, spontaneous speech among young 3M/House subjects is still unknown. However, no matter what levels of speech perception and production are attained by these children, it is apparent that they remain severely communicatively disabled and that the implant does not eliminate the need for special services and for consistent, ongoing training.

Another obvious lack in performance data concerns the enhancement of lipreading with the use of the 3M/House implant. In all of the many publications emerging from HEI, there is no information provided on the contribution of the implant to the lipreading ability of these children. Although difficult with those whose language skills are deficient, it is possible to evaluate lipreading in such children, as described in Chapter 11. Again, several unanswered questions result. Whereas it has been demonstrated that the implant provides lipreading assistance to the most successful 3M/House children (see Chapter 11), what effect, if any, does the level of speech perception achieved by the majority of these children have on lipreading ability? That is, does the ability to make auditory prosodic discriminations contribute to the ability to lipread word, sentence and narrative materials?

A small minority of the 3M/House children has demonstrated some open-set speech recognition, although reports do not permit a calculation of the percentage of the total patient population achieving this level of perception. There is also some question about the choice of materials used to evaluate speech recognition. Although presented in an open-set format, the 12 GASP word items, similar to those of the MTS or the DAT, are rich in syllabic stress information and almost form a closed-set; the sentence material, limited to 10 questions each in a similar format, also appears to reduce the range of possibilities and approach a closed field. It is interesting to note that HEI's 5-year-old Nucleus patient was able to achieve limited open-set whole-word recognition on the GASP, but was unable to do so with the more difficult monosyllabic items from a PBK word list.

Several characteristics of the population demonstrating better performance with the 3M/House implant have been identified. Most, if not all, of those children achieving open-set recognition have experienced acquired hearing loss as a result of meningitis. In recent reports, statistical analysis correlates better results with the duration of implant use or months of stimulation; that is, improvement over time is observed and better performance occurs with increased experience. However, because the implanted children were not compared to control groups in which age, training, and other factors were matched, it is not possible to isolate and identify the implant as the sole cause of change over time. Such improvement could conceivably result from maturation or rehabilitative intervention. Other factors that might contribute to improved results are a later age at onset of deafness, a shorter period of auditory deprivation prior to implantation, and auditory/verbal training and education. These elements have been targeted by the Nucleus children's program as factors that are predictive of success with the implant. In contrast to the 3M/House program, the Nucleus' patient selection protocol considers these elements and seeks "optimal" implant candidates who presumably have a higher chance of success.

Generalizations about children implanted with the Nucleus multi-electrode system are not yet possible because too little data are available. Given such limited information, only a few tentative observations are offered. Results suggest that for those who are recently deafened prior to implantation, the Nucleus device provides immediate assistance and the ability to achieve high levels of speech perception. This is demonstrated both by one adolescent and the 5-year-old implanted at HEI. Of the two children implanted at HEI, it appears that even with long-standing deafness and prelingual loss, the multichannel device affords rapid progress. Recall that in a 3-year followup study of 21 3M/House subjects, a mean of 9.2 was attained on the DAT at the 3-year postimplant test interval. In contrast, the 5-year-old Nucleus patient had achieved a DAT level of 12 at 3-months postimplant; the 9-year-old, who was prelingually deafened, with a duration of deafness of approximately 8 years, had obtained a

DAT level of 8 at 7 weeks postimplant. Based on the Nucleus case reports providing postimplant data for at least 1 year followups, it might be anticipated that these young children will demonstrate improvement over time.

For postlingually deafened teens, it appears that the Nucleus implant will result in a wide range of performance, just as it does with postlingually deafened adults (see Chapter 3). Among both the younger and older children, pre- or postlingually deaf, are those who are unable to take advantage of the enriched signal and spectral information provided by this multichannel system. However, barring a complete lack of response to electrical stimulation, timing and intensity information, similar to that transmitted by a single-channel system, are still available to such patients.

It might reasonably and justifiably be argued that comparisons between 3M/House and Nucleus results ignore individual patient differences. It is assumed that individual differences in surviving auditory neural elements, in intelligence and cognition, in inherent language abilities, and in educational and verbal levels, all have some impact on performance with an implant. For children, the family support system, mode of communication, the history of hearing-aid use, and educational and training methods might also exert an influence on results.

Presently, a new consideration has emerged: the comparison of the benefits provided by a multichannel versus a single-channel system. A determination of the implant providing the greatest benefits to young children can only be made with comparative, longitudinal studies in which an effort is made to match the numerous variables that might impinge on performance and in which the same evaluation protocols are applied. Until such findings are available, it may be appropriate to decrease the rate at which young deaf children are being implanted, so that, when implanted, it is known that they will receive the best currently available system.

REFERENCES

Allsman, C. S., & Tonokawa, L. L. (1987, November). *Single-channel cochlear implants in children: A three-year follow up* [ASHA Scientific Exhibit]. Presented at the annual convention of the American Speech-Language-Hearing Association, New Orleans, LA.

Banfai, P., Karczag, A., Kubik, S., Luers, P., & Surth, W. (1986). Extracochlear sixteen-channel electrode system. *Otolaryngologic Clinics of North America, 19,* 371–408.

Bell, B. A., & Tonokawa, L. L. (1987, November). *Comparative study of hearing aids and cochlear implants in children* [ASHA Scientific Exhibit]. Presented at the annual convention of the American Speech-Language-Hearing Association, New Orleans, LA.

Bender, L. (1938). *A visual motor gestalt test and its clinical use* (Research Monograph 3). New York: American Orthopsychiatric Association.

Berliner, K. I. (1982). Risk versus benefit in cochlear implantation. *Annals of Otology, Rhinology and Laryngology, 91* (Suppl. 91), 90–98.

Berliner, K. I., & Eisenberg, L. S. (1985). Methods and issues in the cochlear implantation of children: An overview. *Ear and Hearing, 6* (Suppl.), 6S–13S.

Berliner, K. I., & Eisenberg, L. S. (1987). Our experience with cochlear implants: Have we erred in our expectations? *American Journal of Otology, 8,* 222–229.

Berliner, K. I., Eisenberg, L. S., & House, W. F. (Eds.) (1985). The cochlear implant: An auditory prosthesis for the profoundly deaf child. *Ear and Hearing, 6* (Suppl.), 4S–69S.

Berliner, K. I., Eisenberg, L. S., & House, W.F. (1986). Reply to Geers and Moog, and Owens [Letter to the Editor]. *Ear and Hearing, 7,* 127–129.

Berliner, K. I., Tonokawa, L. L., Hill–Brown, C. J., & Dye, L.M. (1987, November). *Results of cochlear implants in children* [ASHA Scientific Exhibit]. Presented at the annual convention of the American Speech-Language-Hearing Association, New Orleans, LA.

Busby, P. A., Dowell, R. C., Nienhuys, T. G., & Clark, G. M. Audiological assessment of profoundly hearing-impaired children. *Annals of Otology, Rhinology and Laryngology, 96* (Suppl. 128), 85–86.

Carrow, E. (1973). *Test for Auditory Comprehension of Language* (Ed. 5). Boston, MA: Teaching Resources Corp.

Cassel, R. N. (1962). *The Child Behavior Rating Scale.* Los Angeles, CA: Western Psychological Services.

Chouard, C. H., Fugain, C., & Meyer, B. (1985). Technique and indications for the French multichannel cochlear implant "Chorimac-12" for deafness rehabilitation. *American Journal of Otology, 6,* 291–294.

Chouard, C. H., Fugain, C., Meyer, B., & Chabolle, F. (1986). The Chorimac 12: A multichannel intracochlear implant for total deafness. *Otolaryngologic Clinics of North America, 19,* 355–370.

Chute, P. M., Kretschmer, R., Wang, H. S., & Parisier, S. C. (1987, November). *The use of the 3M/House single channel cochlear implant in teenagers.* Presented at the annual convention of the American Speech-Language-Hearing Association, New Orleans, LA.

Clark, G. M. (1986). The University of Melbourne/Cochlear Corporation (Nucleus) program. *Otolaryngologic Clinics of North America, 19,* 329–354.

Clark, G. M., Blamey, P. J., Busby, P. A., Dowell, R. C., Burkhard, K. F., Musgrave, G. N., Nienhuys, T. G., Pyman, B. C., Roberts, S. A., Tong, Y. C., Webb, R. L., Kuzma, J. A., Money, D. K., Patrick, J. F., & Seligman, P. M. (1987a). A multi-electrode intracochlear implant for children. *Archives of Otolaryngology, 113,* 825–828.

Clark, G. M., Busby, P. A., Roberts, S. A., Dowell, R. C., Tong, Y. C., Blamey, P. J., Nienhuys, T. G., Mecklenburg, D. J., Webb, R. L., Pyman, B. C., & Franz, B. K. (1987b). Preliminary results for the Cochlear Corporation multielectrode intracochlear implant in six prelingually deaf patients. *American Journal of*

Otology, 8, 234–239.

Clark, G. M, Shepherd, R. K., Patrick, J. F., Black, R. C., & Tong, Y. C. (1983). Design and fabrication of the banded electrode array. In C. W. Parkins & S. W. Anderson (Eds.), Cochlear prostheses: An international symposium. *Annals of the New York Academy of Sciences, 405,* 191–210.

De Filippo, C. L., & Scott, B. L. (1978). A method for training and evaluating the reception of ongoing speech. *Journal of the Acoustical Society of America, 63,* 1186–1192.

Dowell, R. C., Seligman, B. E., Blamey, P. J., & Clark, G.M. (1987). Evaluation of a two-formant speech-processing strategy for a multichannel cochlear prosthesis. *Annals of Otology, Rhinology and Laryngology, 96* (Suppl. 128), 132–134.

Dunn, L. M. (1965). *Peabody Picture Vocabulary Test.* Circle Pines, MN: American Guidance Service.

Eisenberg, L. S. (1982). Use of the cochlear implant by the prelingually deaf. *Annals of Otology, Rhinology and Laryngology, 91* (Suppl. 91), 62–66.

Eisenberg, L. S. (1985). Perceptual capabilities with the cochlear implant: Implications for aural rehabilitation. *Ear and Hearing, 6* (Suppl.), 60S–69S.

Eisenberg, L. S., Berliner, K. I., Thielemeir, M. A., Kirk, K. I., & Tiber, N. (1983). Cochlear implants in children. *Ear and Hearing, 4,* 41–50.

Eisenberg, L. S., & House, W. F. (1982). Initial experience with the cochlear implant in children. *Annals of Otology, Rhinology and Laryngology, 91* (Suppl. 91), 67–73.

Eisenberg, L. S., Kirk, K. I., Berliner, K. I., & Thielemeir, M. A. (1986a). Response to Popelka and Gittelman (1984): Audiologic findings in a child with a single-channel cochlear implant [Letters to the Editor]. *Journal of Speech and Hearing Disorders, 51,* 180–182.

Eisenberg, L. S., Kirk, K. I., Thielemeir, M. A., Luxford, W. M., & Cunningham, J. K. (1986b). Cochlear implants in children: Speech production and auditory discrimination. *Otolaryngologic Clinics of North America, 19,* 409–421.

Eisenberg, L. S., Luxford, W. M., Becker, T. S., & House, W. F. (1984). Electrical stimulation of the auditory system in children deafened by meningitis. *Otolaryngology — Head and Neck Surgery, 92,* 700–705.

Erber, N. P. (1982). *Auditory training.* Washington, D.C.: Alexander Graham Bell Association for the Deaf.

Erber, N. P., & Alencewicz, C. M. (1976). Audiologic evaluation of deaf children. *Journal of Speech and Hearing Disorders, 41,* 256–267.

Fretz, R. J., & Fravel, R. P. (1985). Design and function: A physical and electrical description of the 3M House cochlear implant system. *Ear and Hearing, 6* (Suppl.), 14S–19S.

Geers, A. E., & Moog, J. S. (1986). Comment on "The cochlear implant: An auditory prosthesis for the profoundly deaf child." [Letters to the Editor]. *Ear and Hearing, 7,* 122–125.

Geers, A. E., & Moog, J. S. (1987). Predicting spoken language acquisition of profoundly hearing-impaired children. *Journal of Speech and Hearing Disorders, 52,* 84–94.

Geers, A. E., & Moog, J. S. (1988). Predicting long-term benefits from single-channel cochlear implants in profoundly hearing impaired children. *American Journal of Otology, 9,* 169–176.

Hill–Brown, C. J. (1987, November). *Comparison of speech productions of implanted and unimplanted deaf children* [ASHA Scientific Exhibit]. Presented at the annual convention of the American Speech-Language-Hearing Association, New Orleans, LA.

House, W. F., Berliner, K. I., & Eisenberg, L. S. (1983). Experiences with the cochlear implant in preschool children. *Annals of Otology, Rhinology and Laryngology, 92,* 587–592.

Jastak, J. F., & Jastak, S. (1978). *Wide Range Achievement Test.* Wilmington, DE: Jastak Associates.

Johnson, J. S. (1987a, November). *Auditory discrimination abilities of cochlear implant children.* Presented at the annual convention of the American Speech-Language-Hearing Association, New Orleans, LA.

Johnson, J. S. (1987b, November). *Speech production performance of children with cochlear implants.* Present at the annual convention of the American Speech-Language-Hearing Association, New Orleans, LA.

Kirk, K. I., & Hill–Brown, C. (1985). Speech and language results in children with a cochlear implant. *Ear and Hearing, 6* (Suppl.), 36S–47S.

Ling, D. (1976). *Speech and the hearing-impaired child: Theory and practice.* Washington, DC: Alexander Graham Bell Association for the Deaf.

Los Angeles County, Office of the Los Angeles County Superintendent of Schools. Audiolgic Services, and Southwest School for the Hearing Impaired. (1980). *Test of auditory comprehension.* North Hollywood, CA: Foreworks.

Luxford, W. M., Berliner, K. I., Eisenberg, L. S., & House, W. F. (1987). Cochlear implants in children. *Annals of Otology, Rhinology and Laryngology, 96* (Suppl. 128), 136–138.

Luxford, W. M., & House, W. F. (1985). Cochlear implants in children: Medical and surgical considerations. *Ear and Hearing, 6* (Suppl.), 20S–23S.

Luxford, W. M., & House, W.F. (1987). House 3M cochlear implant: Surgical considerations. *Annals of Otology, Rhinology and Laryngology, 96* (Suppl. 128), 12–14.

McGarr, N. (1983). The intelligibility of deaf speech to experienced and experienced listeners. *Journal of Speech and Hearing Research, 26,* 451–458.

Mecklenburg, D. J. (1987). The Nucleus children's program. *American Journal of Otology, 8,* 436–442.

Mecklenburg, D. J. (1988, January). *Device fitting in children.* Paper presented at the Symposium for Cochlear Implants, Denver, CO.

Mecklenburg, D. J., Busby, P. A., Roberts, S. A., Dowell, R. C., Musgrave, G. N., Blamey, P. J., Tong, Y. C., Nienhuys, T. G., Staller, S. J., & Clark, G. M. (1987, September). *Results of multiple-electrode cochlear implants in children.* Paper presented at the International Cochlear Implant Symposium, Duren, West Germany.

Mecklenburg, D. J., Staller, S. J., Beiter, A. L., & Brimacombe, J. A. (1988, May). *Experiences of the Cochlear Corporation children's section.* Paper presented at the National Institutes of Health Consensus Development Conference on Cochlear Implants, Washington, DC.

Millar, J. B., Martin, L. F. A., Tong, Y. C., & Clark, G. M. (1987). Temporal coding of speech information for cochlear implant patients. *Annals of Otology, Rhinology and Laryngology, 96* (Suppl. 128), 62–64.

Moog, J. S., & Geers, A.E. (1979). *Grammatical analysis of elicited language —simple sentence level.* St. Louis, MO: Central Institute for the Deaf.

Moog, J. S., & Geers, A. E. (1980). *Grammatical analysis of elicited language — complex sentence level.* St. Louis, MO: Central Institute for the Deaf.

Moog, J. S., & Geers, A. E. (1983). *Grammatical analysis of elicited language — presentence level.* St. Louis, MO: Central Institute for the Deaf.

Moore, B. C. J. (1985). Speech coding for cochlear implants. In R. F. Gray (Ed.), *Cochlear implants* (pp. 163–179). San Diego, CA: College-Hill Press.

Nienhuys, T. G., Musgrove, G. N., Busby, P. A., Blamey, P.J., Nott, P., Tong, Y. C., Dowell, R. C., Brown, L. F., & Clark, G. M. (1987). Educational assessment and management of children with multichannel cochlear implants. *Annals of Otology, Rhinology and Laryngology, 96* (Suppl. 128), 80–82.

Northern, J. L., Black, F. O., Brimacombe, J. A., Cohen, N. L., Eisenberg, L. S., Kuprenas, S. V., Martinez, S. A., & Mischke, R. E. (1986). Selection of children for cochlear implantation. *Seminars in Hearing, 7,* 341–347.

Owens, E. (1986). Questions and comments on "The cochlear implant." [Letters to the Editor]. *Ear and Hearing, 7,* 125–127.

Owens, E., Kessler, D. K., Raggio, M. W., & Schubert, E. D. (1985). Analysis and revision of the Minimal Auditory Capabilities (MAC) battery. *Ear and Hearing, 6,* 280–290.

Pfingst, B. E. (1986). Stimulation and encoding strategies for cochlear prostheses. *Otolaryngologic Clinics of North America, 19,* 219–236.

Popelka, G. R., & Gittelman, D. A. (1984). Audiologic findings in a child with single-channel cochlear implant. *Journal of Speech and Hearing Disorders, 49,* 254–261.

Reitan, R. M., & Davison, L.A. (1974). *Clinical neuropsychology: Current status and applications.* New York: Wiley.

Robbins, A. M., & Miyamoto, R. T. (1987, November). *Communicative development in hearing-impaired children: Language growth in children with cochlear implants.* Presented at the annual convention of the American Speech-Language-Hearing Association, New Orleans, LA.

Selmi, A. (1985). Monitoring and evaluating the educational effects of the cochlear implant. *Ear and Hearing, 6* (Suppl.), 52S–59S.

Thielemeir, M. A., Tonokawa, L. L., Petersen, B., & Eisenberg, L. S. (1985). Audiological results in children with a cochlear implant. *Ear and Hearing, 6* (Suppl.), 27S–35S.

Tiber, N. (1985). A psychological evaluation of cochlear implants in children. *Ear and Hearing, 6* (Suppl.), 48S–51S.

Tonelson, S., & Watkins, S. (1979). *The SKI*HI Language Development Scale.* Logan, UT: University of Utah, Project SKI*HI.

Tong, Y. C., Blamey, P. J., Dowell, R. C., & Clark, G. M. (1983). Psychophysical studies evaluating the feasibility of a speech processing strategy for a multiple-channel cochlear implant. *Journal of the Acoustical Society of America, 74,* 73–80.

Tong, Y. C., Clark, G. M., Blamey, P. J., Busby, P. A., & Dowell, R. C. (1982). Psychophysical studies for two multiple-channel cochlear implant patients. *Journal of the Acoustical Society of America, 71,* 153–160.

Tonokawa, L. L., Berliner, K. I., & Dye, L. M. (1987, November). *Nucleus multichannel cochlear implant in children* [ASHA Scientific Exhibit]. Presented at the annual convention of the American Speech-Language-Hearing Association, New Orleans, LA.

Tonokawa, L. L., & Dye, L. M. (1987, November). *Open-set speech recognition in children with the 3M/House cochlear implant* [ASHA Scientific Exhibit]. Presented at the annual convention of the American Speech-Language-Hearing Association, New Orleans, LA.

Tyler, R. S., Davis, J. M., & Lansing, C. R. (1987). Cochlear implants in young children. *Asha, 29,* 41–49.

Yin, L. & Segersen, D. A. (1986). Cochlear implants: Overview of safety and effectiveness; The FDA evaluation. *Otolaryngologic Clinics of North America, 19,* 423–433.

C H A P T E R **11**

ANN E. GEERS
JEAN S. MOOG

Evaluating Speech Perception Skills: Tools for Measuring Benefits of Cochlear Implants, Tactile Aids, and Hearing Aids

The term *profoundly deaf* is commmonly applied to children with unaided pure tone threshold averages of 90 dB or greater. For children with unaided threshold averages in the moderate and severe ranges, a conventional hearing aid can result in greatly improved speech perception ability which, when combined with appropriate training, should enable most of these children to acquire spoken language. For children with unaided threshold averages in the profound range, the benefits of hearing aids are less clear cut. A variety of alternative devices, either commercially available or under development, are designed to transmit more speech information to the profoundly deaf ear than conventional hearing aids. These include both single and multichannel tactile aids and cochlear implants that vary in terms of frequency coding strategies, placement on the body, method of stimulation, and other practical considerations such as wearablity and durability.

Although none of the devices developed to date restores normal hearing, a device may be judged effective if it offers some children greater benefit than they obtain from acoustic hearing aids. If benefit is ultimately to be assessed in terms of improvement in the ability to perceive speech, evaluation instruments that are sensitive to small differences in speech perception skills must be used. Because important decisions regarding the selection of devices and educational approaches must often be made when the child is quite young, evaluation procedures must be applicable to children who cannot read and whose spoken vocabulary is limited. It is these children, under 10 years of age with hearing thresholds in the profound range, who are the focus of evaluation techniques described in this chapter.

AIDED SPEECH PERCEPTION ABILITIES OF CHILDREN WHO ARE PROFOUNDLY HEARING IMPAIRED

For many years, profoundly hearing impaired children were considered a homogeneous group who could not understand even amplified speech. However, with technological advances in hearing aids and hearing aid fitting procedures, and with educational advances in auditory skill development, a range of speech perception abilities have been demonstrated in these children. When they are given the benefit of appropriate early amplification, auditory training, and intensive instruction in lipreading and speech production, many have the potential for normal or near-normal language and academic development (Moog & Geers, 1985). This potential is greatly affected by small amounts of residual hearing that can be trained to interpret a degraded speech signal. The more speech a child can perceive, the easier it is to teach him to understand and produce it.

When hearing is trained and when appropriate tests are utilized, these children exhibit significant differences in their ability to perceive speech through appropriately fitted hearing aids. Four aided speech perception categories have been proposed to describe differences observed among children within the profoundly hearing-impaired range, as follows:

CATEGORY 1: NO PATTERN PERCEPTION. At the lower end of category 1 are those children who cannot even detect amplified speech. This category also includes children who can detect speech, but have not developed the ability to discriminate speech patterns. They are unable to discriminate auditorally between words or phrases that differ in gross durational pattern (e.g., "cup" versus "lunchbox").

CATEGORY 2: PATTERN PERCEPTION. This category includes children who have developed minimal skills in perceiving speech. At the lower end are children who are just beginning to discriminate words or phrases that differ in durational pattern. They are able to do this only in a closed or limited set. At the upper end are children who can make these pattern differentiations rather easily and can also differentiate units that differ in stress (e.g., "chicken" versus "lunchbox"). However, children in category 2 do not demonstrate the ability to make use of spectral information to discriminate among vowel or consonant sounds.

CATEGORY 3: SOME WORD IDENTIFICATION. This category includes children who demonstrate some minimal ability to make use of spectral or intonational information. These children are able to discriminate among words or phrases of similar stress and durational patterns provided that they are presented in a small closed set of two to three choices and that the words contain highly differentiable vowels (e.g., "cowboy" versus "bathtub"). However, the task is difficult for them and their performance is dependent upon the degree to which the vowels differ.

CATEGORY 4: CONSISTENT WORD IDENTIFICATION. This category includes children who demonstrate greater facility in using spectral information for discrimination. They consistently discriminate among words and phrases that contain different vowel sounds. These words may be presented in slightly larger closed sets (e.g., 4- to 12-choices).

SPEECH PERCEPTION ABILITY AND SPOKEN LANGUAGE DEVELOPMENT

A series of studies (Geers & Moog, 1988) demonstrated that the four proposed aided speech perception categories are associated with differences in profoundly deaf children's aptitudes for acquiring intelligible speech and spoken English skills. Speech and language development were examined in two samples of profoundly deaf children in oral programs. The CID group consisted of 44 children between 8 and 14 years of age enrolled in the Central Institute for the Deaf (CID). The Oral Adolescent group consisted of 100 deaf students between 16 and 18 years of age from oral and mainstream programs across the country. The CID children were fairly homogeneous in that they had been selected as good candidates for oral instruction and were all enrolled in the same educational program, one providing intensive speech training. Because they were similar in their educational experiences and other factors contributing to spoken language development, the impact of differences in speech perception abilities on the development of speech and language may be more clearly evidenced. Being a more heterogeneous sample of deaf children, the group of oral adolescents serves to substantiate the CID findings.

Vocabulary quotient scores on the Peabody Picture Vocabulary Test (PPVT) (Dunn, 1981) and speech intelligibility scores on the Speech

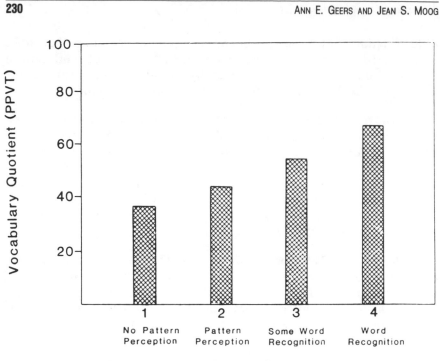

FIGURE 11-1. Mean vocabulary quotient scores on the Peabody Picture Vocabulary Test (PPVT) are plotted for children in four speech perception categories. From Geers, A. E., and Moog, J. S. (1988). Predicting long-term benefits from single-channel cochlear implants in profoundly hearing-impaired children. *American Journal of Otology, 9,* 169–176. Reprinted with permission.

Intelligibility Evaluation (SPINE) (Monsen, 1981) were examined for the 44 profoundly deaf children enrolled in classes at CID. Average vocabulary quotient scores for children in each of the four speech perception categories are plotted in Figure 11-1. The average vocabulary quotient score for eight children in speech perception category 1 was 37. This represents a dramatic delay, with the acquisition of vocabulary proceeding at about one-third the rate of the normal hearing child. Results for 12 children in category 2 (pattern perceivers) were only slightly better with an average quotient of 44. A greater increase in vocabulary for age was observed in the 14 children whose auditory skills placed them in category 3, partial speech identifiers. Their average vocabulary quotient of 55 indicates that new words are being acquired at slightly better than half the normal rate. The 10 children in category 4 achieved an average quotient of 68 — more than two-thirds of the normal rate and over one and one-half times the rate of those in categories 1 and 2.

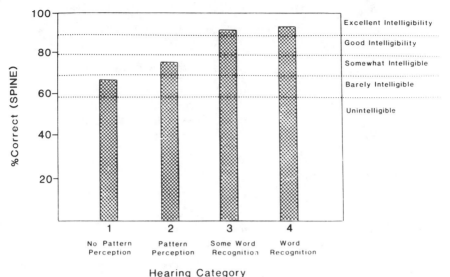

FIGURE 11-2. Mean speech intelligibility scores plotted for children in four speech perception categories. From Geers, A. E., and Moog, J. S. (1988). Predicting long-term benefits from single-channel cochlear implants in profoundly hearing-impaired children. *American Journal of Otology, 9,* 169–176. Reprinted with permission.

Similar results are presented in Figure 11-2 for the speech intelligibility measure (SPINE). Children in speech perception category 1 achieved an average speech intelligibility score of 67 percent, indicating that their speech was barely intelligible. Children in category 2 had slightly better speech with an average percent-correct score of 75 percent, in the somewhat intelligible range. Children whose speech perception test scores placed them in categories 3 and 4, however, had speech intelligibility scores above 90 percent on the SPINE, indicating that their speech was largely intelligible, even to a naive listener.

Results for the 100 oral adolescents are summarized in Table 11-1. Since only three subjects scored in speech perception category 1, average scores are presented for children in categories 2, 3, and 4 only. The Visual Enhancement subtest of the Minimal Auditory Capabilities (MAC) battery (Owens, et al., 1985) is a direct measure of improvement in speech reading as a result of wearing a hearing aid. Lipreading of sentence material with and without amplification is compared. The 36 subjects whose single-word speech perception scores placed them in category 2 averaged only 6 percent improvement with audition. Ten of these subjects actually scored better in the lipreading-alone condition. This suggests that pattern perception skill is not helpful as an aid to lipreading

TABLE 11–1

Average Test Scores of Profoundly Deaf Children in Three Speech Perception Categories

	Speech Perception Rating		
Test	Category 2 Pattern Perception (n = 36)	Category 3 Some Word Recognition (n = 46)	Category 4 Word Recognition (n = 15)
Visual enhancement* (% improvement)	6%	21%	32%
PPVT† (Age score)	8–4	10–4	10–7
SPINE‡ (% intelligible)	76%	88%	93%
Phonetic inventory	75%	84%	88%

    * Minimal Auditory Capabilities Battery.

    † Peabody Picture Vocabulary Test

    ‡ Speech Intelligibility Evaluation.

From Geers, A. E., and Moog, J. S. (1988). Predicting long-term benefits from single-channel cochlear implants in profoundly hearing-impaired children. *American Journal of Otology, 9*(2), 171. Reprinted with permission.

connected speech. In contrast, word recognition ability is quite helpful, with 21 percent improvement with audition for 46 subjects in category 3 and 32 percent improvement for 15 subjects in category 4.

Average vocabulary age scores for children in category 2 on the PPVT was 8 years 4 months (about half their chronologic age). However, children in categories 3 and 4 were at the 10-year level. A similar pattern was observed on the two speech measures. SPINE scores for children in category 2 averaged in the somewhat intelligible range (76 percent). Children in categories 3 and 4, however, attained excellect speech intelligibility (88 percent and 93 percent respectively). The percent of phonemes produced on the CID Phonetic Inventory (Moog, 1988) averaged 75 percent for those in category 2, while those in category 4 produced an average of 88 percent of the phonemes.

The data obtained from this sample of older subjects from a variety of educational programs appear to confirm results from the younger CID sample. The results indicate that the proposed speech perception categories do represent an important factor in the profoundly deaf child's ability to acquire spoken language. Futhermore, these results suggest that even limited vowel discrimination ability, such as that exhibited by children in category 3, is of substantial importance for the acquisition of spoken language. However, the perception of temporal patterns, although allowing children to discriminate words and phrases of different syllabic length, provides only a small benefit with regard to the acquisition of spoken language.

EVALUATION OF SPEECH PERCEPTION SKILLS IN CHILDREN WHO ARE PROFOUNDLY HEARING IMPAIRED

A number of audiologic procedures can be used to evaluate differences in speech perception ability in children who are profoundly hearing-impaired. However, they are not routinely administered because they are not familiar to audiologists. The number of profoundly hearing impaired children is relatively small; thus, audiologists have limited experience evaluating such children. Furthermore, the small differences observed among children with minimal hearing have not been considered important. In its extreme, this is evidenced by children in this range who are not even fitted with hearing aids.

Some speech perception tests for children have recently achieved recognition as a result of current interest in evaluating tactile aids and cochlear implants. These include the Test of Auditory Comprehension (TAC) (Los Angeles, 1980), the Speech Patterns Contrast Test (SPAC) (Boothroyd, 1984), the Discrimination After Training Test (DAT) (Thielemeir, 1982), the Monosyllable, Trochee, Spondee (MTS) Test (Erber & Alencewicz, 1976), the Auditory Numbers Test (ANT) (Erber, 1980), and the Glendonald Auditory Screening Procedure (GASP) (Erber,1982).

The TAC provides normative data for children from a wide range of age and hearing impairment categories. However, it does not provide for distinctions in speech perception abilities among children who are profoundly deaf. The SPAC provides detailed information regarding the type of speech information perceived by a hearing-impaired individual, but it is applicable only to children who can read the response alternatives. Items on the DAT correspond to the speech perception categories described earlier and are applicable to young hearing-impaired children. However, an insufficient number of items are available at the top of the scale to distinguish clearly between children in categories 3 and 4 and to define abilities that exceed category 4. The MTS, the ANT, and the GASP were all designed to evaluate the deaf child's ability to perceive durational and stress patterns in speech and to discriminate words on the basis of vowel sounds. These tests served as a basis for much of the speech perception battery described in this chapter.

For a child who has not yet developed verbal skills, the aided articulation index (AI) (Gittleman & Popelka, 1987) may be used to predict speech perception ability. This value represents the percent of the amplified speech spectrum available to a child when wearing a hearing aid. Calculation of the aided AI requires only aided and unaided thresholds. A comparison between the aided AI and the four categories of speech perception resulted in sufficient agreement to recommend cautiously the aided AI as a means of categorizing the speech perception abilities of profoundly hearing impaired children who are unable to respond to speech tests (Geers and Moog, 1987). However, the validity of the aided AI for predicting speech discrimination ability through tactile aids or cochlear implants has not been determined. Aided thresholds across the frequency range through these devices may not reflect the child's ability to perceive differences in pitch (Eisenberg, 1985; see also Chapter 2).

Adequate comparisons of the benefits obtained from tactile aids and cochlear implants with those obtained from conventional amplification requires the evaluation of speech perception and cannot be made from threshold information. The Early Speech Perception (ESP) Test battery was developed at CID to obtain increasingly more accurate information regarding speech discrimination skills as the profoundly deaf child's verbal abilities develop.

THE EARLY SPEECH PERCEPTION (ESP) TEST BATTERY

The Early Speech Perception (ESP) test battery has been designed for young profoundly hearing-impaired children with limited vocabulary and language skills. The criteria for items in the battery were as follows:

1. The words used would be known by the majority of hearing impaired children by the age of 6.
2. The words used would be "pictureable" so that they could be identified by children who were not yet able to read.
3. The test would be short enough to be administered in at least three conditions in less than 1 hour.

The ESP can be used to place children in the speech perception categories described previously and to define in greater detail their abilities within a category. In order to separate speech perception skills from language ability, each subtest is first administered using both lipreading and listening to ascertain that the child can easily identify the words before testing the ability to identify them through listening alone. Only after the child has indicated comprehension of all of the words is that subtest administered in the listening only condition.

For children who do not understand all of the vocabulary in the standard battery, items have been developed that require the child's comprehension of only a few words. Although these "low-verbal" items provide a more accurate estimate of speech perception ability than does the aided AI, the most reliable information is obtained when the child has sufficient vocabulary to take the standard ESP battery.

The ESP battery is administered by "monitored live voice" (75 dB SPL) and as such is subject to tester variability not present in tests with prerecorded stimuli. Nevertheless, the young age and minimal hearing capabilities of the subjects for whom this test is intended requires complete tester control over stimulus presentation. The examiner must be able to determine when the child is ready to listen and must present the stimuli at a pace appropriate to each individual child. The battery should be administered by a skilled pediatric audiologist who is sensitive to nonverbal cues to the correct response that may be given by glance or a body movement. Care must be taken to insure that the only stimulus to which the child can respond is the spoken word.

The standard ESP battery consists of a pattern perception subtest and two word-identification subtests. Following a description of the standard battery, the low-verbal battery is discussed.

Pattern Perception Test

The Word Categorization subtest of the Glendonald Auditory Screening Procedure (GASP) (Erber, 1982) has been adapted to measure the child's ability to recognize temporal patterns in speech. In this test 12 words in four different durational or stress patterns are presented in a 3 × 4 grid on a picture card shown in Figure 11–3. There are three each of monosyllables, trochees, spondees and 3-syllable words. The examiner names a picture with mouth covered and the child is expected to point to the picture named. As this test is administered live voice, the examiner must monitor the production of each word to be sure that the desired stress pattern is being properly delivered so that the four patterns are clearly differentiable from one another. One method of training examiners in controlled production is to have them present the stimuli to a normal hearing subject through a bone conduction vibrator. These patterns should be perceived through the vibrator with close to 100 percent accuracy by a listener who is prevented from actually hearing the words.

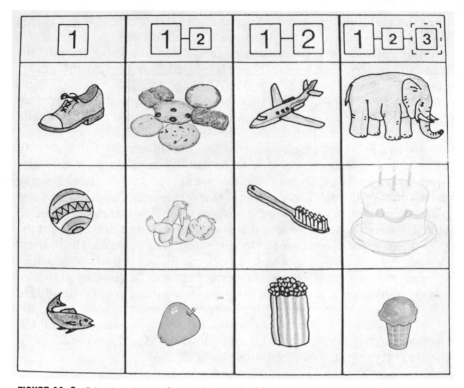

FIGURE 11–3. Stimulus pictures for words in each of four stress categories that form the Pattern Perception subtest have been adapted from the Glendonald Auditory Screening Procedure (Erber, 1982).

SCORING. A word is counted correct for pattern perception if a word with the same stress pattern is selected. For example, if the word given is "popcorn" and the child selects "airplane", the response would be counted as correct for pattern perception. The word need not be correctly identified in order to be scored as correct because only identification of temporal pattern is being evaluated.

Each word is presented twice, so a perfect score is 24 words correctly categorized. Chance performance is 6 words correctly categorized (25 percent). A score of 17 correct out of 24 trials is required to credit the child with discriminating speech patterns (category 2).

SPONDEE IDENTIFICATION TEST

The Spondee Identification Test evaluates differences in word recognition abilities of profoundly deaf children who demonstrate the ability to perceive durational patterns in words (i.e., they scored at least 17 correct out of 24 on the pattern perception subtest). Once it has been determined that a child can perform in speech perception category 2, the Spondee Identification subtest is used to evaluate whether that child can perform in category 3.

The 12 spondees pictured in Figure 11–4 have widely differing vowel sounds. After the child's comprehension of these words has been confirmed by 100 percent audio-visual performance, the words are presented auditory-only in random sequence until each word has been presented twice. The child is expected to point to the picture of the spoken word.

SCORING. A perfect score on this test is 24 words correctly identified. A chance score, obtained by guessing, is 2 correct. A child who identifies 8 out of 24 words correctly demonstrates sufficient word recognition skills to be placed in speech perception category 3. A child who correctly identifies 19 of the 24 presentations demonstrates sufficient word recognition skills to be tested on monosyllabic words in order to determine if his or her skills can be rated in category 4.

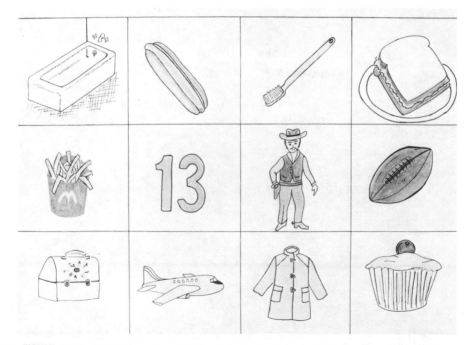

FIGURE 11–4. Stimulus pictures for the 12 words that comprise the Spondee Identification subtest.

MONOSYLLABIC WORD IDENTIFICATION TEST

The closed set of monosyllabic words pictured in Figure 11–5 was designed to provide a more difficult test of word recognition ability for children who demonstrate good identification skills on the Spondee test. Twelve quite similar words are included in this set and identification of the words requires finer vowel discriminations than were required in the spondee set. In this set, all words begin with /b/ and most end with a plosive. Identification is based primarily on vowel recognition. The administration procedures are the same as those described for the Spondee Identification Test.

SCORING. If a child scores better than 50 percent on the Monosyllabic Word Identification Test (i.e., at least 13 correct), sufficient speech discrimination ability has been demonstrated to place the child in speech perception category 4.

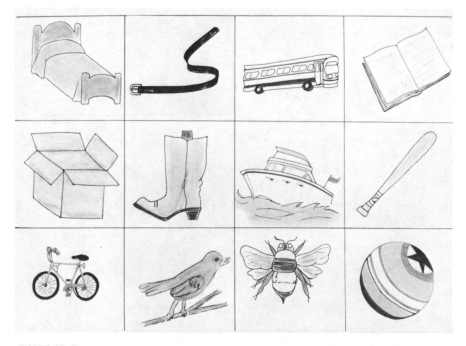

FIGURE 11–5. Stimulus pictures for the 12 words that comprise the Monosyllabic Word Identification subtest.

FURTHER SPEECH PERCEPTION TESTING

Children who score above 75 percent correct on the monosyllabic vowel identification test demonstrate auditory skills beyond category 4. Testing may then proceed with the Word Intelligibility by Picture Identification (WIPI) (Ross & Lerman, 1971), a closed-set speech discrimination test that also uses a picture pointing response. The WIPI requires a more extensive vocabulary (e.g., the child must know such words as "sheep," "queen," "green," "wheel," "seal," "screen") than the Monosyllabic Word Identification Test. Further, the WIPI evaluates consonant discrimination which is more difficult than vowel discrimination. Children who do well on the WIPI are ready for an open-set task such as the Kindergarten Phonetically Balanced (PBK) Word list (Haskins, 1972). By this point the child's auditory functioning is more like that of a child with severe or moderate hearing impairment than a child who is profoundly deaf.

LOW-VERBAL EARLY SPEECH PERCEPTION TEST

With the standard ESP test battery, speech perception skills ranging from discrimination of temporal patterns through discrimination of highly similar spectral features can be measured in most profoundly deaf children over the age of 6. However, decisions regarding training procedures and assistive hearing devices must often be made for children younger than 6 and often for children as young as 2 or 3 years of age. Therefore, the following procedures have been devised for obtaining similar information on very young children who have such extremely limited verbal ablities that they are unable to perform the tasks required in the standard ESP battery. The activities have been appropriately modified for very young children with limited vocabularies.

The following criteria were used in developing the Low-Verbal version of the Early Speech Perception Test:

1. Real objects are used instead of pictures.
2. The objects selected are ones that are of interest to a young child and that are likely to be among the first words learned.
3. The closed sets are very small, consisting of two to three objects.

PATTERN PERCEPTION

Children who do not have sufficient vocabularies to identify the 12 pictures on the standard ESP battery are administered the low-verbal ESP. This level consists of a set of three tasks that require very minimal comprehension of words. These tasks do, however, provide some information about the child's ability to discriminate durational patterns with speech stimuli.

AAAHHH VERSUS HOP HOP. In this task a long continuous sound is contrasted with a short choppy sound. The examiner says "aaahhh" and the child is taught to respond by moving a toy train along a wooden track. The examiner says "hop hop" and the child is expected to make a toy rabbit hop. The child demonstrates understanding of the task by performing the task 10 times with at least 90 percent accuracy using lipreading and listening. Once the association has been established audiovisually, the examiner presents a series of 20 randomly selected stimuli without visual cues and the child responds by making the train glide or the rabbit hop.

MONOSYLLABLE VERSUS THREE-SYLLABLE WORD. This task involves the more difficult discrimination of a one-syllable from a three-syllable word. The examiner may choose either "shoe" or "fish" as the monosyllable item and either "ice cream cone" or "birthday cake" as the three-syllable stimulus, depending on which words the child seems to know best.

The examiner places two objects, one representing each item, on a table in front of the child. The child is expected to point to or pick up the object named. The items are named in random order, with both lipreading and listening provided, until the child correctly identifies six in a row. If the child is unable to identify either of the items with lipreading and listening, the alternate words should be tried. Once the child can perform the task with 90 percent accuracy audiovisually, the listening alone condition is administered for 12 trials.

MONOSYLLABLE VERSUS TWO-SYLLABLE WORD. A similar procedure is followed for the one- versus two-syllable discrimination task in which the child must discriminate between the monosyllable ("shoe" or "fish") and a spondee ("airplane" or "hot dog").

SCORING. An average number correct score is determined for the three tasks. Chance performance on these two-choice tasks is 50 percent. An average score of 10 correct on the three sets of 12 trials is required in order to be reasonably confident (that is, statistically above the 90 percent confidence level) that the child is indeed discriminating speech patterns and may be rated in speech perception category 2.

Word Identification Subtest

A child who can discriminate among speech patterns is administered the World Identification subtest. In this test the child is required to discriminate among 3 one-syllable words and among 3 two-syllable words.

THREE SPONDEES. The two-syllable words are "airplane," "popcorn," and "french fries." The alternates are "lunch box," and "hot dog." One of each object is placed on the table between the child and the examiner. Audiovisual training is used to associate each of the three spondees with the corresponding object using the same procedure described for pattern discrimination. Once this association has been established with 6 correct consecutive responses, the examiner presents 20 trials in the auditory-only condition.

THREE MONOSYLLABLES. The one syllable words are "shoe," "cup," and "ball." The alternates are "fish," "hat," and "boat." The same procedure used for three spondees is repeated for the three monosyllables.

SCORING. Chance performance on these 3-choice tasks is 7 correct responses out of 20 presentations. However, the 90 percent confidence level is 14 correct out of 20 presentations. Therefore, the child's average number correct on the Spondee and the Monosyllable task must be at least 70 percent in order to be rated in speech perception category 3 (some word identification). In order to be placed in category 4 (consistent word identification), nearly perfect performance on the spondees and monosyllables is required (at least 18 out of 20 presentations).

Table 11–2 presents the three levels of tests used to estimate speech perception ability in the young child. This table summarizes the number of correct responses on each task required for placement in the four speech perception categories.

For the preverbal child, who cannot perform the low-verbal tasks in the audiovisual condition, the aided articulation index provides a gross estimate of speech perception ability for children wearing acoustic hearing aids. However, once children are trained to understand the six words needed for the Low-Verbal ESP battery, pattern discrimination and word identification abilities may be estimated with actual speech stimuli. As the child's receptive vocabulary grows, speech perception abilities can be assessed in larger sets. The larger the set of words to which the child can respond, the better the speech perception estimate. Once the child has developed sufficient verbal skills to make reliable audiovisual responses

TABLE 11–2
Estimating Speech Perception Ability in Profoundly Hearing-Impaired Children

Child	Test	Number of Trials	Speech Perception Category			
			1 No Patterns	**2** Speech Identification	**3** Some Word Identification	**4** Consistent Word Identification
Pre-Verbal	Aided AI		0–20%	21–49%	50–69%	70–100%
Low Verbal	"Aaaa" vs. "Hop"	12				
	1 vs. 3-syllable	12	0–9†	10–12†		
	1 vs. 2-syllable	12				
	3-Spondees	20				
	3-Monosyllables	20			14–16†	18–20†
Verbal	Pattern perception	24	0–16†	17–24†		
	Spondee identification	24			8–18†	
	Monosyllable identification	24				13–18† >18†*

† Scores = number correct.
* Further abilities should be evaluated using standard speech discrimination tests (e.g., WIPI, PBK).

to the standard ESP battery, speech perception abilities may be assigned to one of the four speech perception categories with good confidence. For those children who score above category 4 on the Monosyllabic Word Identification Test, more difficult tests with still larger sets are appropriate for evaluating further auditory abilities (e.g., the WIPI and the PBK list).

Visual Enhancement Battery for Children

After the child's auditory speech perception skills have been measured, the next consideration is the degree to which the child's assistive listening device (hearing aid, tactile aid, or cochlear implant) enhances the ability to lipread. Audition may be a helpful adjunct to lipreading and contribute to improved comprehension even for children who are unable to demonstrate comprehension through audition alone. Furthermore, measured improvements in auditory perception may not be beneficial for language development unless face-to-face comprehension of speech is affected.

The procedures for the assessment of visual enhancement are only appropriate for evaluating a device with which the child has been trained extensively. It is probably safe to assume that benefits of visual enhancement for any device will not be evident until the child has had a year or more of consistent use and training with the device. Furthermore, children whose language skills are so minimal that they require the Low-Verbal Early Speech Perception battery are not yet ready for an evaluation of visual enhancement.

Careful selection of materials is necessary to effectively measure how a device enhances lipreading. If the materials used are too easy, an inflated lipreading-alone score will be achieved, and there will not be sufficient points remaining to estimate the full benefit gained from the listening device. On the other hand, if the material selected is too difficult linguistically, the child will be unable to understand it and any enhancement provided by a device will not result in a higher score when compared to lipreading alone. Therefore, it is necessary to provide test materials representing a hierarchy of linguistic difficulty in order to evaluate the child's performance at a level most sensitive to visual enhancement. The hierarchy of tests in the CID Visual Enhancement Battery includes the following:

1. Closed-set word identification (Craig, 1975)
2. Closed-set sentence identification (Craig, 1975)
3. Open-set simple sentences (Monsen, 1981)

4. Open-set complex sentences (Owens et al., 1985)
5. Connected discourse tracking (DeFillipo & Scott, 1978)

Each level of difficulty is first administered in a lipreading-only condition. If the child's performance exceeds 75 percent correct, visual enhancement is not evaluated with that level of material because it is too easy. Testing then proceeds with lipreading-only assessment at the next most difficult level. If the child's performance is less than 40 percent correct, the material is deemed too difficult, and testing proceeds with a lipreading-only assessment of the next easier level. When a level is reached at which the child scores in an optimal range (between 40 percent and 75 percent), testing proceeds in one or more aided conditions and a percent visual enhancement score is obtained by subtracting unaided from aided performance.

CLOSED-SET WORD IDENTIFICATION

The material used to assess visual enhancement at the lowest level of difficulty is the Craig Lipreading Test-Word Level (Craig, 1975). In this test, the examiner presents a word and the child selects the item named out of a choice of four pictures (e.g., kite, fire, white, and light), for a total of 33 test items. Because there are four pictures in each set, it is possible to have four forms of the test so that it can be administered in each of four conditions if necessary (i.e., lipreading alone, lipreading plus hearing aid, lipreading plus implant, and lipreading plus hearing aid plus implant). This test is used to measure enhancement only for those children who score between 40 percent and 75 percent correct in the lipreading-alone condition. Children who score below 40 percent are not yet ready for visual enhancement testing. Children who score above 75 percent should move to the next highest level in the battery, the Craig Lipreading Test-Sentence Level (Craig, 1975).

CLOSED-SET SENTENCE IDENTIFICATION

In the sentence identification test, the examiner says one of four sentences and the child points to the correct picture. Within each set of pictures, critical elements are manipulated, as in the following example: "a drum is on a chair"; "a coat is on a table"; "a drum is on a table"; "a coat is on a chair." Thus, the child must demonstrate an understanding of key words presented in a sentence context. Children who score above 75 percent on this closed-set of 24 sentences in the lipreading-only condition are given the next level of difficulty, open-set simple sentences.

OPEN-SET SIMPLE SENTENCES

A set of sentences devised by Monsen (1981) for evaluating speech intelligibility in children who are deaf consists of four lists of 10 simple sentences. They comprise a well-balanced set of materials both phonemically and linguistically (e.g., "I like ice cream"; "He plays baseball"; "Can you tell us?"). The task is somewhat more difficult than the Craig Sentences because the child is required to imitate sentences presented out of context rather than to select from a closed-set. Each word correctly imitated receives 1 point. Children who score at or above 75 percent correct on all tests through this level in the lipreading-alone condition are given the Visual Enhancement (VE) subtest of the Minimal Auditory Capabilities (MAC) Battery (Owens et al., 1985).

OPEN-SET COMPLEX SENTENCES

The VE subtest of the MAC consists of four sets of 10 CID Everyday Sentences which range from very simple (e.g., "Look out!") to very complex (e.g., "They ate enough green apples to make them sick for a week."). The child's task is to imitate the sentence after the examiner. Only key words in the sentences are scored. For children who score above 75 percent correct lipreading-alone on the VE subtest of the MAC, connected discourse tracking must be used to assess the benefits they derive from a device.

CONNECTED DISCOURSE TRACKING

In the tracking procedure developed by De Filippo and Scott (1978), the examiner reads a passage to the child phrase by phrase and the child is required to repeat back word-for-word what the examiner said. The examiner is allowed to present a word or phrase as many as five times until the child has correctly repeated it. After five repetitions, the examiner may skip the word and proceed with the text. These repetitions lower the child's overall performance because the score is the average number of wpm accurately repeated by the child in a 5-minute segment.

Three 5-minute segments is ideal for one test session. Segments should be alternated between lipreading only and lipreading with the device in the on condition. Because there is some initial improvement in the child's score as he learns the tracking task, assessment requires more than one test session. Evaluation of a single device should consist of a minumum of four sessions resulting in a words per minute score for six lipreading-only segments and six lipreading plus device segments. The visual enhancement score is the increase in wpm with the device under evaluation.

The material selected for connected discourse tracking must be at an appropriate level of difficulty for the particular child in order to observe enhancement. If the child's lipreading-only score during the first session is less than 30 wpm, an easier level of material must be selected and testing started over at the next session. If the child's lipreading-only score during the first session is greater than 70 wpm, a more advanced level of material must be selected. Because all children tested with tracking are selected on the basis of success on the MAC VE sentences, tracking may begin with material at the 4th grade reading level.

USE OF SPEECH PERCEPTION AND VISUAL ENHANCEMENT TESTS FOR DEVICE EVALUATION

EARLY SPEECH PERCEPTION (ESP) TEST BATTERY

In order to illustrate the applicability of the Early Speech Perception Test Battery for device evaluation, results are presented for 12 children with the 3M/House single-channel cochlear implant. These children represented the most successful of the House Ear Institute (HEI) child implant recipients: they were preselected on the basis of having attained word identification ability on the Discrimination After Training Test (Berliner, Eisenberg, & House, 1985; Berliner & Eisenberg, 1987). Six of these children no longer wore hearing aids and were tested in the implant-only condition. The remaining 6 children wore hearing aids on the unimplanted ear and were tested in the following conditions:

BINAURAL: BOTH IMPLANT AND HEARING AID. This condition provides a measurement of the child's ability to perceive speech in a manner typical of the child's daily usage. It also provides information regarding the integration of speech perception through two devices.

LISTENING THROUGH IMPLANT-ONLY. Comparison of the implant-only score with the binaural score reveals information regarding the benefits provided by the hearing aid. If the implant-only score is higher than when listening with both ears, it indicates that the hearing aid may be interfering with perception through the implant. If the implant-only score is the same as in the binaural condition, the contralateral hearing aid ear may be contributing little to the child's perception through the implant. If the implant-only score is poorer than the binaural score, then it demonstrates that the hearing aid provides additional information.

LISTENING THROUGH HEARING AID-ONLY. Comparison of the hearing aid-only score with the binaural score provides information regarding the benefits obtained from the implant. If the hearing aid-only score is higher than that in the binaural condition, it may indicate that the implant is interfering with perception through the hearing aid. If the scores are the same, then the implant may be contributing little to the child's perception with the hearing aid. If the hearing aid-only score is poorer than the binaural score, then the implant is adding useful information.

RESULTS

Results are presented in Table 11–3. Scores for each child on the Pattern Perception Test, the Spondee Identification Test, and the Monosyllabic Word Identification Test are given for the implant-only condition, the hearing aid-only condition, and the binaural condition. Only one child, Subject H, demonstrated category 2 pattern discrimination ability with his hearing aid. None of the children demonstrated category 3 word identification abilities with a hearing aid. In contrast, with the implant, all children achieved better than 40 percent Spondee Identification scores (category 3) and 8 of the children scored at or above 75 percent in Spondee Identification (category 4).

For these 8 children, scores on the Monosyllabic Word Identification Test exceeded 50 percent. Two children, Subjects A and D, scored above 75 percent on the monosyllables, indicating speech perception abilities above the category 4 level. Binaural scores obtained with the hearing aid and implant together were generally no better than implant-only scores, indicating that the hearing aid was not adding significant information.

VISUAL ENHANCEMENT BATTERY

Results for the 12 HEI children with cochlear implants on the Visual Enhancement Battery are presented in Table 11–4. Five of these children were also tested with a hearing aid, allowing comparisons of their performance across four conditions: lipreading alone, lipreading plus implant, lipreading plus hearing aid, lipreading plus hearing aid plus implant. In the last three columns, the lipreading-alone score has been subtracted from each of the aided conditions to produce an enhancement score.

The amount of enhancement achieved with the implant ranged from 10 percent for Subject H to 40 percent for Subject A, with an average enhancement of 26 percent. The amount of enhancement achieved through a hearing aid ranged from −6 percent for Subject L to 25 per-

TABLE 11–3.
Speech Perception Scores of Successful Implant Users

Child	Test	Cochlear Implant		Hearing Aid		Binaural	
		No. Correct	Sp. Cat.	No. Correct	Sp. Cat.	No. Correct	Sp. Cat.
A	Patterns	24					
	Spondees	24					
	Monosyllables	21	>4	NA*		NA	
B	Patterns	24					
	Spondees	24					
	Monosyllables	17	4	NA		NA	
C	Patterns	23					
	Spondees	24					
	Monosyllables	17	4	NA		NA	
D	Patterns	23		0		23	
	Spondees	24		DNT†		22	
	Monosyllables	18	4	DNT	1	19	>4
E	Patterns	22					
	Spondees	20		NA		NA	
	Monosyllables	13	4				
F	Patterns	22		7		22	
	Spondees	21		DNT		21	
	Monosyllables	17	4	DNT	1	18	4

G	Patterns	22		0		23	
	Spondees	18		DNT		16	
	Monosyllables	13	4	DNT	1	11	3
H	Patterns	20		17		22	
	Spondees	18		5		18	
	Monosyllables	12	3	DNT	2	12	3
I	Patterns	17		NA		NA	
	Spondees	13					
	Monosyllables	DNT	3				
J	Patterns	18		NA		NA	
	Spondees	17					
	Monosyllables	DNT	3				
K	Patterns	17		5		17	
	Spondees	13		DNT		14	
	Monosyllables	DNT	3	DNT	1	DNT	3
L	Patterns	17		2		17	
	Spondees	10		DNT		12	
	Monosyllables	DNT	3	DNT	1	DNT	3

* NA = Not applicable.
† DNT = Did not test.

TABLE 11–4
Visual Enhancement Scores of Successful Implant Users

Child	Condition	Pct. Lipreading Alone	Lipreading Plus			Pct. Enhancement		
			+IMP	+HA	BIN	IMP	HA	BIN
A	Monsen sentences	79						
	MAC sentences	22	62	NA	NA	40	NA	NA
B	MAC sentences	42	79	NA	NA	37	NA	NA
C	Craig sentences	100						
	Monsen sentences	76						
	MAC sentences	49	72	NA	NA	23	NA	NA
D	Craig words	85						
	Craig sentences	87						
	Monsen sentences	75						
	MAC sentences	70	100	66	94	30	−4	24
E	Craig words	100						
	Craig sentences	97						
	Monsen sentences	85						
	MAC sentences	79	98	NA	NA	19	NA	NA
F	Craig sentences	46	79	66	87	33	20	41
G	Craig words	66	91	DNT	88	25	DNT	22

H	Craig words	95						
	Craig sentences	83						
	Monsen sentences	53	63	62	62	10	9	9
I	Craig words	75						
	Craig sentences	41	66	NA	NA	25	NA	NA
J	Craig words	78						
	Craig sentences	83						
	Monsen sentences	75						
	MAC sentences	41	72	NA	NA	31	NA	NA
K	Craig words	48	73	73	70	25	25	22
L	Craig words	39	57	33	66	18	−6	27

cent for Subject K, with an average enhancement of 9 percent. Children L and F appear to be benefitting more from the implant and hearing aid together than from either device alone. Children K and H appear to be benefitting about equally from either device. Child D appears to be benefitting the most from his implant.

CHARACTERISTICS OF THE SUCCESSFUL IMPLANT USERS

Table 11-5 summarizes the characteristics of the 12 successful implant users who were tested at the House Ear Institute. The 7 children with speech perception abilities in category 4 are listed followed by those in category 3. These children ranged in age from Subject B, who was not quite 6 years old, to Subject H who was 10 years 6 months old. The age at onset of deafness ranged from 10 months to 3 years. None of these children was congenitally deaf. All of them had acquired their profound hearing loss as a result of meningitis.

Although it might be argued that some of these children were not prelingually deaf (e.g., Subjects C, D, E, and I), there was no sharp dichotomy between implant performance of early or late acquired deafness. Two children with the best speech perception through the implant, Subjects A and F, acquired deafness before 1 year of age, and one of the poorer implant users, Subject I, contracted meningitis at 2 years 11 months.

The next column lists the age at which the children were implanted. For the most part, all of these implants occurred before 6 years of age. The next column lists the time elapsed between loss of hearing and activation of an implant. This duration ranged from 5 months to 4 years 9 months. Although age at time of implantation does not appear to be related to performance, there is a tendency for children who were implanted within two years of the onset of deafness to perform somewhat better than those implanted after more than 2 years. Next, the amount of time each child had worn a cochlear implant is given. All of the children in this sample had used an implant for 3 years or longer.

One of the most striking differences between the seven category 4 children and the five category 3 children was that the top performers were enrolled in programs with an emphasis on speech training (oral or cued), while those performing in category 3 were all in total communication programs. Perhaps the potential for consistent word identification ability observed in category 4 children could only be realized with the intensive auditory training more typically provided in oral programs than in total communication programs.

TABLE 11–5
Characteristics of Successful Implant Users

Child	Category	Age	Age at Onset of Deafness	Age Implanted	Time Elapsed	Duration of Implant Use	Communication Mode
A	4	7–0	0–10	3–3	2–5	3–3	Oral
B	4	5–11	1–3	2–6	1–3	3–5	Oral
C	4	9–6	2–11	3–4	0–5	6–2	Oral
D	4	9–9	3–0	4–5	1–5	5–4	Oral
E	4	8–5	2–11	4–4	1–5	4–1	Oral
F	4	8–3	0–10	3–4	2–6	5–9	Cued speech
G	4	7–3	1–10	2–8	0–10	4–7	Oral
H	3	10–6	0–10	5–5	4–7	5–1	TC
I	3	9–6	2–11	4–7	1–8	4–11	TC
J	3	9–1	1–4	6–1	4–9	3–0	TC
K	3	6–9	1–2	3–2	2–0	3–7	TC
L	3	7–6	1–3	4–6	3–3	3–0	TC

CONCLUSION

The Early Speech Perception (ESP) Test Battery and the Visual Enhancement Battery described in this chapter provide a means of comparing and documenting benefits of assistive hearing devices for young children who are profoundly hearing impaired. The Low-Verbal Early Speech Perception battery permits this type of evaluation in children under 5 years of age.

Because many children who are profoundly hearing impaired derive considerable benefit from conventional hearing aids, these acoustic devices comprise the standard against which any new instrument must be compared. A tactile aid or cochlear implant may be considered beneficial for an individual child if the ability to perceive speech through audition alone or in combination with lipreading is improved significantly when compared with hearing aid performance.

Data presented in this chapter for children with conventional hearing aids suggests that, for the purposes of acquiring spoken language, significant improvement in speech perception through audition alone must exceed the ability to perceive durational patterns in speech. Thus, children whose aided performance is in speech perception categories 1 or 2 will derive significant spoken language benefits only from devices which can provide them with the ability to identify some words presented in a closed-set, thereby moving them to category 3. Data obtained from 12 of the most successful children implanted with the 3M/House single-channel implant indicates that improvement in word identification abilities of this magnitude were, indeed, obtained with the implant. However, all of these children were characterized by an etiology of early childhood meningitis and 3 or more years of implant use. There is not yet evidence that similar benefits are exhibited by the majority of children implanted with this device (Berliner & Eisenberg, 1987; Berliner, Eisenberg, & House, 1985). On the other hand, the proportion of implanted children who do achieve word identification ability with the single-channel implant appears to be increasing as the duration of implant use becomes longer. Data from Thielemeir and colleagues (1985) on the Discrimination After Training (DAT) test showed only 20 percent of the children demonstrating word identification ability through the implant compared to 5 percent through their hearing aids. More recent data reported by Berliner and Eisenberg (1987) showed 40 percent demonstrating word identification through the implant.

At the present time, very few children with category 3 or 4 word identification abilities through hearing aids have been implanted. Children who can use spectral cues to identify words with a hearing aid (categories 3 and 4) should not be considered candidates for an implant unless that device is likely to make it possible to boost their hearing capacity into the severely hearing impaired range. For children in category 3 with hearing aids, an effective device would permit them to obtain above chance scores on difficult closed-set tasks such as the Monosyllabic Word Identification Test or the Word Intelligibility by Picture Identification (Ross & Lerman, 1971). Children who are able to demonstrate category 4 speech perception scores with hearing aids should be considered implant candidates only if such a device would permit substantial open-set word recognition on a test such as the Kindergarten Phonetically Balanced Word List (Haskins, 1975).

Tests that are sensitive to subtle changes in speech perception skills will be needed to demonstrate benefits as more children experience longer periods of practice with their implants. In order to provide valid speech perception scores, such tests must reflect auditory abilities separate from linguistic abilities. The battery of tests described in this chapter is designed to insure that valid estimates of speech perception ability are obtained with children at the youngest possible age.

REFERENCES

Berliner, K. I., Eisenberg, L. S., & House, W. F. (Eds.). (1985). The cochlear implant: An auditory prosthesis for the profoundly deaf child. *Ear and Hearing, 6,* (Suppl.), 1S–69S.

Berliner, K. I., & Eisenberg, L. S. (1987). Our experience with cochlear implants: Have we erred in our expectations? *American Journal of Otology, 8,* 222–229.

Boothroyd, A. (1984). Auditory perception of speech contrasts by subjects with sensorineural hearing loss. *Journal of Speech and Hearing Research, 27,* 134–144.

Craig, W. M. (1975). *Craig Lipreading Test* (1964). Pittsburgh, PA: Western Pennsylvania School for the Deaf.

De Filippo, C. L., & Scott, B. L. (1978). A method for training and evaluating the reception of ongoing speech. *Journal of the Acoustical Society of America, 63,* 1186–1192.

Dunn, L. M. (1981). *Peabody Picture Vocabulary Test* (rev. ed.). Circle Pines, MN: American Guidance Service.

Eisenberg, L. S. (1985). Perceptual capabilities with the cochlear implant: Implications for aural rehabilitation. *Ear and Hearing, 6* (Suppl.), 60S–69S.

Erber, N. P. (1980). Use of the auditory numbers test to evaluate speech perception ability of hearing-impaired children. *Journal of Speech and Hearing Research, 17,* 194–202.

Erber, N. P. (1982). *Auditory training.* Washington, DC: Alexander Graham Bell Association for the Deaf.

Erber, N. P., & Alencewicz, C. M. (1976). Audiologic evaluation of deaf children. *Journal of Speech and Hearing Disorders, 41,* 256–267.

Geers, A. E., & Moog, J. S. (1987). Predicting spoken language acquisition of profoundly hearing-impaired children. *Journal of Speech and Hearing Disorders, 52,* 84–94.

Geers, A. E., & Moog, J. S. (1988). Predicting long-term benefits from single-channel cochlear implants in profoundly hearing-impaired children. *American Journal of Otology, 9,* 169–176.

Gittleman, D., & Popelka, G. (1987). The dynamic range configruation audiogram. *Volta Review, 89,* 69–83.

Haskins, H. L. (1972). Kindergarten PB Word Lists. In H. A. Newby, *Audiology* (3rd ed., pp. 404–405). New York: Appleton-Century-Crofts.

Los Angeles County. Office of the Los Angeles County Superintendent of Schools. Audiologic Services, and Southwest School for the Hearing Impaired. (1980). *Test of Auditory Comprehension.* North Hollywood, CA: Foreworks.

Monsen, R. B. (1981). A usable test for the speech intelligibility of deaf talkers. *American Annals of the Deaf, 126,* 845–852.

Moog, J. S. (1988). *The CID Phonetic Inventory.* St. Louis, MO: Central Institute for the Deaf.

Moog, J. S. & Geers, A. E. (1985). EPIC: A program to accelerate academic progress in profoundly hearing impaired children. *Volta Review, 87,* 259–277.

Owens, E., Kessler, D. K., Raggio, M. W., & Schubert, E. D. (1985). Analysis and Revision of the Minimal Auditory Capabilities (MAC) Battery. *Ear and Hearing, 6,* 280–290.

Ross, M., & Lerman, J. (1971). *Word intelligibility by picture identification.* Pittsburgh, PA: Stanwix House, Inc.

Thielemeir, M. A. (1982). *Discrimination After Training Test.* Los Angeles: House Ear Institute.

Thielemeir, M. A., Tonokawa, L. L., Petersen, B., & Eisenberg, L. S. (1985). Audiological results in children with a cochlear implant. *Ear and Hearing, 6* (Suppl.), 27S–35S.

M A R Y   J O E   O S B E R G E R

Speech Production in Profoundly Hearing-Impaired Children with Reference to Cochlear Implants

T he purpose of this chapter is to describe the characteristics of the speech of children who are profoundly hearing-impaired, to discuss the factors that affect its development, and to present preliminary data on the speech of implanted children. A question that might be raised by some individuals not familiar with this population is "Why study the speech production skills of children who use a cochlear implant?" It would seem that the most direct way to determine benefit from an auditory prosthesis is to measure the child's perceptual abilities. Deafness, however, also affects the ability of the child to acquire intelligible speech. Thus, an auditory prosthesis must serve as an aid for production as well as perception. Indeed, a major purpose of any auditory prosthesis is to assist the profoundly hearing-impaired child in developing intelligible speech. The need for access to auditory information for speech production is not restricted to children with prelingual deafness. Binnie, Daniloff, and Buckingham (1982) and Plant (1982) have shown rapid deterioration of certain features of speech in children who are classified as *postlingually deaf.* Thus, the speech production skills of all implanted children, including adolescents, must be examined in order to obtain a comprehensive view of the benefits of cochlear implants.

The largest body of data on the speech of children who are profoundly hearing-impaired has been gathered on children who use hearing aids. Much of this information is relevant in evaluating the speech of children who use a cochlear implant. In this chapter, research findings on the speech production skills of children with hearing aids will be reviewed. Preliminary data on the speech production skills of implanted children will then be presented.

Speech Characteristics of Hearing-Impaired Children Who Use Hearing Aids

The majority of data have been collected on speech samples subjected to phonetic transcription and subsequent error analyses. Only a brief review of this literature will be provided (see Osberger & McGarr, 1982, for a comprehensive overview) in terms of segmental and suprasegmental patterns and intelligibility.

Segmental Errors

The type of vowel and consonant errors that occur in the speech of children who are profoundly hearing-impaired reflects an inability to execute the rapid and coordinated articulatory gestures characteristic of normally produced speech. The most common vowel error is neutralization (e.g., /ʌ/ as in cup and /ə/ as in about) which results from inadequate tongue movement (Monsen, 1978). Achieving correct vowel targets is difficult for profoundly hearing-impaired children because one of the primary acoustic cues that differentiates the vowels occurs in the frequency region where most of these children have little or no residual hearing (i.e., above 2000 Hz). Also, the tongue movements associated with vowels are relatively invisible and a speaker receives negligible tactile–kinesthetic feedback from these sounds.

The most common consonant error is omission of word-final sounds (Smith, 1975). Substitution errors involving manner of articulation also are frequent. These errors typically result because the speaker is unable to coordinate the sequence of articulatory gestures needed to effect the distinctions. Common errors in this category involve confusion between voiced and voiceless cognates or substitution of a consonant with the same place of production as the intended consonant (Smith, 1975). A typical substitution error of this type is production of a stop consonant for a fricative (e.g., /p/ for /f/) or substitution of an oral sound for a nasal one (e.g., /b/ for /m/).

It has been shown that the degree of hearing loss has a greater effect on the frequency of errors than on the type of errors in the speech of the hearing impaired (Gold, 1980); that is, as the hearing loss increases, the frequency of errors increases but the type of errors made remains unchanged. An exception is the frequent use of glottal stops by children who are profoundly deaf, but not by children with moderate or severe hearing losses (Levitt & Stromberg, 1983). One explanation for this may be that the child receives tactile–kinesthetic feedback when producing the glottal stop and this may be the most reinforcing feedback available. Binnie and colleagues (1982) noted that changes in the speech of a 5-year-old, who suffered sudden deafness from meningitis, appeared to reflect the child's attempts to maximize interoceptive feedback and to slow the rate of movement to maintain articulatory control. Use of glottal stops has been shown to have a detrimental effect on overall intelligibility (Levitt & Stromberg, 1983). The presence of this error suggests that the child does not have adequate control of basic phonatory processes. If this is the case, then it is likely that many features of the child's speech will be distorted. Clinical observations by Osberger and her associates suggest that frequent use of glottal stops is characteristic of the speech of children who are implant candidates, especially those with congenital loss.

SUPRASEGMENTAL ERRORS

Suprasegmental errors involve the characteristics of speech that extend over units composed of more than one phonetic segment. Prolongation of speech segments often occurs, resulting in slow or labored speech that, in turn, distorts the rhythm of the utterance and causes segmental errors (Osberger & McGarr, 1983). Children who are hearing-impaired have been shown to distort the relationship between vowel duration and the voicing characteristic of the following consonant (Monsen, 1974). Also, the proportional shortening of unstressed vowels and syllables relative to stressed ones is smaller, on the average, in the speech of children who are hearing-impaired than in the speech of children with normal hearing (Osberger & McGarr, 1983). Another manifestation of poor timing control is the reduced coarticulation between speech sounds. It appears that children who are profoundly hearing-impaired learn to produce the phonemes of English as invariant targets rather than as segments that vary with phonetic context.

Intonation and pitch problems are frequent in the speech of the hearing-impaired and reflect poor control and coordination of laryngeal and phonatory processes (McGarr & Osberger, 1978). Common problems are insufficient variation in fundamental frequency ($f0$) throughout an utterance resulting in a restricted $f0$ range, excessive and inappropriate variations in $f0$, and failure to produce a fall in pitch at the end of a phrase.

The works of Binnie, Daniloff, and Buckingham (1982) and Leder and colleagues (1986) supported clinical observations by Osberger and associates of deviations in segment duration and fundamental frequency in the speech of children and adults with acquired deafness who are implant candidates. Because these individuals have little or no access to acoustic speech information via their hearing, they lose the ongoing auditory feedback necessary to preserve these features of speech. Leder and associates (1986) show improvement in control of fundamental frequency in a postlingually deafened adult after regaining access to auditory speech information via a cochlear implant. Furthermore, the difficulty that children who are congenitally deaf demonstrate in acquiring normal control of duration and pitch indicates that auditory feedback is necessary to develop these features of speech, and that the amount of residual hearing needed for this development is greater than that possessed by children whose losses exceed 90 dB HL. Because control of fundamental frequency and timing appear to require auditory feedback, any changes noted in these aspects of speech following implantation presumably would be due to the auditory information received from the device. Analysis of these features of speech pre- and postimplant should provide data that will permit evaluation of a cochlear implant in promoting the development and maintenance of speech skills.

INTELLIGIBILITY

The intelligibility of a profoundly hearing-impaired child's speech will be affected by the number of segmental errors present as well as the type of errors that occur. Segmental errors that have been found to have a negative effect on intelligibility are omission of phonemes in the word-initial position, consonant substitutions involving a change in the manner of articulation, substitutions of nonEnglish phonemes such as the glottal stop, and unidentifiable or gross distortions of the intended phoneme (Levitt & Stromberg, 1983). At the suprasegmental level, errors resulting in an incorrect temporal relationship between stressed and unstressed syllables and errors involving poor phonatory control have been found to have a negative effect on intelligibility (Osberger & Levitt, 1979; Smith, 1975).

The largest body of data on the intelligibility of hearing-impaired children's speech is based on a procedure that requires a panel of listeners to write down what they think the child has said. The samples are then scored for the percentage of words understood by the listeners. Assessing intelligibility in this manner requires that the child be able to read (or imitate) short phrases. Even though a substantial effort is required to obtain the intelligibility data with a write-down procedure, information suggests that this approach is more valid and reliable than other procedures, such as rating scales (Samar & Metz, in press) that take less time to administer and score. The average intelligibility of the speech of profoundly hearing-impaired children to listeners who are unfamiliar with this population has been reported to be about 20 percent (Smith, 1975), whereas the intelligibility of the speech of children who are hard-of-hearing is 70 percent or higher (Gold, 1980). In addition to the speaking proficiency of the talker, intelligibility is affected by the complexity of the word (e.g., polysyllabic words) and articulatory targets (e.g., consonant clusters) (Monsen, 1983). Monsen also observed an interaction between a listener's prior experience in hearing the speech of the deaf and the degree of intelligibility of talkers, listener experience having the greatest effect on the scores of the least intelligible talkers. McGarr (1983) found that experienced listeners always assigned higher scores than did the inexperienced ones. Other factors found to affect intelligibility scores are repetition of the utterance, presence of linguistic context, and the ability of the listener to see as well as hear the speech of the deaf talker (Monsen, 1983). All of these factors need to be taken into consideration when assessing the speech intelligibility of children with implants. The reader is referred to Carney (1986) for a more thorough review of this topic.

FACTORS AFFECTING SPEECH DEVELOPMENT IN HEARING-IMPAIRED CHILDREN WITH HEARING AIDS

DEGREE OF HEARING LOSS

Previous research has revealed a seemingly simple relationship between hearing level and speech intelligibility in the hearing impaired. All things being equal, the greater the hearing loss, the more unintelligible the speech will be (Boothroyd, 1969; Monsen, 1978; Smith, 1975). An exception to this trend has been reported for children with profound hearing losses, in which there is no clear-cut relationship between hearing level and intelligibility (Monsen, 1978; Smith, 1975). This situation is reflected in the common observation that some deaf children develop intelligible speech whereas others do not.

The reason for the breakdown in the relationship between production and perception skills in children who are profoundly hearing-impaired has eluded researchers and clinicians for many years. The divergent speech production skills of these children (PTA 90 dB HL or greater) seems less of a mystery when research on their auditory capabilities is examined. The work of Boothroyd and Cawkwell (1970) first suggested that some children might be responding vibrotactually to auditory stimuli. Later research by Erber (1972a, 1972b) contributed significantly in identifying which children are "feelers" and which ones actually hear the stimuli. If a child does not possess residual hearing, then perception will be limited to the time-intensity cues that can be felt. These cues are inadequate for speech understanding. In contrast, children who do possess a certain amount of residual hearing should be able to understand some speech through auditory cues because they can discriminate spectral changes in the acoustic signal.

The recent work of Boothroyd (1984; see also Chapter 6) has delineated further the auditory capabilities of children with profound hearing losses. Boothroyd found that children with losses as great as 105 dB HL were able to identify aspects of speech that required some discrimination of spectral cues. In contrast, the features of speech identified by children with losses greater than 105 dB HL were limited to those that could be made on the basis of time-intensity patterns (i.e., syllabic number and vowel height). Boothroyd also noted a significant difference in the mean intelligibility between subjects with hearing losses of 105 to 114 dB HL and those with losses in excess of 114 dB HL. Data reported by Levitt, McGarr, and Geffner (1987) substantiate this finding.

Even though differentiation between "hearers" and "feelers" cannot be predicted from hearing level alone, clinical and research observations suggest that thresholds at or near the audiometric limits in the low frequencies with no measurable hearing above 1000 Hz are highly suggestive of vibrotactile rather than auditory responses. This is because the skin acts as a low-pass filter and is not sensitive to frequencies above this range (see Chapter 7).

Keeping in mind the divergent auditory capabilities of children classified as profoundly hearing impaired, it seems reasonable to assume that those children who obtained the most reduced speech intelligibility scores in previous studies might have been "feelers" rather than "hearers." Evidence for this notion can be found by examining the speech performance of individual subjects in some of these studies. Using the criterion of no response to pure-tones above 1000 Hz, examination of the individual data in Smith's classic study (1972) show that of the 20 children with the highest intelligibility scores (i.e., those in quartiles 1 and 2), 60 percent had measurable hearing above 1000 Hz. In contrast, only 25 percent of the 20 children with the poorest intelligibility (i.e., those in quartiles 3 and 4) had measurable hearing above 1000 Hz. The difference between subjects in terms of high frequency hearing and speech intelligibility might have been even more striking had the audiometric limits used by Smith exceeded 110 dB HL.

The discussion of the relationship between hearing level and speech is incomplete without addressing the relationship between perception and production skills. The relationship is a complex one that is not completely understood in normally developing children. It is known, however, that perception and production are not simply different sides of the same coin and, as a consequence, production skills cannot simply be inferred from perception skills.

Smith (1975) found that deaf children's performance on a phoneme recognition test was more highly correlated with intelligibility than with hearing level. Stark and Levitt (1974), examining production and perception of selected suprasegmental contrasts in children who are profoundly hearing-impaired, found that those who scored high on the perception test did not necessarily score well on the production test. Children who did well on the production test, however, always scored at an average-to-above-average level on the perception test. Thus, good perceivers did not always turn out to be good producers, but good producers were almost always good perceivers.

Investigators have made little attempt to compare directly the relationship between the perception and production skills of implanted children. Identification of speech features perceived and produced correctly demonstrates the effectiveness of the aid in promoting speech development. However, some features of speech might be perceived but not produced correctly. For example, a child might be able to distinguish a voiced from a voiceless stop in a perception task, but might not be able to execute the rapid and coordinated articulatory gestures necessary to effect the voiced–voiceless distinction. Information of this type will help to identify features of speech that might require additional forms of sensory information (e.g., from a visual display) for learning to occur.

It is also important to keep in mind that procedures used to assess perception skills may not reveal how well the child who is profoundly hearing-impaired is able to make use of acoustic information in everyday situations to learn speech. For example, a common observation is the inability of children who are profoundly hearing-impaired to perform successfully on auditory speech tasks when the stimuli are presented in a recorded format via loudspeaker. Presentation of the same stimuli in a face-to-face setting (with visual cues removed) often produces successful performance. Furthermore, some children may discriminate auditory changes in the speech signal but fail to pair the perceived changes with their associated features. It is conceivable that some of these children can learn to talk by combining and pairing acoustic and visual cues.

AGE AT ONSET OF DEAFNESS

Most of the information on the speech of deaf children has been obtained from children with congenital hearing losses. Relatively little is known about the effects of sudden deafness on maintaining previously acquired skills or developing new ones. This is unfortunate because most of the children who have received a cochlear implant have an acquired deafness. This also presents a problem in evaluating the effect of cochlear implant use on speech production.

A further complication is the use of the terms *prelingual* and *postlingual* with respect to age of onset of deafness. This binary classification implies that there is a definable age at which speech development is complete. Even though a child has developed phonetically correct and intelligible speech during early childhood, refinements in speech motor control apparently continue to at least adolescence (Kent, 1976, 1981). The immature status of the child's speech production system is demonstrated by the relatively rapid deterioration that occurs in the speech of children with acquired deafness, even though the onset occurred as late as 5 years of age (Binnie, Daniloff, & Buckingham, 1982; Plant, 1984). When the deafness occurs during the first 3 or 4 years of life, it not only disrupts development but appears to result in regression to an earlier stage of development (Stoel-Gammon & Otomo, 1986). This regression has been observed by Osberger and her associates in children at the time they are evaluated for an implant. Some of them who lost their hearing before age 3 are able to produce few recognizable sounds of English or intelligible words even after 1 or more years of intensive training.

It is not clear whether some features of speech are more susceptible to deterioration than others. Recent data (Levitt, McGarr, & Geffner, 1987) revealed higher speech intelligibility scores for postlingually than for prelingually deaf children having the same degree of hearing loss. Experience with implant candidates, on the other hand, has shown little difference between the speech skills of children with congenital or acquired deafness during the first 3 years of life. The age of onset of the hearing loss for the postlingually deaf subjects in the study by Levitt, McGarr, and Geffner (1987) is not stated.

RATE OF ACQUISITION OF SPEECH

Relatively little is known about the rate of acquisition of speech skills in profoundly hearing-impaired children, the effectiveness of training in improving speech production skills, or the length of time required to correct specific types of errors. A longitudinal study of the speech skills of 80 deaf children in state-supported schools for the deaf in New York State revealed no significant change in segmental production or intelligibility during a 4-year period (McGarr, 1987). Several studies have shown improvement in production of vowels (Monsen & Shaughnessy, 1978; Osberger, 1987) and selected nonsegmental features of speech with training (Osberger et al., 1978; Osberger, 1983) in children who are profoundly deaf. This group of studies has also shown that the rate and extent of improvement varies considerably among children even when they are exposed to the same kind of training. Moreover, only limited improvement occurs in speech production skills after about 12 years of age (Boothroyd, 1985a; Osberger, 1986). The importance of residual hearing in learning to talk is highlighted by the data of Boothroyd (1985b) which indicated that 5 dB of hearing is worth 1.5 years of instruction in terms of the influence on speech intelligibility.

In summary, although a large body of data has been gathered on the speech production abilities of hearing-impaired children with hearing aids, there appears to have been no systematic investigation of the differences in the production patterns between children who have residual hearing and those who do not. Information on the speech production abilities of "nonauditory" children must be extracted from other studies in which they have been included as part of the subject pool with children who are profoundly hearing-impaired who do have residual hearing. Unfortunately, it has not been until the advent of implants that attention has been focused on this subgroup of profoundly hearing-impaired children (i.e., those who have no residual hearing). In fact, there exists no body of data to which the performance of subjects before or after implantation might be compared. Changes in speech production abilities following implantation are determined by using wihin-subject analyses. The problem with this approach is the difficulty in determining the significance of the changes in an individual child's speech after implantation relative to an unimplanted child. As a consequence, it is difficult to establish whether and to what degree the child has improved with the device. Because of this situation, baseline data on the production abilities of nonauditory children are being gathered by Osberger and her associates while simultaneously attempting to determine the effectiveness of a device in improving these skills.

PRELIMINARY FINDINGS ON THE SPEECH SKILLS OF CHILDREN WITH COCHLEAR IMPLANTS

The data to be reported have been obtained through collaborative research by the author and the staff of the cochlear implant team at the

Indiana University School of Medicine in Indianapolis. The team is directed by Richard T. Miyamoto, M.D. and consists of professionals in the areas of audiology, speech-language pathology, and psychology. This group began implant work with children in 1983, using the 3M/House single-channel device. Currently, the Indiana team is also evaluating the speech skills of children who have received the Nucleus 22-channel device, but data with this implant system are limited at this time.

It is important to note that the children who have received an implant were nonauditory. They typically demonstrated neither unaided nor aided responses to pure tones, or they responded only to low frequency sound at high levels. Preoperatively, all of the children were in educational settings in which aural/oral training was provided. Postimplant, the children return to their previous educational placements and continue intensive auditory training. Thus, although the ongoing therapy varies and consistency in method is not maintained from child to child, emphasis is placed on aural/oral training for each of the children. In addition, during the first year postimplant, the children return to the implant center once a month for a day of intensive, directed therapy. This training, totaling approximately 40 hours, stresses global communication techniques and does not specifically concentrate on speech production.

The initial challenge in evaluating the speech of the implanted children was the need to develop protocols that would permit a fine-grained analysis of the changes that might occur in the children's speech over time. In particular, the necessity of a new approach to assess the speech of children with the most limited production abilities was acute. For the most part, these were preschool or young school-age children who did not read. The procedures developed for use with these children are referred to as Protocol One, whereas the procedures used for the older children or children with better speech skills are referred to as Protocol Two. Preliminary data are reported for both protocols.

PROTOCOL ONE

A number of samples obtained from children with the most reduced speech skills demonstrated that procedures typically used to assess the speech of profoundly hearing-impaired children were not adequate to describe the characteristics of their speech. The speech of these young children, even after 2 or 3 years of intensive training, consisted of isolated sounds or single-syllable utterances with an extremely limited phonetic repertoire. There was no evidence of consonant vowel (CV) strings or anything resembling babbling behavior. Although many of their utterances had a vocalic quality, no identifiable vowel sound could be assigned to what was heard. The children used inappropriate vocal gestures that were not tied to any communicative intent (e.g., strings of glottal stops) or inappropriate gestures for intended sounds (e.g., lip smacking). Also, inappropriate articulatory gestures, such as exaggerated mouth and jaw opening, were used without phonating. Whereas some of these gestures are used by deaf children who do have residual hearing, they constituted a major part of the nonauditory children's speech behavior. Improvement in speech production in these children was viewed as consisting of the elimination of undesirable vocal and articulatory gestures as well as the development of the sounds of English. It was also hypothesized that the emergence of phonemes might be preceded by an increase in "speechlike" sounds that gradually would assume more of the aspects characteristic of intelligible speech.

To describe adequately the changes in these children's speech, a scheme of analysis based on that used to study the speech of normally developing infants was adapted (Kent & Murray, 1982). A speech sample, elicited from the child during a play situation, is video- and audio-recorded and subsequently analyzed by two listeners who classify independently the child's utterances as *speech, speechlike,* or *nonspeech.* Utterances classified as *speech* are recognizable phonemes of English or reasonable approximations of phonemes. *Nonspeech* sounds are those that do not at all represent speech sounds (e.g., grunts, growls). All other sounds are classified as *speechlike.* A broad definition has been used to describe the sounds in the speechlike-category to avoid excluding utterances that might represent precursors of recognizable phonetic elements. A category referred to as *other* denotes articulatory behaviors that should be eliminated from the child's productions (e.g., lip smacking). These data are then analyzed to determine the relative frequency of occurrence of each category type over time. Ultimately, acoustic analyses will be performed on the speech and speechlike tokens to obtain a finer grained analysis of changes in the children's speech.

Table 12–1 summarizes the characteristics of a group of children's preimplant speech using the classification scheme described above. The age of onset of deafness for these children ranged from birth to 2 years 9 months. The four children in Group 1 were born deaf; the age of onset of deafness for the two children in Group 2 was 16 months; and the two children in Group 3 experienced later onset of deafness, one at age 2 years and the other at 2 years 9 months. The most striking feature of the data is the similarity among the speech of the children irrespective of age of onset. The two children who lost their hearing after 2 years of age (Group 3) produced slightly more speech and speechlike sounds than did the children with losses of earlier onset, but the difference was small.

TABLE 12-1

Frequency of Occurrence of Percent in Four Categories of Vocalizations for Children Grouped According to Age at Onset of Deafness

Age at Onset	Speech	Speechlike	Nonspeech	Other
Group 1* (n = 4)	32	38	11	10
Group 2† (n = 2)	35	36	15	16
Group 3‡ (n = 2)	42	46	2	10

* Age at onset: birth.

† Age at onset: 16 months.

‡ Age at onset: 2 years and 2 years 9 months.

The greatest difference between the children with later onset of deafness (Group 3) and earlier onset (Groups 1 and 2) was in the use of nonspeech vocalizations. The children with later onset of deafness, however, did use inappropriate articulatory gestures, indicated by the *other* category.

These data show the dramatic impact that the sudden loss of auditory feedback has on speech development in young children. Not only is development arrested, but the child's speech behavior shows regression. The regression does not result in vocal behaviors comparable to those of younger children with normal hearing, but rather to those of their peers who are congenitally deaf with no residual hearing. It appears that the effect of some period of normal auditory experience is not reflected in the speech abilities of the children with acquired deafness prior to implantation. Because of prior auditory experience and retention of some minimal degree of auditory memory, it is hypothesized that the speech skills of children with acquired deafness will ultimately exceed those of their congenitally deaf peers once these children are again given access to acoustic speech information via a cochlear implant. Speculation about the extent or rate of their speech improvement is not possible.

Figure 12-1 shows the longitudinal data from preimplant to 3 years postimplant for one child. This subject was congenitally deaf due to Mondini malformation of the inner ear. He received the 3M/House single-channel implant at age 4 after being followed by the team at Indiana University School of Medicine for over 1-and-a-half years. His loss was identified during the second year of life, and, since that time, he has been enrolled in a cued speech program with heavy emphasis on the develop-

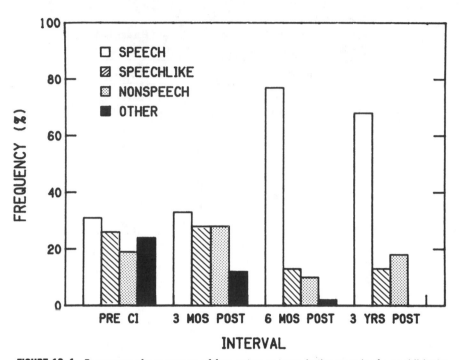

FIGURE 12-1. Frequency of occurrence of four category-types in the speech of one child who is totally deaf before receiving a single-channel implant and at three intervals postimplant.

ment of oral communication skills. The preimplant data reflect his level of performance after approximately 2-and-one-half years of intensive oral training with conventional hearing aids. A 6-minute sample of speech was analyzed at each test interval.

The data in Figure 12-1 show a fairly equal distribution of all 4 types of categories in his speech prior to receiving the implant. Only about 30 percent of the tokens at this time could be classified as sounding like speech. The number of different types of speech sounds that he used were extremely limited, as shown by the summary of his phonetic repertoire in Table 12-2. In particular, the behaviors classified as *other* were distracting when he was engaged in a communicative situation in that he often substituted lip-smacks for vocalizations.

There is negligible change in his speech 3 months following surgery, except for a reduction in the frequency of occurrence of the behaviors in the *other* category. Six months postsurgery, however, there is a dramatic increase in the number of vocalizations categorized as speech and a reduction in the number of other types of sounds. Unfortunately, record-

TABLE 12-2

Summary of Phonetic Repertoire in the Pre- and Postimplant
Conditions for One Subject

Preimplant		3 Years Postimplant	
Phoneme	**Number of Occurrences**	**Phoneme**	**Number of Occurrences**
b	4	n	39
m	4	d	29
n	1	b	27
d	1	p	20
ə	20	m	14
i	3	h	8
		j	8
		r	7
		f	4
		t	3
		v	2
		d	1
		w	1
		ə	57
		a	18
		æ	11
		ɛ	10
		aU	3
		aI	3
		i	3
		u	2

ings of his speech between 6 months and 3 years postimplant are not available. The data obtained 3 years postimplant continue to show that the majority of the sounds that he makes can be recognized as phonemes of English. Note, however, the continued presence of *speechlike* and *nonspeech* sounds in his vocalizations. The use of other inappropriate articulatory gestures appears to have been eliminated from his speech.

A summary of his phonetic repertoire at 3-years postimplant appears in Table 12-2. There has been a tremendous increase in the number of different consonants and vowels in his speech, but an obvious absence of continuant sounds. Frequent use of the schwa vowel (/ə/), both pre- and postimplant, is characteristic of the speech of all children who are profoundly hearing-impaired.

To date, longitudinal data has been obtained for only a few children. Not all of the subjects show the dramatic change in their speech in the relatively short period of time that this child did, and the changes appear to be highly individualized, not lending themselves to group analysis. Some of the observed changes include an increase in frequency of speech sounds with a more limited increase in phonetic repertoire or change in type of syllable (e.g., vowel (V), vowel-consonant (VC), consonant-vowel (CV), and so forth). The latter is reflected in the use of CV-syllable strings and consonant-vowel-consonant (CVC) monosyllabic words rather than isolated vowels or consonant-vowel combinations.

PROTOCOL TWO

A range of procedures is used to assess the speech production skills of more intelligible talkers. Data from only one of these measures, the Speech Pattern Contrast (SPAC) test, will be presented. Developed by Boothroyd (1985a; see also Chapter 6), the purpose of this test is to examine the ability of speakers to convey phonetic contrasts to listeners using a forced-choice response task. The test consists of monosyllabic words that the child, provided with a visual and auditory sample, produces on an imitative basis. This format is used to maintain uniformity in eliciting samples across children because not all of them can read the stimulus words. In obtaining a sample of each child's best speech, it is desirable to control the elicitation process.

The recorded speech samples are digitized, randomized, and played to a panel of three judges who must decide which word among a four-word set the child has produced. The four response-alternatives provide the possibility of independent errors along two phonetic contrasts (chance performance for each dimension is 50 percent). Four subtests are used to evaluate the following contrasts: vowel height, vowel place, initial consonant voicing, initial consonant continuance (i.e., stop versus fricative), initial consonant place, final consonant voicing, final consonant continuance, and final consonant place. The listener responses are scored in terms of the percentage of time that a contrast is perceived correctly. Alternatively, the scores can be viewed as the percentage of time that a child is able to convey correctly a particular contrast to the listeners. The scores reported here are based on each child's production of six words, each in a four-choice set containing the targeted contrasts. Scores have been averaged across the three judges and across word position (i.e., initial and final) for the contrasts.

Before presenting data on the performance of the implanted children, data will be presented for one nonauditory child at two intervals following the onset of deafness at age 6 years 10 months as the result of meningitis. This child obtained no responses to pure tones under earphones or in the sound-field with powerful hearing aids. The time of

TABLE 12–3
SPAC Production Scores in Percent Obtained by One Subject at Two Intervals After the Onset of Deafness at 6 Years 10 Months of Age*

Contrast	8 Months Post-Onset	11 Months Post-Onset
Vowel height	98	99
Vowel place	95	88
Voicing	74	67
Continuance	91	90
Place	95	85

* Chance performance = 50 percent.

onset is one that many professionals might label *postlingual*. The data in Table 12–3, however, suggests otherwise. The first set of data was obtained 8 months post-onset, and the second set was collected 3 months later. Scores have been averaged across the word-initial and word-final positions for each of the three consonant contrasts. A striking finding is the rapid deterioration in the child's ability to convey the voicing contrast to listeners. Her ability to convey vowel place and consonant place also appears to be deteriorating as evidenced by the decreased scores for these contrasts 11 months post-onset. The dramatic effect that the loss of auditory feedback has had on her ability to produce a distinction between voiced and voiceless phonemes implies that maintenance of this feature requires some access to the acoustic speech signal. This is not surprising because there are essentially no visual or tactile–kinesthetic cues that a speaker can use for feedback. The voiced–voiceless confusion occurs frequently in the speech of children who are congenitally deaf and has been found to have a significant negative effect on overall speech intelligibility.

Table 12–4 shows three more sets of SPAC data. The first column lists the scores obtained by Boothroyd (1985a) at the time when the SPAC items were produced by a group of 16 deaf children between the ages of 13 to 19 years who wear hearing aids. Better ear pure-tone thresholds (3-frequency average) ranged from 82 dB HL to 110 dB HL, with a median of 102 dB HL. The age of onset is not reported by Boothroyd, but presumably the losses were congenital or of early onset. These data are representative of the performance of profoundly hearing-impaired children who have residual hearing and benefit from hearing aids. The other two columns show the data for two subjects with congenital deafness,

TABLE 12–4
SPAC Production Scores in Percent Obtained by a
Range of Children with Congenital Deafness*

Contrast	Boothroyd†	LD	RG
Vowel height	88	73	47
Vowel place	87	62	47
Voicing	41	54	58
Continuance	59	63	60
Place	64	64	64

* Chance performance = 50 percent.
† Mean for 16 children, aged 13 to 19 years, with hearing aids. Adapted from Boothroyd, A. (1985). Evaluation of speech production of the hearing impaired: Some benefits of forced choice testing. *Journal of Speech and Hearing Research, 28,* 185–196.

neither of whom receives benefit from conventional amplification. The difference between their performance and that of the subjects in Boothroyd's study reflects the impact of the lack of access to acoustic speech information on the production of the speech contrasts under study. Both of these subjects were 11 years old. Presumably the characteristics of each child's speech have been developed via visual or tactile-kinesthetic feedback. Since these data were collected, subject LD has been fitted with a vibrotactile aid (the Tactaid II) and subject RG has received a Nucleus 22-channel cochlear implant.

The data in Table 12–4 demonstrate two important findings. First, note the superior ability of the subjects in Boothroyd's study to convey vowel contrasts to the listeners, suggesting that some degree of residual hearing is necessary to develop these contrasts. This should not imply that the vowels produced by the subjects sound normal, but only that they were able to convey the front–back and high–low distinction to listeners. The importance of residual hearing in learning the high–low and front–back contrasts is highlighted by the reduced scores obtained by RG. This also is not an unexpected in view of the relative invisibility of articulatory gestures used to produce vowels.

The second striking finding is the similarity among the scores for all subjects on the consonant contrasts. All subjects scored at little better than chance. In this case, the presence of residual hearing does not appear to provide the congenitally hearing-impaired talkers an advantage in learning to produce these consonant features.

TABLE 12–5
SPAC Production Scores in Percent Obtained by Two Implant Users with Deafness of Early Onset*

Contrast	DP		SM
	2 Yrs Post	2 Yrs 5 Mos Post	2 Yrs Post
Vowel height	67	88	73
Vowel place	65	75	70
Voicing	49	59	70
Continuance	69	69	60
Place	76	81	50

* Chance performance = 50 percent.

The data in Table 12–5 show SPAC scores obtained by two subjects who use the 3M/House single-channel implant. Subject DP was 16 years old when she received her implant. She had been deaf for approximately 15 years due to meningitis, which she contracted around 10 months of age. The onset of subject SM's loss was also at 10 months of age, but she was only 13 when she received her device. Recordings were obtained from DP at 2 and 2 years 5 months postimplant. Because there is no pre-implant data for these subjects, the data reported in Table 12–4 will be used to infer the effect of implant use on their speech. There is a noticeable increase in DP's ability to convey vowel-height and vowel-place information over time. In particular, the score that she obtained on the vowel-height contrast is similar to that of her peers with residual hearing and substantially better than that of her nonauditory peers (i.e., LD and RG). There is an obvious improvement in her ability to convey consonant-place information. Note the score that she achieved on this feature (81 percent) is substantially higher (1 percent) than that of her peers who have residual hearing as well as those who do not. Considering the change in her speech between the first and second administration of the SPAC, and assuming that here scores were similar to those of LD and RG prior to implantation, the data shown in Table 12–5 indicate that the use of the implant had a direct effect on improving her ability to convey the contrasts of vowel height, vowel place, and consonant place of production. This improvement is quite remarkable when age of onset of deafness and length of deprivation of acoustic speech information are considered. Recall that previous research has shown little, if any, change in speech development in profoundly hearing-impaired children once they reach adolescence (Boothroyd, 1985b).

It is difficult to offer the same conclusions regarding the speech of subject SM. It appears that the voicing contrast might have been improved since obtaining the implant. The score that SM achieved on this contrast (70 percent) is higher than that of her profoundly hearing-impaired peers. It is unlikely that she would have received a score of 70 percent on this subtest before implantation, especially when recalling the rapid deterioration of this feature in the speech of the subject whose onset of deafness occurred when she was almost 7 years old (see Table 12–3).

Table 12–6 provides SPAC production data for two totally deaf subjects, both of whom lost their hearing at 18 months of age. TA is 12 years old and BC is 14. At the time that BC was tested, he had been using the 3M/House implant for approximately 3 years. TA's scores in Table 12–6 were obtained in the unaided condition, although he has since been fitted with a vibrotactile aid. Because preimplant SPAC data for BC is lacking, the performance of TA, a nonauditory child, will be used to infer the status of BC's speech prior to receiving his implant. Comparing the two columns of data, only minimal differences are observed for all features except for consonant continuance and place. BC was able to produce these features substantially better than TA. Assuming that BC's speech was similar to TA's prior to implantation, his superior performance on the continuance and place features is most likely due to the use of the implant. Production of the place feature might have been enhanced by the use of both auditory and visual cues in the elicitation of the speech samples. However, it seems improbable that the ability to produce this

TABLE 12–6

SPAC Production Scores in Percent Obtained by Two Subjects with Onset of Deafness at 18 Months of Age. One Subject (BC) is an Implant User Whose Data were Obtained 3 Years Postimplant. The Other Subject (TA) is Nonauditory

Contrast	TA	BC
Vowel height	72	61
Vowel place	73	73
Voicing	47	56
Continuance	51	72
Place	60	82

* Chance performance = 50 percent.

feature is due strictly to the use of visual cues. If this were true, then this feature should be conveyed equally as well by the nonauditory subjects (i.e., TA, LD, and RG).

Table 12–7 gives SPAC data for three subjects who lost their hearing between 5 and 6 years of age. RJ lost his hearing at age 5 years 2 months and he had been deaf for only about 1 year 2 months. RS lost his hearing at age 5, but was 10 at the time of the study. The similarity in the performance between RJ and RS demonstrates the rapid rate at which speech can deteriorate in children of this age group. Subject HC lost his hearing at age 5 years 9 months and received an implant approximately 1 year later. It is assumed that his SPAC scores would be comparable to those of RG and RS prior to implantation. The first testing interval for HC was 2 years postimplant and the second was 3 years postimplant. At the 2-year test date, the scores for all features are higher for HC than for the other two subjects. At 3 years postimplant, continued improvement is shown in his ability to convey all the consonant contrasts. It is highly unlikely that the superior production abilities of HC would have occurred without the cochlear implant. These data demonstrate the importance of evaluating the change in speech production abilities in these children on a longitudinal basis.

Longitudinal data are available for only one user of the Nucleus 22-electrode device. The subject, who has a congenital hearing loss, received her implant when she was 11 years of age. SPAC production data, which were obtained only 6 months postimplant, showed about a 40 percent improvement in her ability to convey vowel height contrasts and a 25 percent improvement in her ability to convey vowel place information.

TABLE 12–7

SPAC Production Scores in Percent Obtained by 3 Subjects with Onset of Deafness at 5 Years of Age. Subject HC is an Implant User*

Contrast	RJ	RS	HC	
			2 Yrs Post	3 Yrs Post
Vowel height	72	86	92	96
Vowel place	87	72	96	92
Voicing	54	56	71	83
Continuance	54	64	85	91
Place	52	74	78	91

* Chance performance = 50 percent.

The extent of the speech change of this subject exceeds that observed for any of the adolescent users of the 3M/House device whose deafness was of early onset with a long period of acoustic deprivation. Additional data are needed to determine if large changes in speech production abilities typically occur in the speech of those children who use a multichannel system.

DISCUSSION

The preliminary data with respect to the effect of cochlear implants on the speech production abilities of totally deaf children are encouraging. The data reported have dealt with changes at the feature or phoneme level only. An issue of interest is whether the overall intelligibility of the children's speech has improved. Only clinical impressions are possible at this time because analysis of speech intelligibility is still underway. The degree to which these children's speech can be understood covers a wide range, and it is inappropriate to describe their speech as simply "intelligible" or "unintelligible". The child with the most intelligible speech, HC (see Table 12–7), can be completely understood by all listeners. In contrast, the speech of the other four implanted children probably could not be understood by listeners who are unfamiliar with the speech of deaf talkers. However, in a face-to-face interaction with contextual cues, approximately 75 percent of the speech produced by SM and DP (Table 12–5) and about 50 percent of the speech of the congenitally deaf subject (Figure 12–1 and Table 12–2) and subject BC (Table 12–6) could be understood by persons who have experience in listening to the speech of the deaf.

Longitudinal data must be collected from a wide range of children before generalizations about the effects of cochlear implants on speech production abilities are possible. The changes in the abilities of the few children described here appear to be highly individualized with large learning effects. Some children do not demonstrate noticeable changes in their speech until 12 to 18 months postimplant, which no doubt reflects maturation as well as device use. Accordingly, it is crucial that adequate time for learning be allotted before judgments are made about the effectiveness of a cochlear implant in promoting speech skills. Nonauditory children, unlike postlingually deaf adults who may demonstrate large improvement in their performance immediately after receiving an implant, must be given time to learn how to make use of the auditory information to which they are given access. Indeed, no one would expect profoundly hearing-impaired children with residual hearing to reach their potential in speech development during the first year or two of device use whether the device is a tactile aid, a hearing aid, or an implant.

Although performance results with multichannel systems are expected to exceed those obtained with single-channel devices, there is a need to continue to study the performance of children who use single-channel implants. First, a large number of children have received single-channel devices and relatively little is known about their performance, especially with respect to individual patterns of speech production. Second, differences in performance between users of single- and multichannel devices cannot be inferred from adult data, but must be demonstrated empirically in children. Some children with acquired deafness are performing open-set speech recognition tasks with the 3M/House implant. In fact, these children appear to be achieving higher levels of performance than postlingually deaf adults who use the same device. Such findings are difficult to explain in view of the signal provided by the 3M/House implant, although recent research suggests that some phonemic information may be available in the waveform envelope (Van Tasell et al., 1987). Further research is needed to resolve this question.

How significant are the changes that have occurred in the speech of these implanted children? This question raises an important issue concerning the criteria that are used to evaluate device success. Unfortunately, no criteria have been established. There appears to be a trend toward using the highest level of success attained by adult implant users, that of open-set speech recognition, to judge the success of children who use the same device. If this were the criterion used to evaluate hearing aid success in profoundly hearing-impaired children with residual hearing, few successful users would be found. It is conceivable that some children with an implant will achieve high levels of speech performance, especially with improvement in implant devices. Even with the most sophisticated devices, however, children will require a number of years of use and training to achieve their highest level of performance, especially if the loss is congenital or of very early onset (i.e., less than 1 year of age). The point to be stressed is that observations are being made on the speech performance of developing children. Until more data are accumulated, the benefits that they will receive from any cochlear prosthesis cannot be predicted.

An approach adopted by Osberger and colleagues in determining device success is to define the highest level of communication performance of which these children are capable. Given the limitations of any cochlear prosthesis at this time, it can be predicted that the performance levels of nonauditory children might match, but not exceed, those of profoundly hearing-impaired children with residual hearing who use hearing aids (i.e., those children with unaided thresholds between 90 to 105 dB HL through 4000 Hz). The hearing aid users will provide the baseline data for determining the optimal level of performance for the implant users. Not all children will achieve this level of performance, just as all adult implant users do not attain open-set speech recognition. If the highest level of performance is not achieved, it does not mean that the device has failed to provide benefit. On the contrary, the benefits from a sensory aid should be viewed as falling along a continuum. The minimum amount of change in performance that constitutes benefit from the device must be defined. That is, in order to determine whether a child is better off with or without an implant, the minimal changes that must be observed in the child's communication abilities need to be specified. This is not an easy task. It is hoped that future research efforts will provide the data to answer these questions.

ACKNOWLEDGMENTS

The assistance of Richard T. Miyamoto and the staff (Catherine Carotta, Wendy Myres, Amy Robbins, and Julia Renshaw) at the Indiana University School of Medicine in obtaining the speech samples from the children with cochlear implants is greatfully acknowledged. The assistance of Maureen Dolan, Lori Tschernach, Tristen Sato, and Elizabeth Pick in analyzing the data is greatly appreciated. This work was supported by the Spencer Foundation (through the School of Education of the University of Wisconsin-Madison), the Deafness Research Foundation, and the National Institutes of Health (NS25043).

REFERENCES

Binnie, C. A., Daniloff, R., & Buckingham, H. (1982). Phonetic disintegration in a five-year-old following sudden hearing loss. *Journal of Speech and Hearing Disorders, 47,* 181--189.

Boothroyd, A. (1969). *Distribution of hearing levels in the student population of the Clarke School for the Deaf.* Northampton, MA: Clarke School for the Deaf.

Boothroyd, A. (1984). Auditory perception of speech contrasts by subjects with sensorineural hearing loss. *Journal of Speech and Hearing Research, 27,* 134–144.

Boothroyd, A. (1985a). Evaluation of speech production of the hearing impaired: Some benefits of forced-choice testing. *Journal of Speech and Hearing Research, 28,* 185–196.

Boothroyd, A. (1985b). Residual hearing and the problem of carry-over in the speech of the deaf. *ASHA Reports, 15,* 8–14.

Boothroyd, A., & Cawkwell, S. (1970). Vibrotactile thresholds in pure-tone audiometry. *Acta Otolaryngologica, 69,* 384–387.

Carney, A. E. (1986). Understanding speech intelligibility in the hearing-impaired. *Topics in Language Disorders, 6,* 47–59.

Erber, N. P. (1972a). Auditory, visual, and auditory-visual recognition of consonants by children with normal and impaired hearing. *Journal of Speech and Hearing Research, 14,* 496–512.

Erber, N. P. (1972b). Speech envelope cues as an acoustic aid to lipreading for profoundly deaf children. *Journal of the Acoustical Society of America, 51,* 1224–1227.

Gold, T. (1980). Speech production in hearing-impaired children. *Journal of Communication Disorders, 13,* 397–418.

Kent, R. D. (1976). Anatomical and neuromuscular maturation of the speech mechanism: Evidence from acoustic studies. *Journal of Speech and Hearing Disorders, 19,* 421–447.

Kent, R. D. (1981). Sensorimotor aspects of speech development. In R. N. Aslin, J. R. Alberts, & M. R. Peterson (Eds.), *Development of perception* (pp. 161–189). New York: Academic Press.

Kent, R. D., & Murray, A. (1982). Acoustic features of infant vocal utterances at 3, 6, and 9 months of age. *Journal of the Acoustical Society of America, 72,* 353–365.

Leder, S. B., Spitzer, J. B., Milner, P., Flevaris-Phillips, C., Richardson, F., & Kirchner, J. C. (1986). Reacquisition of contrastive stress in an adventitiously deaf speaker using a single-channel implant. *Journal of the Acoustical Society of America, 79,* 1967–1974.

Levitt, H., McGarr, N. S., & Geffner, D. (1987). Language and communication skills of deaf children. *ASHA Monographs, 26.* Washington, DC: American Speech-Language-Hearing Association.

Levitt, H., & Stromberg, H. (1983). Segmental characteristics of the speech of the hearing impaired: Factors affecting intelligibility. In I. Hochberg, H. Levitt, & M. J. Osberger (Eds.), *Speech of the hearing impaired: Research, training, and personnel preparation* (pp. 53–73). Baltimore, MD: University Park Press.

McGarr, N. S. (1983). The intelligibility of deaf speech to experienced and inexperienced listeners. *Journal of Speech and Hearing Research, 26,* 451–458.

McGarr, N. S. (1987). Communication skills of hearing-impaired children in schools for the deaf. In H. Levitt, N. S. McGarr, & D. Geffner (Eds.), Language and communication skills of deaf children. *ASHA Monographs, 26.* Washington, DC: American Speech-Language-Hearing Association.

McGarr, N. S., & Osberger, M. J. (1978). Pitch deviancy and the intelligibility of deaf speech. *Journal of Communication Disorders, 11,* 237–247.

Monsen, R. B. (1978). Toward measuring how well hearing-impaired children speak. *Journal of Speech and Hearing Research, 21,* 197–219.

Monsen, R. B. (1983). The oral speech intelligibility of hearing-impaired talkers. *Journal of Speech and Hearing Disorders, 48,* 286–296.

Monsen, R. B., & Shaughnessy, D. H. (1978). Improvement in vowel articulation of deaf children. *Journal of Communication Disorders, 11,* 417–424.

Osberger, M. J. (1983). Development and evaluation of some speech training procedures for hearing-impaired children. In I. Hochberg, H., Levitt, & M.J. Osberger (Eds.), *Speech of the hearing-impaired: Research, training, and personnel preparation* (pp. 333–348). Baltimore, MD: University Park Press.

Osberger, M. J. (1986). Language and learning skills of hearing-impaired students. *ASHA Monographs, 23.* Washington, DC: American Speech-Language-Hearing Association.

Osberger, M. J. (1987). Training effects on vowel production by two profoundly hearing-impaired speakers. *Journal of Speech and Hearing Research, 30,* 241–251.

Osberger, M. J., & Levitt, H. (1979). The effect of timing errors on the intelligibility of deaf children's speech. *Journal of the Acoustical Society of America, 66,* 1316–1324.

Osberger, M. J., & McGarr, N. S. (1982). Speech production characteristics of the hearing-impaired. In N. Lass (Ed.), *Speech and language: Advances in basic science and research* (pp. 221–283). New York: Academic Press.

Osberger, M. J., Johnstone, A., Swarts, E., & Levitt, H. (1978). Evaluation of a model speech training program for deaf children. *Journal of Communication Disorders, 11,* 293–313.

Plant, G. (1984). The effects of an acquired profound hearing loss on speech production. *British Journal of Audiology, 18,* 39–48.

Samar, B. J., & Metz, D. E. (in press). Criterion validity of speech intelligibility procedures for the hearing-impaired population. *Journal of Speech and Hearing Research.*

Smith, C. R. (1972). *Residual hearing and speech production in deaf children.* Unpublished doctoral dissertation, City University of New York.

Smith, C. R. (1975). Residual hearing and speech production in deaf children. *Journal of Speech and Hearing Research, 18,* 795–811.

Stark, R., & Levitt, H. (1974). Prosodic feature reception and production in deaf children. *Journal of the Acoustical Society of America, 55,* S23.

Stoel-Gammon, C., & Otomo, K. (1986). Babbling development of hearing-impaired and normally hearing subjects. *Journal of Speech and Hearing Disorders, 51,* 33–41.

Van Tasell, D., Soli, S. D., Kirby, V. M., & Widin, G. P. (1987). Speech waveform envelope cues for consonant recognition. *Journal of the Acoustical Society of America, 82,* 1152–1161.

CHAPTER 13

PAULA TALLAL

AUDITORY PROCESSING AND SPEECH PERCEPTION: IMPLICATIONS FOR COCHLEAR IMPLANTS IN YOUNG CHILDREN

T here are presently several viable theories and models that have been developed to account for auditory processing and speech perception. Included are (1) those based on neurophysiologic studies of the manner in which acoustic signals are represented in activities of the auditory nerves; (2) those based on psychoacoustic investigations; (3) and those concerned with such factors as perceptual confusions, delineation of the acoustic correlates of speech sounds, and categorical perception (see Sloan, 1986, for a general review). Even distinctions between the terms *processing* and *perception* are imprecise and exact definitions are lacking. According to Sloan (1986),

> auditory processing refers to everything that occurs from the moment a sound enters the external ear canal to the moment that that particular acoustic event is experienced by a listener ... the signal is transformed, coded, and recoded by the auditory pathways, so that what is actually experienced is not a direct replica of the acoustic event but a representation of that event constructed by the processing that occurs as the signal is transmitted through the auditory system. In short, real sound events are processed before they become conscious experience .... Auditory perception is the outcome of auditory processing. Sensations are the components of our experience, but they do not simply add up together to form that experience. Rather, they are integrated and organized by the auditory system into perceptual events. (p. 1)

Conversely, "In broad terms, an auditory processing difficulty can be defined as a difficulty in processing the acoustic speech signal that interferes with accurate and efficient perception of speech" (p. 35).

Through research, considerable advances in knowledge have been made in recent years. Nonetheless, it is difficult to address issues pertaining to abnormal auditory processing and speech perception, because the normal mechanisms are not yet understood. It is known that certain aspects of speech perception can be demonstrated almost from birth in normal infants. The investigations of Eimas and colleagues (1971), Kuhl (1977), and Eilers and Minifie (1975), for example, have certainly demonstrated what would previously have been considered amazing speech discrimination abilities in very young infants. At the other end of the continuum, however, some language impaired children, even much later in life, have difficulty discriminating the same kinds of signals that are readily discriminated by normal infants (Tallal & Piercy, 1974, 1975). Tallal and colleagues hypothesized that the study of such differences might reveal some of the mechanisms underlying normal speech perception. Some results of their subsequent experimental work seem applicable to the question of cochlear implants in young children.

THE ACOUSTIC WAVEFORM

The initial step in investigating the prerequisites for normal speech perception is an examination of the psychoacoustics of sound. The acoustic waveform is composed of just a few major physical properties: intensity or amplitude, frequency, and time. However, Liberman and his associates (1967) have demonstrated that when speech is heard it is not the actual sounds of the acoustic waveform that are perceived, but rather an abstract code. That is, at the central or neurological level, it seems probable that what is perceived is a transformation of those initial acoustic cues that occurred at the periphery. If the acoustic waveform is not received adequately at the periphery (as in the case of sensorineural hearing loss), then presumably sounds are not encoded into this abstract form necessary for speech perception at the central level. If the ultimate goal in designing cochlear implants is to improve speech perception, then knowledge of those aspects of the acoustic waveform that are most critical at the periphery for further transformation and encoding of speech centrally is essential; that is, the minimal acoustic cues necessary for adequte speech perception must be determined.

Not all elements of the acoustic signal are equally salient for speech perception. Certain aspects of the signal mask others. One of the primary aspects of the acoustic waveform required for adequate speech perception is change over time (Cutting, 1973; Stevens, 1980; Studdert-Kennedy & Shankweiler, 1970). Tallal and Piercy (1973a, 1973b) have suggested that temporal cues, particularly the rate at which the acoustic waveform changes within ongoing speech, may be one of the most important features that must be encoded for normal development of speech and language functions. It is important to distinguish here between the temporal elements of speech prosody and the fine temporal structure of speech sounds. The prosodic or suprasegmental cues of duration and timing refer to those characteristics of speech that extend over more than one phonetic unit or segment, such as syllabic pattern or stress. This discussion focuses on the fine temporal cues that refer to very rapid timing changes within a single sound or phonetic segment, such as voicing or continuance.

A MODEL OF AUDITORY PROCESSING

In order to determine the extent to which, and manner in which, central processing abilities relate to speech perception, Tallal and colleagues have studied normal hearing children and adults, as well as those with language deficits. They employed a specific model of processing as follows. Given an acoustic signal, the first requirement in the hierarchy of information processing is the ability to detect the occurrence of that signal. Obviously several processing stages occur between the initial detection of a signal and its final processing into something meaningful, such as speech. In examining these possible stages, the presentation of a single event must first be considered. When a single event is perceived it can only be detected. It cannot be described as loud, or short, or high because there is nothing with which to compare it. Thus, if there is only a single event, the highest possible level of processing is achieved once it has been detected.

To proceed past the level of detection, the next processing stage must include the detection of more than a single event. These events must occur far enough apart in time in order for them to be processed as distinct rather than fused, but they cannot be so distant in time that they are incapable of being stored for comparison. Only after it has been perceived that two distinct pieces of information have occurred can higher levels of processing be engaged. That is, questions of comparison or discrimination can then be asked. Thus, the detection of "twoness" as separate from "oneness" is a prerequisite to more complex acoustic analysis such as discrimination. The ability to detect the occurrence of two events involves a function called temporal resolution, which depends on the perception of a silent gap between the offset of the first signal and the onset of the second. When that gap is too short to be detected, only a continuous or single event is perceived. When the gap becomes somewhat longer, the listener is able to perceive that one event ends and the next begins. The precise duration necessary for this temporal resolution depends on the neurophysiological system of the listener.

Once the listener has perceived two events, further information processing can then occur to determine whether the events are the same or different. If it is determined that the two events are the same, then the highest processing stage possible for these events has been achieved and no further information can be extracted. Proceeding beyond the stage of temporal resolution depends on having some difference on which to base a comparison. Only when it is determined that a signal consists of two events that are not the same can the listener proceed to discrimination, the next level of processing. At this level, a variety of processing strategies may be invoked. Initially, the listener attempts to determine how the signals differ. The ability to discriminate difference will depend on the actual amount of physical difference between the signals, the duration of the signals to be discriminated, and the duration of the interval between the signals. The ability of subjects to discriminate just noticable differences (JNDs) between sounds defines the limits of the auditory system for a given species. Finally, when the listener knows that two signals are different and how they differ, the next level of processing is engaged, namely the determination of the temporal order in which the sounds entered the nervous system. The whole series is then begun again, processing three or more signals, which also engages short-term and serial memory functions.

A critical aspect of this model is that it is hierarchical, with prerequisite stages of processing determining the ultimate level that can be achieved in any analysis. For example, the listener would be unable to determine the temporal order in which two signals were presented unless it had previously been perceived that two events had occurred and that the two signals were different from each other. Once the hierarchical stages of processing two events have been accomplished, then additional events can be processed through the use of storage and memory mechanisms. Although this is a hierarchical model composed of prerequisite stages, it is important to note that the possibility of these stages being accessed either serially or in parallel is not precluded. That is, several stages of processing may occur simultaneously rather than in serial order.

One of the most salient aspects of speech, as mentioned previously, is that it changes extraordinarily quickly and requires very rapid analysis of acoustic cues (Cutting, 1973; Studdert–Kennedy & Shankweiler, 1970; Tallal & Piercy, 1973a, 1973b). Even at the cellular level the brain responds best to change in the environment. For example, it has been demonstrated that single cells in the auditory cortex of cats respond better to rapid change over time than they respond to any other physical difference (Andersen, 1988). Single brain cells are "on the alert", as it were, waiting to receive some input. The input that most easily excites the cells and causes them to fire is change over time. Speech, because it is constantly changing, extensively employs this particular neural attention-getting mechanism in the brain.

AUDITORY PROCESSING IN CHILDREN WHO ARE DYSPHASIC

In the majority of the studies by Tallal and colleagues, young children with normal language development were compared with children specifically language impaired (developmentally dysphasic) who, by definition, have normal peripheral hearing and intelligence (Benton, 1964). Because of the serious language deficits of these children, in spite of normal peripheral hearing, it has been suggested that they may be impaired in processing sound at a higher, more central level (Benton, 1964; Eisenberg, 1976; Eisenson, 1966). The studies of Tallal and her associates have focused on assessing the central auditory processing abilities of these children in relation to their speech and language development.

In the course of these investigations a series of techniques for evaluating higher cortical processing of auditory stimuli in children were developed. It is important when testing young children that test instruments not be constrained by higher level conceptual demands and that they allow for the evaluation of information processing in a hierarchical, step-wise, nonverbal fashion so as not to confound nonverbal and verbal processing abilities. The Repetition Method (Tallal, 1980) was developed to meet these needs. In this procedure, children are taught, through operant conditioning techniques, to press buttons on a response box in order to indicate what they perceive. Beginning with a simple signal, the child is trained to press a button to indicate that the signal has been detected. Next, the test evaluates the gap of silence necessary to resolve temporally the occurrence of two events as opposed to one. Then, the subject's ability to discriminate the events as same or different is assessed. If they are different, the subject's ability to determine their temporal order is evaluated. Finally, memory span for an increasingly longer series of signals is assessed. Each processing stage uses a simple button pushing response procedure.

Through these nonverbal testing techniques, Tallal and colleagues have found that dysphasic children actually process sound very well at each central processing level. To date, the only difference that has been demonstrated in these children relates to the rate at which they are able to integrate more than one piece of information converging on the nervous system quickly in time (Tallal & Piercy, 1973a, 1973b, 1974; Tallal, Stark & Mellits, 1985a, 1985b). That is, these children responded normally on all tasks provided that they were not required to process stimulus change quickly.

In order to understand the relationship between central auditory nonverbal processing and speech perception, the acoustic wave forms that characterize individual speech sounds must be examined. Certain speech sounds require rapid processing of acoustic change over time, while other speech sounds do not. The pattern of speech perception and production deficits in dysphasic children revealed that they had greater difficulty both processing and producing those speech sounds that required them to extract rapid acoustic change than those that did not (Stark & Tallal, 1979; Tallal & Piercy, 1975; Tallal & Stark, 1981). For example, two speech sounds that require rapid discrimination of acoustic change are the syllables /ba/ and /da/. The major portion of the signal in these stop-consonant vowel syllables, the vowel /a/, is the same in both stimuli; therefore, it cannot be used to aid in discrimination. In order to discriminate /ba/ from /da/, the very rapid frequency changes that occur at the onset of the syllable must be tracked. Demanding a rapid analysis, these occur over approximately a 40 msec period of time. Other speech sounds, such as the vowels /ɛ/ and /æ/, involve no frequency change over time, because they are produced by placing the vocal apparatus in a static position. It was hypothesized and later demonstrated that dysphasic children cannot discriminate between speech signals such as /ba/ versus /da/, but have no difficulty discriminating between speech signals that change more slowly over time or that are steady state (Tallal & Piercy, 1974).

The critical nature of this rate processing deficit was demonstrated by using a computer to generate speech signals in which the duration of the critical segments of the waveform were extended in time. Children who were unable to discriminate between the normal /ba/ and /da/, containing formant transitions of 40 msec, had no difficulty discriminating between the same speech sounds when the transitions had been computer-extended to 80 msec (Tallal & Piercy, 1975). Thus, it has been demonstrated that these children respond normally at all of the stages of central auditory processing described above if the rate of presentation of information to be processed is slowed down. Subsequent studies showed a direct correlation between the degree of difficulty a dysphasic child has in rapid auditory processing of both nonverbal and verbal stimuli and that child's degree of receptive language impairment (Tallal, Stark, & Mellits, 1985a, 1985b). Parallels between speech perception difficulties and speech production deficits have also been observed (Tallal et al., 1980).

APPLICATION TO COCHLEAR IMPLANTS IN YOUNG CHILDREN

Through the careful assessment of information processing abilities that may be prerequisites for speech perception, and through the subsequent enhancement of the acoustic signal using advanced computer techniques, Tallal and colleagues have demonstrated that significant improvement in children's speech perception abilities can be achieved. Although the reported research has thus far focused on children with central rather than peripheral auditory deficits, it may provide a model for future research on cochlear implants. The test techniques that have been introduced are flexible in that they can assess stages of processing and memory either auditorally, visually, tactually, or cross-modally depending on the stimuli used. Comparisons between performance in different sensory modalities, as well as between nonverbal and verbal processing, can be made by giving the same test with a variety of stimuli. For example, because of the hearing impairment of young cochlear implant candidates, the visual modality may be the most efficient in determining the integrity of their central information processing abilities. Because basic nonverbal central perceptual and memory capacities are so critical for normal speech perception, it is important to ensure that these capacities are intact in young cochlear implant candidates, especially those who may have sustained their hearing loss from known central insult such as meningitis. Assessment in a nonauditory sensory modality, either visual or tactile, might be useful in preoperatively determining the integrity of central processing and memory mechanisms. Such assessment techniques would also be effective for implanted children in the postoperative evaluation, when comparisons between performance across sensory modalities might help assess the success of the implant in basic auditory processing domains.

CONCLUSION

In designing cochlear implants and in selecting appropriate candidates to receive an implant, it is important to assess whether the device can transmit and the candidate can process specific aspects of the acoustic waveform. Because the critical role of temporal processing has been demonstrated, cochlear implants must preserve and enhance the fine temporal components of sound. Further studies of auditory processing can contribute to the development of cochlear implants by isolating and identifying those acoustic cues critical for speech perception. Once known, cochlear implants capable of transmitting those features can be designed. For postimplant patients who cannot discriminate certain acoustic features, the implant device might be constructed so that modifications and adjustments are possible, just as computer-extending specific formant transitions allowed particular discriminations in dysphasic children. With information pooled from all relevant disciplines — speech and hearing sciences, linguistics, engineering, psychoacoustics, neurophysiology, audiology, and speech pathology — the potential for providing young children with the acoustic cues needed for auditory processing and speech perception is highly promising.

REFERENCES

Andersen, R. A. (1988). The neurobiological basis of spatial cognition: Role of the parietal lobe. In J. Stiles–Davis, M. Kritchevsky, & U. Bellugi (Eds.), *Spatial cognition: Brain bases and development.* Hillsdale, NJ: Lawrence Erlbaum Associates.

Benton, A. L. (1964). Developmental aphasia and brain damage. *Cortex, 1,* 40–52.

Cutting, J. E. (1973). Parallel between degree of encodedness and the ear advantage: Evidence from an ear monitoring task. *Journal of the Acoustical Society of America, 53,* 368.

Eilers, R. E., & Minifie, F. D. (1975). Fricative discrimination in early infancy. *Journal of Speech and Hearing Research, 18,* 158–167.

Eimas, P. D., Siqueland, R., Jasczyk, P., & Vigoito, J. (1971). Speech perception in infants. *Science, 171,* 303–306.

Eisenberg, R. B. (1976). *Auditory competence in early life.* Baltimore: University Park Press.

Eisenson, J. (1966). Perceptual disturbances in children with central nervous system dysfunction and implications for language development. *British Journal of Disorders of Communication, 1,* 21–32.

Kuhl, P. K. (1977). Speech perception in early infancy: Perceptual constancy for vowels. *Journal of the Acoustical Society of America, 61,* 539 (A).

Liberman, A. M., Cooper, F. S., Shankweiler, D., & Studdert–Kennedy, M. (1967). Perception of the speech code. *Psychological Review, 74,* 431–461.

Sloan, C. (1986). *Treating auditory processing difficulties in children.* San Diego: College-Hill Press.

Stark, R., & Tallal, P. (1979). Analysis of stop-consonant production errors in developmentally dysphasic children. *Journal of the Acoustical Society of America, 66,* 1703–1712.

Stevens, K. N. (1980). Acoustic correlates of some phonetic categories. *Journal of the Acoustical Society of America, 68,* 836–842.

Studdert-Kennedy, M., & Shankweiler, B. (1970). Hemispheric specialization of speech perception. *Journal of the Acoustical Society of America, 48,* 579–594.

Tallal, P. (1980). Perceptual requisites for language. In R. Schifelbusch (Ed.), *Nonspeech language and communication* (pp. 449–467). Baltimore: University Park Press.

Tallal, P., & Piercy, M. (1973a). Defects of non-verbal auditory perception in children with developmental aphasia. *Nature, 241,* 468–469.

Tallal, P., & Piercy, M. (1973b). Developmental aphasia: Impaired rate of non-verbal processing as a function of sensory modality. *Neuropsychologia, 11,* 389–398.

Tallal, P., & Piercy, M. (1974). Developmental aphasia: Rate of auditory processing and selective impairment of consonant perception. *Neuropsychologia, 13,* 83–93.

Tallal, P., & Piercy, M. (1975). Developmental aphasia: The perception of brief vowels and extended stop consonants. *Neuropsychologia, 13,* 69–74.

Tallal, P., & Stark, R. (1981). Speech acoustic-cue discrimination abilities of normally developing and language-impaired children. *Journal of the Acoustical Society of America, 69,* 568–574.

Tallal, P., Stark, R. E., Kallman, C., & Mellits, D. (1980). Developmental dysphasia: Relation between acoustic processing and verbal processing. *Neuropsychologia, 18,* 273–284.

Tallal, P., Stark, R., & Mellits, D. (1985a). Identification of language impaired children on the basis of rapid perception and production skill. *Brain and Language, 25,* 314–322.

Tallal, P., Stark, R., & Mellits, D. (1985b). The relationship between auditory temporal analysis and receptive language development: Evidence from studies of developmental language disorder. *Neuropsychologia, 23:* 527–536.

CHAPTER 14

SUSAN CURTISS

ISSUES IN LANGUAGE ACQUISITION RELEVANT TO COCHLEAR IMPLANTS IN YOUNG CHILDREN

T his chapter will briefly address some of the issues in language acquisition that are most pertinent to cochlear implants in young children. The first section considers language acquisition in deaf children; the second section discusses maturational constraints on language acquisition in both hearing and deaf children; and the third section concerns factors in normal, spoken language acquisition that may be relevant to cochlear implantation in young children.

LANGUAGE ACQUISITION IN CHILDREN WHO ARE DEAF

Deaf children have normal language learning capacity and readily acquire language when given the opportunity. This fact is attested to by these children's acquisition of sign language as a native language from infancy, a situation that arises only 5 to 10 percent of the time in the deaf population (Hoffmeister & Wilbur, 1980; Liben, 1978). It occurs when a congenitally deaf child has deaf parents who are users of sign, and the child thus has everyday exposure to sign in the home.

A preliminary comment on the status of sign language as a language may be in order. Linguistic description and analysis of sign language has concentrated primarily on American Sign Language (ASL). However, just as the study of a single spoken language can reveal facts that are true of all languages (i.e., language universals), the study of a single sign language reveals much about the nature of sign languages generally. As recently as the early 1960's (Stokoe, 1960; Stokoe, Casterline, & Croneberg, 1965), linguistic work on ASL made it clear that, despite differences in performance modality, sign language shares the defining characteristics of all human languages. It is, in fact, startlingly like spoken language in many of its organizational properties, although quite different from English in structural typology.

Regarding the question of language learning in congenitally deaf children, the data referred to derive from studies investigating the acquisition of ASL as a native language. Briefly, every study conducted to date has found that acquisition of ASL as a native language is, in every respect, an instance of normal language acquisition. The general characteristics of its acquisition (stages for the occurrence and combinatorial possibilities of linguistic categories, stages for the expression of semantic categories and their combinations, componential analysis of complex forms, etc.) conform to the universal characteristics of normal language acquisition (Caselli, 1983; Hoffmeister, 1978; Hoffmeister & Wilbur, 1980; Kantor, 1982; Newport & Ashbrook, 1977). The acquisition of language particular details (e.g., verb agreement morphology) parallels the acquisition of typologically similar phenomena in spoken languages (see Meier, 1981; Newport & Meier, 1985; and Supalla, 1982, for a review). Furthermore, children learning ASL as a native language appear to overlook or ignore the transparency/iconicity of signs (i.e., the similarities between a sign form and its referent; for example, the similarities between the "look" of the ASL sign for *tree* and a *tree*) to which adult learners or observers make reference. Rather, the deaf child performs a formal and abstract analysis on the basis of the *linguistic* properties of the sign system. Particularly convincing data were presented by Jackson (1984) and Pettito (1983) regarding acquisition of personal and possessive pronouns and negation, and by Meier (1981, 1982) regarding verb agreement morphology. Thus, in details of developmental timing and in details of the nature of the "errors" made (grammatically motivated misanalyses), the evidence is strong that the acquisition of sign as a native language by deaf children of deaf parents is characterizable along the same bases as the acquisition of spoken language. It is most like the acquisition of spoken languages that are similar to ASL in linguistic typology.

Another pertinent question concerns the possible effects that learning sign language as a first language might have on the acquisition of spoken language. There are two unrelated pieces of evidence on this issue, both of which make it clear that knowing a sign language has no detrimental effect on learning spoken language or related skills such as lipreading.

The first source of evidence comes from studies of bimodal, bilingual acquisition in hearing children of deaf parents. Such children, who learn sign as well as a spoken language from their everyday environment, show no difficulties or abnormalities in acquiring a spoken language by virtue of their simultaneous acquisition of a sign language (Bonvillian, Orlansky, & Novack, 1983; Jackson, 1984; Prinz & Prinz, 1979, 1981; Schlesinger & Meadow, 1972).

The second source of evidence comes from studies comparing deaf children of deaf parents (*deaf of deaf*) with deaf children of hearing parents (*deaf of hearing*) on tests of spoken and written English competence, speech production and lipreading skills, and general educational performance. These studies uniformly show that the *deaf of deaf*, who have learned ASL as a native language, perform as well or better than other deaf children. *Deaf of deaf*, compared with their *deaf of hearing* peers, have significantly better scores on English reading and writing tests and demonstrate no statistically significant differences on speech production and lipreading skills; they show larger English vocabularies, higher academic achievement scores, and higher levels of attainment in formal education (Charrow & Fletcher, 1974; Meadow, 1966, 1968; Quigley & Frisina, 1961; Stevenson, 1964; Stuckless & Birch, 1966; Vernon & Koh, 1970). It is difficult to separate the effect of early language knowledge from the contribution of social and environmental differences to subsequent linguistic and academic performance. However, the possibility remains that for fostering the potential to learn spoken language, language related, and academic skills during school years, there is an advantage to knowing *any* language over knowing no language during the preschool years. If borne out, this would indicate that acquisition of (spoken or signed) English as a second language may be less problematic than the delayed learning of (spoken or signed) English as a first language. The importance of early linguistic experience for subsequent linguistic and academic achievements is further supported by data from deaf children whose hearing parents signed with them from infancy. These children are also reported to outperform their *deaf of hearing* peers, both linguistically and academically (Schlessinger, 1978).

A Critical Period for Language Acquisition

The importance of the age at which first language acquisition takes place is an issue that may be particularly relevant to the question of whether and when to implant. The central question is whether or not there is a critical period for first language acquisition outside of which language cannot be acquired normally or fully. It is known from animal studies (e.g., see Chapter 2) that there are strong biological constraints on the development of neural systems and on their organization. But it is also known that those biological constraints interact in very important and complex ways with environmental factors. In the study of ontogeny in animals, critical periods have been defined as those points in time where sensory experience and environment exert their major influence in the development of neural systems or their organization. There exists a large animal literature demonstrating that sensory experience has marked effects on neural and behavioral development during a very circumscribed time period — a critical period — in ontogeny.

Given sufficient exposure to language, children normally acquire a first language within a relatively short span of time, attaining near-native competence by approximately age 6. This remarkable feat has led numerous researchers to postulate that children are biologically preprogrammed for language acquisition, in a general cognitive sense, in a specific linguistic sense, or both. The fact that language acquisition occurs at a relatively uniform pace and time cross-culturally, marks it as a maturationally constrained phenomenon. Language thus becomes a good candidate to be a neural system with a developmental critical period.

The hypothesis that there is a critical period for first language acquisition was initially made explicit by Lenneberg (1967). He proposed that the critical period for language learning ends approximately at puberty. Although there have been relatively few opportunities to test this hypothesis, the data on acquisition of both sign and spoken language that address the hypothesis are consistently supportive.

The most thoroughly studied and widely reported test case for the acquisition of spoken language was that of Genie. Found in adolescence after having undergone unprecedented social isolation and experiential deprivation, Genie faced the task of first language acquisition at the age of 13 and-a-half. Based on 8 years of study, her case has been taken as support for Lenneberg's hypothesis; although she has developed some language, she has not acquired language fully or normally. Most important in this regard is the striking contrast between her acquisition of morphology and syntax on the one hand and her acquisition of semantic knowledge on the other. Genie's acquisition of vocabulary and of how to express meaning relations through words, including multipropositionality, steadily progressed and increased, whereas her acquisition of the grammer has remained very limited (Curtiss, 1977, 1981, 1982). In addition, although Genie failed to master many of the social conventions of discourse, she demonstrated impressive communicative competence in most situations.

The data from Genie's case suggest that language embodies distinct modules or components of knowledge, and that these separate components of language are differentially vulnerable to age at acquisition. The lexical and pragmatic modules appear to be the most resilient, while the computational component (the rules of phonology, morphology, syntax, and logical form) seems to be the most vulnerable.

A more recent case, involving a deaf woman in her thirties learning signed and spoken English as a first language, shows the same basic results as the Genie case: good lexical learning, good communicative skills, and little learning of the grammer (Curtiss, unpublished data). Even after 5 years of intensive language intervention, knowledge of the grammar seems elusive. Language learning patterns observed in other recent cases, although not documented in detail, also appear to be consistent with the pattern Genie displayed. Young (1981) and McKinney (1983) reported on first language acquisition in a few hearing-impaired adults who knew only esoteric gestures and, maximally, a few spoken words, before language training in adulthood was begun. From the descriptions provided, these cases appear to demonstrate the same relative vulnerability of grammar acquisition as opposed to the learning of individual vocabulary items, the expression of semantic relations, and the development of communicative competence. These cases all suggest that significantly delayed acquisition of spoken language results in substantial linguistic deficiency, despite the achievement of useful conceptual and communicative abilities.

Age of acquisition has been shown to impinge critically on the character and extent of sign language acquisition as well as spoken language. Mayberry, Fischer, and Hatfield (1983) demonstrated experimentally that those individuals who acquired sign in the teenage years performed worse on sign competence tasks than those who acquired sign in childhood. Moreover, the later sign was learned, the worse the performance. Mayberry (1984) also demonstrated that not only did the signers who had learned sign later (from 8 years of age and older) perform worse on the tasks, but they also performed differently. Additional support for Mayberry's findings comes from work reported by Newport (1984). She investigated the relative effects of age versus number of years signing versus age at acquisition on the production and comprehension of ASL utterances involving grammatically complex verbs of motion. An effect only for age at acquisition was found. The main effect observed was between native and early acquirers on the one hand and "late" learners (those learning sign between the ages of 12 and 21) on the other. Once again, most vulnerable to the effect of age at acquisition were grammatical aspects of the system, with only native signers and early learners demonstrating mastery of the complex grammatical structure of verbs of motion. In addition, the structural analyses entertained by the late learners were very different from those of the native and early learners. Importantly, there were also significant performance differences between native signers and those who had learned sign early in life (before 6 years of age). This finding suggests that even moderately delayed language acquisition can have significant effects on grammar learning, thereby increasing the importance of early (preschool) exposure to a conventional language model (see also Woodward, 1973; Fischer, 1978; and Newport, 1981, 1982, for related findings).

In all of these cases involving later-than-normal acquisition of language, a marked disparity occurs. On the one hand, there is the ability to learn vocabulary and string vocabulary together to express meaningful utterances; on the other hand, there is the ability to learn those aspects of the language that take strings of lexical items and elaborate or reorder them into grammatical sentences. Whereas the former ability is relatively impervious to acquisition age, the latter ability is particularly vulnerable to acquisition age. An additional source of support for such findings comes from an interesting linguistic phenomenon that occurs when adults who speak mutually unintelligible languages need to form a basis for communication. Under such circumstances, they create a system that is called a *pidgin* which, in very simplified terms, is a stock of lexical items and a rule-ordered system of combining that lexicon into sentences. However, the system of language, the *pidgin*, that they create is devoid of many of the morphological and syntactic devices that are found in any natural language. In contrast, when children are in a position to learn this *pidgin* as a native language (i.e., from infancy), they elaborate the *pidgin* into a *creole* — a full-blown language having the grammatical devices and structural complexity present in all other natural human languages. In effect, even when the model language is an impoverished linguistic system, as is a *pidgin*, young children create a full language like other natural languages in its structural richness. This phenomenon compellingly illustrates that language acquisition by the young child is qualitatively and quantitatively different from language learning by the older child or adult, with grammar acquisition most affected by maturational differences in the learner.

A similar phenomenon is repeated in every generation by second-generation deaf children learning ASL (Singleton & Newport, 1987). Their parents, being first generation deaf, do not have native competence in ASL, having been exposed to ASL only in later childhood or beyond. Second-generation deaf children surpass their parents in ASL competence, enriching and elaborating the improverished lingusitic model provided by their parents.

The existence of a critical period for first language acquisition for both sign and spoken language is supported by all of the data discussed. The evidence not only suggests that the effects of age at acquisition may include limitations on what can be learned, but also may involve the utilization of different and inadequate strategies or mechanisms in language processing and production. Moreover, there may be maturational constraints on the point at which auditory experience or stimulation may trigger or lead to normal *inter*hemispheric and/or *intra*hemispheric cerebral specialization. Neville (1977), in her research on hemispheric specialization in the deaf, has found that individuals who did not learn sign and had very little linguistic knowledge of any sort showed no hemispheric specialization in response to either language or nonlinguistic stimuli. Those who had learned sign during childhood showed atypical hemispheric specialization, compared to hearing subjects. These findings led Neville to study the effects on functional brain specialization of such factors as age at acquisition, language modality, and auditory experience. Her findings to date suggest that, if not used for the learning of spoken language, auditory cortex may become committed to other abilities. Neville (1984) and Neville, Schmidt, and Kutas (1983) have demonstrated an increased electrical potential to visual stimuli from the auditory cortex in deaf individuals, suggesting that auditory cortex, when deprived of auditory stimulation, may become organized to process visual information. Confirming data have been obtained from Neville's Event Related Potential (ERP) studies of individuals for whom cochlear degeneration had been delayed until 4 years after birth. These individuals did not display the large visual potentials over auditory cortical areas that subjects who are congenitally deaf had shown. In short, auditory cortex may become committed to the performance of other cognitive functions if not linguistically stimulated at the appropriate time.

Aspects of Spoken Language Acquisition

Neville's findings suggest that early auditory stimulation may be necessary for normal cerebral organization. Early auditory experience is obviously also essential for spoken language acquisition. The key question is whether cochlear implantation can provide or enhance the accessibility of the auditory-linguistic information that appears to play a particularly important role in early spoken language acquisition.

The mechanisms by which a child extracts linguistic information from the acoustic speech signal are not understood at present. Because there is no linguistic structure inherent in the signal itself, however, the ability to extract information from it and impute structure to it must be an inherent property of the child's mind. Because the deaf child demonstrates normal language acquisition and, thus, normal ability to derive linguistic structural information from a physical signal when that signal is readily perceivable, as in sign language, the major obstacle for the deaf child in learning spoken language would appear to be receiving sufficient acoustic input to perceive the speech signal linguistically.

The single-channel devices being implanted in children are reported to provide significant increases mainly in the perception of intensity changes, durational information, and pitch changes limited to a restricted low frequency range (Bilger et al., 1977; Berliner, Eisenberg, & House, 1985; Eisenberg et al., 1983; Shannon, 1983; Thielemeir, Brimacombe, & Eisenberg, 1982). This by no means amounts to increasing the perception of all aspects of the acoustic signal necessary for providing the auditory-linguistic experience that allows for the natural unfolding of spoken language acquisition. However, the aspects of the speech signal that are made more accessible by these single-channel implants may be important ones for enhancing spoken language acquisition in the deaf child, especially for a language such as English.

There is some evidence that the young child may be predisposed to pay particular attention to prosodic information, that is, *pitch, duration,* and *intensity* cues, early in language acquisition (Bever, Fodor, & Weksel, 1965; Kaplan & Kaplan, 1970; Nakazima, 1962). For stress-accent languages such as English, in which pitch and timing patterns are systematically related to constituent structure (Selkirk, 1983) — for example, syntactic boundaries marked by intonational cues — perceiving and attending to such cues may provide important information about constituent structure. This may, in turn, aid in the initial parsing of the speech signal into grammatical units and provide information regarding the target language's linguistic typology. This information may then trigger or play a crucial role in accessing or learning other grammatical information, particularly those aspects of the grammar that may be predictable on the basis of a few key typological facts.

There is also some evidence that linguistic information in stressed units is learned earliest (Slobin, 1973, 1982). Linguistic stress is signalled by a composite of prosodic parameters: duration, pitch, and intensity. It has been suggested that there is a predisposition for an initial analysis of the acoustic signal in such languages as English into units of stressed syllables (Gleitman & Wanner, 1982). Together with other hypotheses concerning innate predispositions of the language learner, this hypothesis fares well in accounting for what appears to be mastered early, both in comprehension and in production of English and other stress-accent languages.

Several studies thus suggested a potential significance of prosodic information in the initial stages of language acquisition in the very young child. It is not yet known, however, whether the same perceptual "strategies" would be at play in language acquisition in a somewhat older child. Along those lines, intonational cues appear to have little or no effect on the comprehension of structurally ambiguous sentences in the mature listener (Lehiste, 1973; Wales & Toner, 1979). Even more importantly, the mechanisms — auditory or otherwise — by which the brain apprehends prosodic structure are not yet understood. Consequently, there is no assurance at this time that cochlear implants, even in a very young child, will provide all or any of the necessary information for recipients to make use of relevant prosodic cues for language acquisition. As an example, the role of *pitch* as a prosodic cue may be crucial, but it is a parameter whose perception with cochlear implants is limited to a severely narrow frequency range, and, at least with single-channel devices, devoid of spectral information. Perception of *duration* and *intensity* differences alone may be insufficient to trigger the effects of prosodic information on language learning. Moreover, prosody, even fully apprehended, contains relatively little information about phonetic or phonological structure, and even less information about an important range of grammatical facts to which a child must be exposed in order to acquire any spoken language. In addition to prosodic information, normal hearing children acquiring spoken language appear to have mastered most phonetic, phonologic, and grammatic information in their preschool years. At least some of this information may indeed become unlearnable beyond that point. In evaluating the effects of cochlear implantation, it would be well to keep in mind this larger perspective on the role of prosody and its relation to other aspects of language acquisition.

SUMMARY

Excluding children who are deaf and who have developmental problems in addition to their deafness, deaf children have normal language learning abilities. As with hearing children, however, the capacity for normal language acquisition is maturationally constrained. It is not merely advantageous to learn language early in life, it may be fully possible only at that time. If learning a spoken language is a goal, adequate and early exposure to spoken language is essential. It is possible that cochlear implantation in young children, who are profoundly deaf may enhance their chances of receiving some important aspects of spoken language input, thereby nurturing their potential for spoken langauge acquisition. Unfortunately, it is too soon to know. Only time and carefully controlled longitudinal studies will permit objective evaluations of the contribution of implants, both single- and multichannel, to the acquisition of language and the development of speech production in young children.

REFERENCES

Berliner, K. I., Eisenberg, L. S., & House, W. F. (Eds.) (1985). The cochlear implant: An auditory prosthesis for the profoundly deaf child. *Ear and Hearing, 6* (Suppl.), 1S–69S.

Bever, T., Fodor, J., & Weksel, W. (1965). Theoretical notes on the acquisition of syntax: A critique of "context generalization." *Psychological Review, 72,* 467–482.

Bilger, R., Black, F., Hopkinson, N., Myers, E., Payne, J., Stenson, N., Vega, A., & Wolf, R. (1977). Evaluation of subjects presently fitted with implanted auditory prostheses. *Annals of Otology, Rhinology and Laryngology, 86* (Suppl. 38), 92–140.

Bonvillian, J., Orlansky, M., & Novack, L. (1983). Early sign language acquisition and its relation to cognitive and motor development. In J. Kyle & B. Woll (Eds.), *Language in sign: An international perspective on sign language* (pp. 116–125). London: Croom Helm.

Caselli, M. C. (1983). Communication to language: Deaf children's and hearing children's development compared. *Sign Language Studies, 39,* 113–144.

Charrow, V., & Fletcher, J. (1974). English as the second language of deaf children. *Developmental Psychology, 10,* 463–-70.

Curtiss, S. (1977). *Genie: A psycholinguistic study of a modern-day "Wild-Child."* New York: Academic Press.

Curtiss, S. (1981). Dissociations between language and cognition. *Journal of Autism and Developmental Disorders, 11,* 15–30.

Curtiss, S. (1982). Developmental dissociations of language and cognition. In L. Obler & L. Menn (Eds.), *Exceptional language and linguistics* (pp. 285–312). New York: Academic Press.

Eisenberg, L., Berliner, K., Thielemeir, M., Kirk, K., & Tiber, N. (1983). Cochlear implants in children. *Ear and Hearing, 4,* 41–50.

Fischer, S. (1978). Sign language and creoles. In P. Siple (Ed.), *Understanding language through sign language research* (pp. 309–331). New York: Academic Press.

Gleitman, L., & Wanner, E. (1982). The state of the state of the art. In E. Wanner & L. Gleitman (Eds.), *Language acquisition: The state of the art* (pp. 3–48). New York: Cambridge University Press.

Hoffmeister, R. (1978). *The development of demonstrative pronouns, locatives and personal pronouns in the acquisition of American Sign Language by deaf children of deaf parents.* Unpublished doctoral dissertation, University of Minnesota, Minneapolis.

Hoffmeister, R., & Wilbur, R. (1980). Developmental: The acquisition of sign language. In H. Lane & F. Grosjean (Eds.), *Recent perspectives on American Sign Language* (pp. 61–78). Hillsdale, NJ: Erlbaum.

Jackson, C. (1984). *Language acquisition in two modalities: Person deixis and negation in American Sign Language and English.* Unpublished master's thesis, University of California, Los Angeles.

Kantor, R. (1982). Communicative interactions: Mother odification and child acquisition of American Sign Language. *Sign Language Studies, 36,* 233–282.

Kaplan, E., & Kaplan, G. (1970). The prelinguistic child. In J. Eliot (Ed.), *Human development and cognitive processes* (pp. 358–381). New York: Holt, Rinehart, and Winston.

Lehiste, I. (1973). Phonetic disambiguation of syntactic ambiguity. *Glossa, 7,* 107–122.

Lenneberg, E. (1967). *Biological foundations of language.* New York: Wiley.

Liben, L. (1978). The development of deaf children: An overview of issues. In L. Liben (Ed.), *Deaf children: Developmental perspectives* (pp. 3–20). New York: Academic Press.

Mayberry, R. (1984, November). *Early and late learning of sign language: Processing patterns.* Paper presented at the annual convention of the American Speech-Language-Hearing Association, San Francisco.

Mayberry, R., Fischer, S., & Hatfield, N. (1983). Sentence repetition in American Sign Language. In J. Kyle & B. Woll (Eds.), *Language in sign: An international perspective on sign language* (pp. 206–214). London: Croom Helm.

McKinney, V. (1983). *First language learning in deaf persons beyond the critical period.* Unpublished doctoral dissertation, Claremont Graduate School, Claremont, CA.

Meadow, K. (1966). *The effects of early manual communication and family climate on the deaf child's early development.* Unpublished doctoral dissertation, University of California, Berkeley.

Meadow, K. (1968). Early manual communication in relation to the deaf child's intellectual, social, and communicative functioning. *American Annals of the Deaf, 133,* 29–41.

Meier, R. (1981). *Icons and morphemes: Models of the acquisition of verb agreement in ASL.* (Papers and Reports on Child Language Development, No. 20, pp. 92–99). Stanford, CA: Stanford University.

Meier, R. (1982). *Icons, analogues, and morphemes: The acquisition of verb agreement in ASL.* Unpublished doctoral dissertation, University of California, San Diego.

Nakazima, S. (1962). A comparative study of the speech developments of Japanese and American English in childhood. *Studia Phonologica, 2,* 27–39.

Neville, H. (1977). Electroencephalographic testing of cerebral specialization in normal and congenitally deaf children: A preliminary report. In S. Segalowitz & F. Gruber (Eds.), *Language development and neurological theory* (pp. 121–131). New York: Academic Press.

Neville, H. (1984). Effects of early sensory and language experience on the development of the human brain. In J. Mehler & R. Fox (Eds.), *Neonate cognition: Beyond the blooming buzzing confusion* (pp. 349–363). Hillsdale, NJ: Erlbaum.

Neville, H., Schmidt, A., & Kutas, M. (1983). Altered visual-evoked potentials in congenitally deaf adults. *Brain Research, 266,* 127–132.

Newport, E. (1981). Constraints on structure: Evidence from American Sign Language and language learning. In W. A. Collins (Ed.), *Aspects of the develop-*

ment of competence. Minnesota Symposia on Child Psychology (Vol. 14, pp. 93–124). Hillsdale, NJ: Erlbaum.

Newport, E. (1982). Task specificity in language learning? Evidence from speech perception and American Sign Language. In E. Wanner & L. Gleitman (Eds.), *Language acquisition: The state of the art* (pp. 450–486). New York: Cambridge University Press.

Newport, E. (1984). *Constraints on learning: Studies in the acquisition of ASL.* (Papers and Reports on Child Language Development, No. 23, Keynote Address). Stanford, CA: Stanford University.

Newport, E., & Ashbrook, E. (1977). *The emergence of semantic relations in American Sign Language.* (Papers and Reports on Child Language Development, No. 13, pp. 16–21). Stanford, CA: Stanford University.

Newport, E., & Meier, R. (1985). Acquisition of American Sign Language. In D. Slobin (Ed.), *The cross-linguistic study of language acquisition* (pp. 881–938). Hillsdale, NJ: Erlbaum.

Pettito, L. (1983). *From gesture to symbol: The acquisition of personal pronouns in American Sign Language.* Unpublished qualifying paper, Harvard University, Cambridge, MA.

Prinz, P., & Prinz, E. (1979). Simultaneous acquisition of ASL and spoken English (in a hearing child of a deaf mother and hearing father). Phase 1: Early lexical development. *Sign Language Studies, 25,* 283–296.

Prinz, P., & Prinz, E. (1981). Acquisition of ASL and spoken English by a hearing child of a deaf mother and a hearing father. Phase II: Early combinatorial patterns. *Sign Language Studies, 30,* 78–88.

Quigley, S., & Frisina, R. (1961). *Institutionalization and psycho-educational development in deaf children.* Washington, D.C.: Council on Exceptional Children.

Schlesinger, H. (1978). The acquisition of signed and spoken language. In L. Liben (Ed.), *Deaf children: Developmental perspectives* (pp. 69–85). New York: Academic Press.

Schlesinger, H., & Meadow, K. (1972). *Sound and sign.* Berkeley: University of California Press.

Selkirk, E. (1983). *Phonology and syntax: The relation between sound and structure.* Cambridge, Massachusetts: MIT Press.

Shannon, R. V. (1983). Multichannel electrical stimulation of the auditory nerve in man. I. Basic psychophysics. *Hearing Research, 11,* 157–189.

Singleton, J., & Newport, E. (1987). *When learners surpass their models: The acquisition of American Sign Language from impoverished input.* Paper presented at the Society for Research in Child Development, Baltimore, MD.

Slobin, D. (1973). Cognitive prerequisites for the development of grammar. In C. Ferguson & D. Slobin (Eds.), *Studies of child language development* (pp. 175–208). New York: Cambridge University Press.

Slobin, D. (1982). Universal and particular in the acquisition of language. In E. Wanner & L. Gleitman (Eds.), *Language acquisition: The state of the art* (pp. 128–170). New York: Cambridge University Press.

Stevenson, E. (1964). A study of the educational achievement of deaf children of deaf parents. *California News, 80,* pp. 1–3.

Stokoe, W. (1960). *Sign language structure.* (Studies in Linguistics, Occasional Papers 8). Buffalo, New York: University of Buffalo Press.

Stokoe, W., Casterline, D., & Croneberg, C. (1965). *A dictionary of American Sign Language on linguistic principles.* Washington, D.C.: Gallaudet College Press.

Stuckless, R., & Birch, J. (1966). The influence of early manual communication on the linguistic development of deaf children. *American Annals of the Deaf, 111,* 452–460.

Supalla, T. (1982). *Structure and acquisition of verbs of motion and location in American Sign Language.* Unpublished doctoral dissertation. University of California, San Diego.

Thielemeir, M., Brimacombe, J., & Eisenberg, L. (1982). Audiological results with the cochlear implant. *Annals of Otology, Rhinology and Laryngology, 91* (Suppl. 91), 27–34.

Vernon, M., & Koh, S. (1970). Effects of early manual communication on achievement of deaf children. *American Annals of the Deaf, 115,* 527–536.

Wales, R., & Toner, H. (1979). Intonation and ambiguity. In W. Cooper & E. Walker (Eds.), *Sentence processing: Psycholinguistic studies presented to Merrill Garrett* (pp. 135–158). Hillsdale, NJ: Erlbaum.

Woodward, J. (1973). Inter-rule implication in American Sign Language. *Sign Language Studies, 3,* 47–56.

Young, R. (1981). *Sign language acquisition in a deaf adult: A test of the critical period hypothesis.* Unpublished doctoral dissertation, University of Georgia, Athens.

J. W I L L I A M E V A N S

THOUGHTS ON THE PSYCHOSOCIAL IMPLICATIONS OF COCHLEAR IMPLANTATION IN CHILDREN

The psychosocial implication of cochlear implantation in children is a very broad topic. This discussion will focus on a limited number of issues: (1) informed consent; (2) the preoperative assessment process; (3) the role of the mental health clinician in that process; (4) the successful psychological adaptation to cochlear implantation; and (5) problems that might be anticipated from the implant procedure.

INFORMED CONSENT

A significant ethical question is raised with regard to informed consent: who assumes responsibility when children are involved in investigational or experimental procedures? The general public is aware of this question through recent news coverage on cardiac transplantation in children. In the United States, children are to some degree the property of their parents. As such, they do not share equal rights in determining their involvement in elective cochlear implantation procedures. In an informal survey (Evans, unpublished raw data), prelingually deafened adults were asked whether they would choose to have an implant if it were possible that some hearing could be restored. The response was approximately 85 percent negative. The common explanation they offered was that the procedure would be destructive to their social relationships, to the world that they had come to know, and to their adaptive mechanisms. Accordingly, if these adults questioned the beneficial effect of cochlear implantation on their lives, the impact of this kind of surgical intervention in children must be examined carefully.

The primary factor in evaluating the child's involvement in the consent process is that of variable competence, a concept developed by Gaylin (1982). Variable competence includes a consideration of the child's age, intellect, emotional state, language ability, and so forth. A lack of consistency appears in the laws regarding the competence of children. In some states individuals are given adult status at 18 years of age whereas in others adulthood is conferred at age 21 (Guyer, Harrison, & Rieveschi, 1982). In certain situations children are granted adult rights before reaching legal age, but such rights are restricted and specific to a given circumstance. As a dramatic demonstration of legal inconsistency, a 12-year-old girl may legally have an abortion without the knowledge or consent of her parents, but she would be breaking the law if she were to miss school as a result of having that abortion.

The child's capacity to participate in the informed consent process must be assessed, especially with regard to the understanding of risk factors. Before approximately 7 years of age, a child lacks clarity regarding reality and fantasy. Older elementary school-aged children may provide greater input, but it will remain concrete. The development of formal operational thought involving the use of symbols and logic in problem solving does not usually develop until adolescence. The child's conceptual ability can be assessed through a clinical interview and psychological testing. Clearly, the child's capacity to participate actively in a decision regarding elective surgery increases with maturity.

THE ROLE OF THE MENTAL HEALTH CLINICIAN IN PREOPERATIVE ASSESSMENT

Although neither the Nucleus nor the 3M/House groups thoroughly explore the role of the mental health clinician in the implant process, both their children's programs report that preoperative psychological evaluations are required as part of their patient selection procedures (Mecklenburg, 1987; Tiber, 1985). The potential contributions of the psychological/psychiatric team are more fully appreciated in a discussion of the psychosocial issues surrounding the implantation of children conducted at a colloquium on implants in children (Downs et al., 1986). Mental health clinicians, primarily psychiatrists and psychologists, must participate in determining a child's candidacy for a cochlear implant by providing a cognitive evaluation, a linguistic evaluation, and an evaluation of the child's emotional status. Assessment involves interviews and formal test batteries. Specialized techniques, including graphic materials, dream interpretation and storytelling, and play therapy are integral tools in this clinical assessment. An understanding of the child's life experience is necessary in that children often have surprising perceptions of the world (Cohen, 1979). For example, some elementary school-age, deaf youngsters of hearing parents may have a good grasp of deafness and how it effects their lives, but when questioned closely they often reveal a belief that they will acquire hearing when they are adults without anything external happening to alter their sensory state. Obviously, they have never been exposed to adults who are deaf and have only known and observed hearing adults. Only careful clinical intervention can reveal the fantasies and expectations of children.

Sensitive mental health professionals must also provide support to the family as well as to the child undergoing the implant procedure. The outcome of surgery may not be what the child or the family anticipate, and, in addition, untoward effects can occur. The greater the preparation of the child and family in anticipation of the surgical procedure, the better the outcome (Tarnow & Gutstein, 1983). To the extent that children rehearse exactly what is going to happen and what to expect, they are more apt to accept the process and to master the necessary tasks involved.

Children frequently manufacture certain outcomes of surgical intervention of which adults may be totally unaware (Zamorski, Fischhoff, & Cuneo, 1969). For example, in Evans, an unpublished case study, a deaf child of 8, was interviewed at the time his mother was hospitalized for a hysterectomy. The youngster had a congenital absence of his left hand and seemed to have adapted fairly well to his disability. He had become quite upset about his mother's surgery, and it was initially assumed that he was anxious about her welfare. As the interview progressed, however, he revealed his expectations that his absent hand, which he surmised had lain dormant in his mother's body, would be recovered by the surgeon and restored to him. He was particularly concerned that no one had discussed the matter with him. Although not certain of the outcome, he hoped that the hand would be restored, and he suspected that people were planning it as a surprise for him. This child's fantasy, undetected by medical and other personnel, was only discovered after careful questioning and discussion. Because these kinds of fantasies could easily occur with any surgical intervention, an exploration of the child's expectations must be part of the preoperative assessment for cochlear implantation.

Psychological Adaptation to Cochlear Implantation

The general absence of reports on untoward psychological effects as a result of cochlear implantation is of concern. Surgical interventions frequently have either positive or negative psychological outcomes. In particular, surgeries that involve a change in body image, such as the treatment of severe obesity with gastrointestinal bypass (Castelnuovo–Tedesco & Schiebel, 1976) or the restoration of sight (Gregory & Wallace, 1963; Valvo, 1971; Von Senden, 1960), have a statistically significant incidence of psychologically distressing symptoms. There have been no reports of negative psychological difficulties in cochlear implantation, which is a curious phenomenon. Accordingly, clinicians should be alert to the potential for such symptoms as a result of cochlear implantation, especially in the adolescent phase of a child's life.

Essential among the factors that contribute to a successful implant procedure for children is a strong family support system, a requirement well recognized in the implant literature (Boothroyd, 1987; Downs et al., 1986; Nienhuys et al., 1987; Tiber, 1985). The family needs to be involved and well-informed regarding the possible outcomes for the child. Tiber (1985) has noted that in 10 percent of the House Ear Institute cases additional preoperative family counseling was needed, often because of misconceptions and unrealistic expectations regarding the benefits and limitations of the implant. Implant programs also recognize the essential role of the family in pursuing a successful post-implant rehabilitation course. An issue of equal importance, but seldom discussed in the literature, is that the family must remain supportive regardless of the postoperative result. The child who does not obtain significant benefit may experience guilt and assume he is responsible for responding poorly. Parents always wish to have the perfect child, and families of children who are disabled experience a grieving process in which they mourn the loss of the perfect family member (Chess, Fernandez, & Kern, 1980). With cochlear implantation, the desire to have the perfect child may be rekindled, and any outcome that is not ideal may result in a renewal of depression and grief. These feelings must be recognized, acknowledged and worked through; they are not to be avoided.

Another factor contributing to a successful postoperative conclusion is the absence or minimizing of stigmatizing equipment. In present implant devices, the external wearable processor and transmitter are obvious mechanical devices that in combination tend to be more conspicuous than hearing aids. The result may be strong feelings of difference and isolation, particularly among adolescents. The teen-aged population will tend to be a more difficult group among cochlear implant patients, because identity is crystallized during the adolescent years. This crystallization process involves a desire to conform and identify with peers. Stigmatizing equipment interferes with this process. The unique problems of adolescence have been acknowledged in the implant community (Downs et al., 1986), and difficulties occurring among those teenagers who have discontinued or restricted their use of the device have already been noted in some implant programs (Berliner & Eisenberg, 1985). These adolescents have been characterized (Berliner & Eisenberg, 1985) as being concerned with cosmetic issues or influenced by peer group pressures. Downs and colleagues (1986) state that, during the preoperative assessment, the motivations of prospective adolescent candidates must be evaluated independently from those of their parents.

Other factors related positively with postoperative outcome include intelligence, communicative capacity, and language capability. Language is utilized for mastery; it is a necessary prerequisite for discussion of disappointment and the resolution of frustration. The child who is capable of using language in order to indicate and describe the presence of untoward effects, whether emotional or sensory, for example, is certainly going to adjust better than the child who lacks such language facility.

Presumably, some children receiving implants will have been educated in oral programs, others in manual programs, and others in total communication programs. Total communication has certainly been helpful to deaf youngsters, and some studies indicate that the use of a simultaneous manual and oral approach optimizes language development (Greenberg, 1980). Cochlear implantation in children need not result in an alteration of whatever linguistic approach has been chosen by the family. Rather, the implant appears to supplement existing communication strategies; at the present time, it is not a substitution for one communication approach over another. Psychologically, the goal of language is to establish reciprocal relationships. That is, language initially allows for interactions with parents and, later, with others. Whatever mode of communication fosters reciprocal relationships should be encouraged. Parents of children receiving cochlear implants must still accept their children's hearing impairment, whether or not the implant is successful. They will still need to make the efforts and sacrifices that are necessary in order to establish the reciprocal interactive process. At present, cochlear implantation does not eliminate the parental responsibility to determine the linguistic mode most appropriate for the child. By definition, that determination must be based on the child's needs and not the family's wishes.

POTENTIAL PROBLEMS

Thoughts on two issues that potentially affect all professionals involved in implant work need to be introduced. First, as many clinicians are aware, the face of deafness is changing. More multiple-handicapped infants now survive their first few years of life. Because deafness is involved in many of these infants, there has been a concomitant increase in the population of deaf multiple-handicapped youngsters. A number of studies indicate that among children with multiple disabilities the incidence of psychiatric disorder increases dramatically as the number of handicapping conditions increases (Rutter, Tizard, & Whitmore, 1970; Werner, Bierman, & French, 1971). When these children become candidates for cochlear implants, the clinical presentation will become increasingly complex. It is essential that psychiatrists, psychologists, and other mental health clinicians be included not only in the assessment process, but also in followup evaluations. Communication with such children is, of course, determined by the level and mode of communication of the individual child. Professionals should possess the ability to use sign language, which is frequently the only available mode of communication. A less satisfactory alternative is the use of an interpreter.

Finally, it has been suggested (see Chapter 6) that current cochlear implants may result in the audiologic shift of the population of young children who are totally deaf to the level of aided profoundly or severely hearing-impaired. A large group of individuals who are hard-of-hearing may thus be created. These individuals may present as youngsters who can use speech, but who may be heavily dependent on lipreading and who may still use sign language. Although at first glance this population shift appears desirable, hard-of-hearing adolescents experience particularly noteworthy difficulties; they tend to be culturally homeless, belonging to neither the deaf nor to the hearing communities. The typical clinical and social picture is that of an individual who achieves moderate academic success, who may be intellectually bright, who has a fairly solid family relationship, but who is socially miserable. One example (Evans, unpublished case study) was a 16-year-old boy with profound hearing loss who was quite successful from his parents' perspective. He was a mainstreamed B student who participated on his hearing school's basketball team. Although his family was cohesive and he was successful in school, he was quite depressed. His depression stemmed from his feelings of isolation and the knowledge that there was no one else in school like him. He felt that the other students treated him with condescension and that he was included in group activities only because he was different and not because of any positive attributes. The possibility of creating a large group of children mirroring this adolescent exists with cochlear implantation.

As the implantation of children rapidly proceeds, the need for support services becomes mandatory. These services must include consultation and counseling with mental health clinicians who understand hearing impairment and have the capability of interacting in the appropriate linguistic mode. Present-day cochlear implants do not eliminate disability. Rather, they appear to change and modify the particular stress within a child's life. Strong attention to those stresses will be a continued need.

References

Berliner, K. I., & Eisenberg, L. S. (1985). Methods and issues in the cochlear implantation of children: An overview. *Ear and Hearing, 6* (Suppl.), 6S–13S.

Boothroyd, A. (1987). Management of profound sensorineural hearing loss in children: Possibilities and pitfalls of cochlear implants. *Annals of Otology, Rhinology and Laryngology, 96* (Suppl. 128), 84.

Castelnuovo–Tedesco, P., & Schiebel, D. (1976). Studies of superobesity: II Psychiatric appraisal of Jejuno-Ileal bypass surgery. *American Journal of Psychiatry, 133,* 26.

Chess, S., Fernandez, P., & Kern, S. (1980). The handicapped child and his family: Consonance and dissonance. *Journal of the American Academy of Child Psychiatry, 19,* 56–67.

Cohen, R. (1979). The clinical examination. In Call, J.D., Noshpitz, J. D., Cohen, R. L., & Berlin, I. N. (Eds.), *Basic handbook of child psychiatry: Vol. 1. Development* (pp. 505–508). New York: Basic Books, Inc.

Downs, M. P., Campos, C. T., Firemark, R., Martin, E., & Myres, W. (1986). Psychosocial issues surrounding children receiving cochlear implants. *Seminars in Hearing, 7,* 383–405.

Gaylin, W. (1982). The "competence" of children. *Journal of the American Academy of Child Psychiatry, 21,* 153–162.

Greenberg, M. (1980). Hearing families with deaf children: Stress and functioning as related to communication method. *American Annals of the Deaf, 125,* 1063–1071.

Gregory, R. L., & Wallace, J. G. (1963). *Recovery from early blindness, a case study* (Monograph No. 2). Cambridge, England: Experimental Psychology Society.

Guyer, M., Harrison, S., & Rieveschi, J. (1982). Developmental rights to privacy and independent decision making. *Journal of the American Academy of Child Psychology, 21,* 298–302.

Mecklenburg, D. J. (1987). The Nucleus children's program. *American Journal of Otology, 8,* 436–442.

Nienhuys, T. G., Musgrave, G. N., Busby, P. A., Blamey, P. J., Nott, P., Tong, Y. C., Dowell, R. C., Brown, L. F., & Clark, G. M. (1987). Educational assessment and management of children with multichannel cochlear implants. *Annals of Otology, Rhinology and Laryngology, 96* (Suppl. 128), 80–82.

Rutter, M., Tizard, J., & Whitmore, K. (1970). *Education, health and behavior: Psychological and medical study of childhood development.* New York: Wiley.

Tarnow, J., & Gutstein, S. (1983). Children's preparatory behavior for elective surgery. *Journal of the American Academy of Child Psychology, 22,* 365–369.

Tiber, N. (1985). A psychological evaluation of cochlear implants in children. *Ear and Hearing, 6* (Suppl.), 48S–51S.

Valvo, A. (1971). *Sight restoration after long-term blindness: The problems and behavior patterns of visual rehabilitation.* New York: American Foundation for the Blind.

Von Senden, M. (1960). *Space and sight: The perception of space and shape in congenitally blind patients, before and after operation.* London: Methuen.

Werner, E. E., Bierman, J. M., & French, F. E. (1971). *The children of Kauai.* Honolulu: University of Hawaii Press.

Zamorski, E., Fischhoff, J., & Cuneo, R. (1969). Body image and amputations: A psychological investigation of children. *American Journal of Orthpsychiatry, 39,* 254.

CHAPTER 16

DORCAS K. KESSLER
ELMER OWENS

CONCLUSIONS:
CURRENT CONSIDERATIONS
AND FUTURE DIRECTIONS

T he contributions in this volume reflect the controversies surrounding cochlear implantation in young children. Given the subject matter — the welfare of deaf children — controversies are not surprising. Indeed, the history of the care and education of young deaf children has been consistently characterized by debate and contention (see Rapin, 1986, for a brief review). Following early reports of the House Ear Institute implants in children, several of the problems associated with the implantation of children were identified by Simmons (1985); many of these problems remain unresolved at the present time. In the following discussion, the pertinent issues related to cochlear implantation in young children are considered in light of current knowledge and only with respect to children who are deaf and who are not multihandicapped. Unless otherwise indicated, references to contributors relate directly to their offerings in this book.

CURRENT CONSIDERATIONS: ISSUES AND QUESTIONS

EARLY ASSESSMENT

Probably least controversial is the paramount importance of delineating at as early an age as possible the nature and extent of residual hearing in a child with suspected hearing impairment (Fria & Shallop,

Chapter 5; Wilson, Chapter 4). Auditory Brainstem Response (ABR) can serve as an early indicator and provide useful estimates of loss within the first few months of life. It is generally agreed, however, that such results must be corroborated by behavioral responses. Electrophysiological testing evaluates a different function than does behavioral testing and both must be used in conjunction with one another. Given appropriate facilities and equipment in combination with skilled practitioners, Wilson states that behavioral pure-tone thresholds for children with hearing loss should be attainable by the age of 6- to 12-months. He also points to successful testing of speech discrimination, binaural fusion, and masking effects in very young children.

As techniques become more sophisticated, behavioral audiometric results will possibly be obtainable earlier than 6 months of age. Skilled audiologists using appropriate equipment are basic requirements; all facilities interested in implantation and working with young children who are deaf must verify that their clinicians have received the most advanced training and have had experience in evaluating an infant population. Otologic, pediatric, psychologic and neurologic examinations, as well as parental interviews, should be part of the evaluative procedure.

EARLY STIMULATION AND CRITICAL PERIODS

Once a hearing loss is suspected, there is good agreement on the need for auditory stimulation as early as possible. Structures ordinarily devoted to central processing of auditory input may atrophy or fail to develop in the absence of peripheral stimulation (Shannon, Chapter 2), and areas of auditory cortex may be usurped by other modalities (Curtiss, Chapter 14). Conversely, electrical stimulation of the auditory system at an early age may prevent atrophy (Loeb, Chapter 8). It is generally acknowledged that there are critical periods for the development of auditory processing and the acquisition of language and speech (Curtiss; Jackler & Bates, Chapter 9; Loeb; Shannon).

As defined by Curtiss, a critical period is a point in time during which sensory experience and environment exert a major influence on the development and organization of neural systems. The concept of a critical period is a complex one however. Ruben (1986) reports that various models for critical periods exist and range along a continuum. For example, one model suggests that there is a single time period during which a stimulus has an effect; another model asserts that the stimulus is always effective, but there is a period of time during which it has its maximum effect. Both animal (Shannon) and human (Curtiss) studies indicate that there may be varying critical periods for specific components of a single general function (e.g., auditory localization in animals and language in humans). Although critical periods for audition have been less well studied than those for visual perception, mounting evidence from animal studies suggests that the central auditory pathways will fail to develop normally if there is a lack of auditory stimulation (Eggermont & Bock, 1986; Ruben & Rapin, 1980; Stark et al., 1986).

Wilson notes that in a normal hearing child it cannot be assumed that there is a free period of time during which auditory learning is not taking place. Several of the contributors (Loeb; Shannon; Tallal, Chapter 13) stress the necessity for an intact central auditory processing system as well as a functioning peripheral system for normal language and speech development. It seems that those postlingually deafened adults who have successfully achieved speech recognition with an implant (Owens, Chapter 3) are able to use the impoverished signal they receive because they can make closure with an intact central auditory and language base (Loeb; Shannon). They have a complete and mature reference system against which to compare the signals provided by the implant; this process of comparison and closure probably involves the use of what has been commonly referred to as an "auditory memory for speech." Although the reporting is scanty, indications of relatively minimal benefit, if any, from the auditory stimulation supplied by an implant among congenitally deaf adults (Owens) suggests additional evidence of the need for an intact auditory processing system. Presumably, these adults who were prelingually deaf possessed neither the processing skills to utilize the implant signal nor the neural plasticity required to learn to use these signals. Stark and associates (1986) state that neural plasticity in the human decreases as a function of age, probably beginning at about 4 years of age and gradually reaching a plateau after puberty. They note both clinical and behavioral evidence indicating that the earlier sensory stimulation begins, the more effective it will be. The concept of a critical period or "window of time" in which neural plasticity is greatest pervades and influences all considerations of implantation in young children.

DEGREE OF LOSS AND DIAGNOSTIC TRAINING

On the assumption that early language and speech stimulation is necessary for all children, it follows that consensus exists on the need to determine within the deaf child's very first years the kind of sensory device and educational program that will best provide such stimulation. This determination must consider information from all the evaluative personnel including parents and teachers. The hearing parents of young deaf children are typically confronted with a host of difficult and emotionally laden questions focusing on whether the best approach to the child's development is to be found in an aural/oral, total communication, or manual educational program. Evans (Chapter 15) points out that the family's decisions regarding linguistic mode and educational methods must first consider the needs of the child over and above the desires of the family. Cochlear implantation, controversial in itself, unfortunately steps into the very center of these long-standing issues on educational methods and deaf life style. Viewed as simply another form of amplification for purposes of auditory stimulation, cochlear implantation in children should entail a strong and ongoing commitment to auditory/verbal training and the belief that even limited audition is ultimately beneficial.

Although the audiogram, per se, is limited as a predictor of progress in language and speech acquistion, a consideration of children who are deaf must include the degree of hearing loss as an index of potential implant candidacy. Considerable advances have been made in defining distinctions within the larger category of profound hearing impairment that are predictive of the potential for speech perception and production (Boothroyd, Chapter 6; Geers & Moog, Chapter 11; Osberger, Chapter 12). The usefulness of a hearing aid (Boothroyd) or a tactile aid (Roeser, Chapter 7) must be thoroughly explored in this context. Emphasis is placed on the functional benefits of any sensory aid, and the child's ability to perceive speech with the device and make use of residual hearing must be carefully evaluated (Boothroyd et al., 1986; Geers & Moog). To fully explore these distinctions and the possible benefits of non-invasive aids, a substantial period of diagnostic teaching is required (Boothroyd et al., 1986; Roeser).

Boothroyd classifies children with losses ranging from 91 to 110 dB HL as likely to benefit from a hearing aid and by habilitative methods emphasizing acoustic stimulation. Such children have access to the intonation patterns of speech and to some frequency dependent contrasts, including vowel place, voicing, continuance, and talker sex. Both Boothroyd and Osberger suggest that for the majority of children with losses greater than 110 dB HL, the 3M/House cochlear implant can offer information similar to that provided by hearing aids in profoundly deaf children with losses in the 100 to 110 dB range, or similar to the subcategory of profoundly deaf "with a little residual hearing." However, in considering recent information on a small number of 3M/House children with acquired hearing loss who have achieved some open-set phoneme recognition, Boothroyd estimates that approximately 10 percent of the children implanted with the 3M/House device will have access to information similar to that found in the severely hearing impaired with losses ranging from 60 to 90 dB HL. Based on adult findings with the Nucleus multi-electrode implant, Boothroyd estimates that children implanted with this device will have a 50 percent chance of attaining information available to those in the severely hearing impaired category.

LANGUAGE AND SPEECH ACQUISITION

Prelingually deaf children with losses greater than 110 dB HL, for whom a hearing aid is of questionable benefit and who may thus be potential implant candidates, should probably be enrolled in a *total communication* program emphasizing language acquisition and including tactile stimulation in addition to acoustic amplification. The probability of a critical period for language acquisition, whether spoken or signed, suggests the need for the immediate introduction of signing, assuming that "there is an advantage to knowing any language over knowing no language during the preschool years" (Curtiss). This would, of course, require special and intensive counseling and orientation of parents regarding the desirability of their learning to sign and thereby opening an immediate avenue of communication with the child. The aim would be to provide the child with concepts of language and communication as early as possible on the assumption that a language base can facilitate and enhance the value of any subsequent habilitative efforts, including an implant.

Numerous studies have demonstrated that the acquisition and use of sign language in no way impedes, and may enhance, the development of other language skills, including speech production, lipreading, reading, and writing (Curtiss; Rapin, 1979). In a recent investigation comparing the deaf children of deaf parents (i.e., native signers) with the deaf children of hearing parents (Geers & Schick, 1988), it was found that at ages 5 and 6, the two groups were comparable in their expressive English language ability. By age 7, however, the deaf of deaf demonstrated significant advantages in both their spoken and signed English.

Boothroyd is strongly critical of the lack of focus on auditory/verbal training in most educational programs for the deaf. Geers and Moog also note that total communication programs fail to provide strong aural/oral training. However, it should be recalled that the ideal total communication program places equal emphasis on all aspects of communication; enrollment in a total program should in no way preclude auditory/verbal stimulation and exposure to sign language would not be expected to inhibit the development of auditory/verbal skills.

Assuming the validity of a critical period, the issue of the earliest age at which implant surgery can be undertaken relates to how long an implant can be delayed without the loss of potential for language and speech acquisition through auditory stimulation. Because exact knowledge on this point is lacking, and because there is no assurance that language and speech can be acquired through audition after age 2 or 3 years with little or no previous experience of sound, it seems imperative that children who are prelingually deaf be provided as early as possible with the tools to acquire a language system. Through exposure to a *total communication* approach, valuable time critical for language development will not have been lost if auditory stimulation with an implant should be unproductive of speech. Moreover, sign will have been introduced when the organism is most receptive to the acquisition of a language. At the same time, the acquisition of a language base by this means should increase the likelihood of learning spoken language through audition if an implant is applied at a later date.

MEDICAL, SURGICAL, AND BIOENGINNERING CONSIDERATIONS

Given the present state of technology and knowledge, the age of 2 or 3 years seems to be the earliest time for implantation for those children showing little evidence of speech acquisition despite extensive use of amplification or tactile stimulation. Ideally, potential candidates should have been carefully evaluated and received extensive diagnostic training by that age. Jackler and Bates indicate that concerns about such factors as the effects of head growth on the implant are substantially reduced after age 2.

A number of issues related to the development of an appropriate pediatric cochlear implant continue to require attention. A device fully capable of accommodating head growth and of precluding the medial spread of middle ear infection has yet to be developed (Jackler & Bates; Loeb). Methods and techniques for faithfully revealing the status of cochlear patency (Jackler & Bates) and mapping the location and magnitude of auditory neural elements (Loeb; Owens & Kessler, Chapter 1) remain to be found. Concern has been expressed by Loeb and by Jackler and Bates about the durability and stability of devices. Published accounts of the 3M/House implant do not permit accurate calculations of the total number of surgical revisions required because of internal device failures or biological and medical problems (Kessler, Chapter 10; Loeb), and the reliability of this relatively uncomplicated device remains unknown. Although depicted as technically simple, the revision procedure is, in fact, a surgical one, requiring a general anesthetic, and hospitalization. It must be assumed that any surgical procedure has an emotional impact on the young child (Evans). Although revisions of the 3M/House implant have been successfully accomplished and all such undertakings have reportedly resulted in functioning devices, it is essential that clinicians do not lose sight of the psychological welfare of the child and the seriousness of any surgical procedure.

At the present time, the implantation of children must be done with the knowledge that technological advances in the development of implants will, at some future point, render the device being implanted obsolete; reimplantations seem inevitable (Jackler & Bates; Loeb). Given the possibility of additional reimplantations because of mechanical weaknesses and because neither short- nor long-term (over the period of a lifetime) durability can be guaranteed, careful consideration must be given to the type of device being implanted.

TYPE OF IMPLANT

Loeb offers several points in favor of an extracochlear, single-channel device that conceivably might provide a more enhanced range of auditory information than the 3M/House implant while retaining the viability of the scala tympani for improved devices of the future. He further suggests the possibility that, given the greater plasticity of an immature nervous system, the young deaf child compared with an adult may be better equipped to organize and develop the distorted stimulation provided by implants into a "new representation of linguistic sounds." In turn, this implies that the acoustic information or speech features that might be essential for the development of a linguistic and phonologic system cannot be known. Speech processing for the young deaf child, Loeb states, should probably remain simple and should concentrate on providing as full a signal as possible rather than attempting to extract specific features on the basis of normal adult speech perception. With the exception of patients implanted in Austria, results for adults using single-channel extracochlear systems have thus far indicated limited improvement in hearing, similar to that of the 3M/House device. However, a recent study done in Austria by Tyler (in press), employing German speech materials, has supported the Vienna group's reports of open-set speech recognition in their patients with single-channel implants, weighing in favor of Lobe's suggestions (see Owens).

Although recognizing both the need for a device capable of readily allowing replacement of the electrode without damage to the cochlea and the lack of an "ideal" intracochlear multichannel implant, Jackler and Bates favor the use of multichannel devices for young children. They believe that simpler single channel devices, either intra- or extracochlear, may potentially inhibit auditory development. Jackler (personal communication, December 1987) cites evidence from animal models (Clopton & Winfield, 1976) indicating that early exposure to simple or distorted auditory stimuli may restrict the ability of the developing central auditory system to respond to more complex stimuli. Thus, he disagrees with those investigators who advocate the early placement of a simple single-channel unit with a view to subsequent implantation of more complex intracochlear systems after some period of growth has occurred. Because of the apparent perceptual modeling during the critical period, the initial use of simple devices that provide only minimal information may render the eventual use of sophisticated devices, capable of delivering richer stimuli that is more faithful to the speech signal, less fruitful due to restrictions in central auditory responsiveness.

Based on adult implant performance, Boothroyd and Owens also support the use of multichannel implants in young children. Reports of open-set speech understanding with multichannel implants in adults (Owens) and preliminary data on the rapid progress provided by the Nucleus device in children (Kessler) suggest that the potential for speech and language acquisition is greater with a multichannel system. However, as multichannel implants become more complex, offering options in speech coding strategies and the number of stimulating channels, the issue of device adjustment for the best sound quality becomes a major consideration (Loeb). Obviously, this process is more complicated than with single channel units and more complex with prelingual loss children, who are unable to provide feedback and who may never have experienced sound. Initially, the application of this process in children will require trained personnel to extrapolate from adult experiences to children. Settings can be made on the basis of close behavioral observations, much as with hearing aids that are selected and adjusted for young children who are deaf. The objective measures of EABR (Fria & Shallop) and stapedial reflex testing (Jerger, Oliver & Chmiel, 1988) may become increasingly useful in device setting. Potentially, the mapping of cochlear neural elements may provide a guide for establishing channels of stimulation and appropriate processing schemes.

Not all adults achieve open-set speech understanding with multichannel implants, and methods of preoperatively estimating or predicting postoperative benefit are needed. The most common explanation for the wide range of results among adults is the status of the surviving cochlear neurons. An electrophysiological approach has been attempted in the effort to determine the location and magnitude of surviving neurons and psychophysical investigations are being undertaken to determine the potential for central auditory processing required for speech perception (Owens & Kessler; Shannon; Tallal). For the young child who is deaf, Tallal suggests that temporal processing might be evaluated through other modalities, such as vision.

Early evidence indicates that children receiving multichannel implants will, like adults, demonstrate a wide range of results (see Kessler). Those children failing to attain open-set understanding appear to receive information similar to that commonly received with a single-channel implant. Presumably, then, those children without nerve tissue adequate to accommodate multichannel stimulation might still obtain any advantages of single-channel stimulation using a multichannel system (Boothroyd; Kessler; Owens). How children use any implant, however, depends much upon their learning ability, upon the state of their peripheral and central auditory systems, and upon the training and education they receive.

Emotional and Psychological Considerations and Counseling

Psychologic/psychiatric evaluation and counseling for both parents and children are mandatory before and after the implant. In addition to an opportunity to explore their fears, anger, guilt, and frustration (Evans), parents need to become fully aware of their options and they require some guidance in arriving at realistic expectations of what an implant can and cannot do. In their own terms, they must accept and acknowledge that, with the 3M/House device, only a very small minority of children are able to achieve recognition of a few phonemes, words, or simple sentence materials and that these children all had acquired deafness as a result of meningitis (Boothroyd; Geers & Moog; Kessler). In contrast, the great majority of children with this implant are limited to an awareness of gross sounds and an appreciation of the intonation and rhythm of speech (Kessler).

Given this limited range of results, parents must question how such stimulation might alter and affect their child's life, specifically the long-range prospects for acquiring academic, social, and vocational/occupational skills. The evidence is still unclear, even after several years of concentrated observation, regarding the acquisiton of intelligible, spontaneous speech by those children who may have previously never heard sound or who had only minimal exposure to sound. There is some argument regarding the potential for speech acquisition when auditory perception is limited to intonation of speech patterns and to some first formant information. On the one hand, Boothroyd and Osberger suggest that access to this level of speech perception provides a chance, given appropriate training, for the development of speech skills, and Osberger has documented various signs of improvement. For example, she describes one of four children implanted with the 3M/House device who achieved almost normal speech intelligibility. Unfortunately, data permitting comparisons of pre- and postimplant intelligiblity are lacking for this child. On the other hand, the investigations of Geers and Moog indicate that, in order to achieve speech intellibility, the level of auditory perception must exceed that of speech pattern perception. Moreover, while acknowledging its position as one of the earliest acquired speech perception skills, Curtiss questions the contribution of prosodic perception to the development of a language system.

In regard to the Nucleus multichannel implant, many of the same cautions and considerations are applicable in counseling parents and children, perhaps with a bit more optimism. Parents must be informed that only preliminary data are available and that expectations are primarily based on adult postlingual performance. Very litte information exists on the progress of pre- or perilingually deaf children with the Nucleus device. While adult performance both with the Nucleus and other multichannel devices suggests that access to second formant and spectral information may afford auditory speech understanding, parents must become fully aware that the range of results with all these devices is wide and apparently dependent on numerous factors that are presently unmeasurable. Presumably, children would also be subject to such variation, and parents must understand that the achievement of speech understanding and spoken language with the implant cannot yet be predicted with any accuracy.

Data on the development of speech production skills and the speech intelligibility of children implanted with the Nucleus device are almost nonexistent at this time, although Osberger has provided preliminary data on one subject indicating rapid improvement in production skills at 6 months postimplant. Osberger points out that perception and production do not have a simple one-to-one relationship and that one cannot be inferred from the other. It is generally acknowledged, however, that deficits in auditory processing and speech perception will effect speech production (Sloan, 1986; Tallal). It might then be assumed that the richer and fuller the auditory signal, such as that provided by a multichannel system, the greater will be the chance of acquiring intelligible speech.

AGE AT ONSET OF DEAFNESS

PRELINGUALLY DEAF CHILDREN OF HEARING PARENTS. The age at onset of deafness cannot be ignored in considering implantation in young children. The foregoing discussion was largely concerned with children who are prelingually deaf. As information on implants in children accumulates, it appears that distinctions between subjects who are prelingually deaf might be made on the basis of whether their losses were acquired or congenital. Those children falling in the category of *perilingual* — those whose losses were acquired after early infancy, but prior to the development of language and speech — seem to have some residual auditory processing system that permits them to attain better implant performance, as demonstrated by the most successful 3M/House children (Boothroyd; Geers & Moog; Kessler). It should also be noted that most of these children were implanted in the preschool years and that length of auditory deprivation may have an impact on any residual auditory processing system. A number of factors have been suggested as predictive of implant success in children (Kessler), and both later age-of-onset and shorter duration of deafness have been identified as possible correlates of better performance. For the most part, the overwhelming majority of children with early, prelingual acquired loss have had meningitis.

In none of the reports to date, from either 3M/House or Nucleus, have congenitally deaf children been identified as among the "better performers". This suggests, again, the presence of a critical period for the acquisition of auditory processing skills and speech perception. According to Ruben (1986), most evidence points to a critical period for speech perception that probably ranges from birth to the 12th through 18th postnatal month. To the extent that this proves to be a valid estimate, and given that implants are presently not contemplated before 2 years of age, the outlook for congenitally deaf children appears to be rather discouraging. Clearly, the earlier that stimulation can be provided for these children, the better their chances of making progress with an implant.

POSTLINGUALLY DEAF CHILDREN OF HEARING PARENTS. Meningitis has been by far the leading cause of postlingual losses in children. If the onset occurs before the age of 5 or 6 years, the child's speech may be rendered unintelligible or lost completely after a period of time (Osberger). There are also suggestions that even though hearing might be lost at age 4 or 5, the child may function as prelingually deaf and cannot properly be labeled as postlingual (Kessler). Nevertheless, as with children who are prelingually deaf, careful evaluation, including a thorough trial with a hearing aid or a tactile device, is mandatory before an implant. It is still not known whether the 3M/House device can be routinely relied upon, even with special training, to maintain the intelligible spontaneous speech of a child under 6 years of age given the limitations of the auditory information it provides. Data on the maintenance of speech intelligibility in children with the Nucleus device are also unavailable. Certainly, the child's intelligence and motivation, the training program in which she or he is enrolled, and the quality and quantity of parental support are all crucial factors.

Among those postlingually deafened children over age 6 or 7 years, psychological factors play an especially significant role, particularly with teenagers. As Evans states, the extreme sensitivity and concern with self-concept, self-image, and peer approval demands that older children participate actively in the decision whether or not to obtain a cochlear implant. For example, they must be informed of any possible untoward effects of surgery and they must be apprised of the appearance and cosmetic aspects of the wearable device. The motivations, feelings, and fantasies of the older child may remain unverbalized and hidden (Evans). Counseling with the prospective implant candidate, as well as with the family, should be a standard part of the patient selection process and the followup protocol.

DEAF CHILDREN OF DEAF PARENTS. The extent to which deaf children of deaf parents have become candidates for the cochlear implant is not known, but, presumably, there have been relatively few. A position paper, "Cochlear Implant Surgery", prepared by the Ad Hoc Committee on Ear Surgery of The Greater Los Angeles Council on Deafness (GLAD) (1985), took issue with assumptions implicit in the publicity surrounding the value of the 3M/House device to a deaf child and appears to reflect the attitude of many manual deaf adults. The authors protest what they perceive as widespread misinformation on the implant procedure and its benefits; they question whether the benefits exceed the costs; and, they decry claims that an implant results in significant enhancement in quality of life and improved educational achievement. In general, they are concerned that publications promote impressions that the lives of the deaf are fraught with fear and disaster and that their cultural existences are trivial or suspended in time until medicine can intervene. The Committee strongly emphasizes the contrary: that the deaf minority in the United States forms a viable language and cultural group although it is devoid of sound. The National Deaf Children's Society of England (NDCS) has raised similar objections to the introduction of cochlear implants for deaf children in England (1984).

A timely review by Sacks (1986), based on publications by Lane (1984) and Groce (1985), adds a valuable perspective on deafness, particularly with respect to signing. Sacks reiterates that American Sign Language (ASL) is a bonafide language with complete syntax and grammar (see also Curtiss); that language must be introduced and acquired as early in life as possible lest its development be permanently retarded (see Rapin, 1979, for an extensive review of acquired cognitive disorders associated with severe language delay resulting from deafness); and that for deaf children the only certain way of ensuring the acquisition of language is by its introduction through signing. The review concludes on an optimistic note in referring to Groce's account of a commmunity where the prevalence of deafness resulted in sign language becoming, in effect, the common language, integrating the deaf with normal hearers who also signed. That is, the deaf were not isolated or stigmatized in any way, because their deafness was not perceived as a handicap, and daily communication and interchange were in no way inhibited.

Although cochlear implants are not mentioned in Sacks' review, the reader is alerted to yet another option for children who are deaf, namely, no implant at all. Such an alternative does not necessarily involve the abandonment of auditory and speech training through conventional amplification or tactile stimulation, but it must be accompanied by a greater acceptance of deafness, the use of sign language, and the deaf community.

Whereas the GLAD paper states that "some individuals may choose to have such a tool [the implant], and others will not," Evans notes that young children, in fact, have no choice; their parents make the choice. Accordingly, the familiar informed consent process assumes a different meaning than that for adult implant patients, creating an unusual ethical and moral dilemma. It is also the parents of young deaf children who, with appropriate guidance, decide upon the educational program for their children. Consequently, parents must be provided with the tools to make an intelligent and free choice. As the GLAD report suggests, this demands the collection and dissemination of accurate information about implant prostheses to those who are deaf as well as to the hearing parents of deaf children so that all parents may have the materials for a reasoned choice.

Parents must be provided with a more complete understanding of language acquisition as distinct from speech production, of deafness in general, and of deaf culture. Those adults who are deaf in the United States and who communicate primarily through sign, although largely isolated from the hearing, have acquired the socialization and vocational skills necessary to create and support a viable culture (Rapin, 1979). Deaf children who are initially taught aurally/orally, and who eventually enter a total or manual program, frequently express relief and gratitude that they are among peers with whom they can freely communicate in a common language (Norris, 1975). Hearing parents who have a child who is deaf must be exposed to all of these facts as early in the life of their child as possible. House (1986) has recognized that young deaf children, particularly those in their early teens, have developed an identity with the deaf culture and are reluctant to alter their self-image. He notes that the hearing parents of such children are seldom aware of the turmoil and conflict that the prospect of an implant might create in these children. All those working in the area of implantation must be particularly sensitive to prelingually deaf adolescents who have become part of the deaf culture, and who do not choose to alter their status.

FUTURE DIRECTIONS

In selecting an implant for a young child, one primary consideration should apply: the child should be provided with the device offering the greatest possible auditory information. Given this imperative, the widespread implantation of multichannel systems in children is apparently forthcoming, and the design and fabrication of sophisticated systems more suitable for children is clearly one major direction in the future of implants. In considering the application of multichannel systems to children, the adjustment of the device poses a greater challenge than for single-channel implants. However, it is precisely the number and flexibility of adjustment options that may permit the achievement of the optimal sound for each patient. Mechanical difficulties and the possibility of surgical complications would still be important factors to consider. The necessity of continuous long-term rehabilitative training, special educational placement, and counseling would still apply.

A tremendous need exists for continued research on all aspects of the cochlear implant. The predictability and location of viable auditory neural tissue, safety factors, accommodation for head growth, the prevention of infection, the stability and reliability of devices, and the delineation of the most promising speech processing techniques continue to be major concerns. Particularly pertinent are studies on critical periods in auditory development and on the long-term effects of early stimulation with "distorted" signals. Almost everything known about the development of speech and language argues for early stimulation; on the other hand, the current state of the development of implants, of the assessment of infants, of the need for a period of diagnostic teaching, and of surgical considerations seem to preclude implantation before 2 or 3 years of age. Thus, a time conflict is perhaps the most significant problem to confront implant investigators and clinicians. Although seldom explicitly offered, the data that can be gleaned from implant literature suggest that children with congenital loss, even when implanted in the preschool years, have less opportunity than those with prelingual acquired loss to develop comparable levels of speech perception and speech production.

A sharp reduction in the rate of implantation with the 3M/House implant commensurate with carefully planned followup studies on controlled groups would seem appropriate. Concomitantly, a thorough followup on the adult recipients of this device would be most helpful for a comprehensive picture of implant results thus far. This research would be greatly enhanced in its objectivity were it done by those not involved in the selection and habilitation of the children and adults being studied. By the same token, objective, independent studies of both children and adults implanted with the Nucleus device are also needed. Most importantly, a comparative, longitudinal investigation of single-channel (both 3M/House and Vienna) and multichannel implants in children, with groups matched as closely as possible, would provide a basis for an intelligent choice.

Loeb's preference for continued study of extracochlear, single-channel devices with respect to their application in children, including research for a better sound signal, suggests another important avenue of investigation. Because the ability to explant a single electrode and reimplant a multielectrode array has been explored in only a few instances, it is not yet definitely known whether the scala tympani of a child will remain intact and receptive to multichannel implantation following the insertion and explantation of a single-channel electrode. There is also a need for continued study of alternative signal processing schemes with intracochlear single-channel systems. At the same time, highly promising and exciting results, primarily the documentation of speech understanding (and steady improvement in this understanding over time) with several easily wearable multichannel implants, compels research on multichannel stimulation. The multichannel results for adults and the auspicious preliminary data on children with the Nucleus device cast serious doubt on the wisdom of continuing to apply single-channel devices if they provide only prosodic cues for the majority of children.

Cochlear implants are receiving increasing acceptance among clinicians as a major tool in the rehabilitation of the deaf. They cannot be regarded as a passing fad, and continued attention to their development and further refinement seems certain. With little doubt, they have proven beneficial for adults. Growing evidence suggests that they will also be beneficial in the rehabilitation of children. In closing, it is urged that the cochlear implant not be viewed as a panacea, but as one more contribution to the continued efforts to reduce and ultimately remove the barriers facing young deaf children.

REFERENCES

Boothroyd, A., Balkany, T. J., Geers, A., Hayes, D., McFarland, W., Miyamoto, R. T., Novak, M., & Shallop, J. K. (1986). Issues of pre- and postimplant evaluation regarding cochlear implants in children. *Seminars in Hearing, 7,* 349–359.

Clopton, B. M., & Winfield, J. A. (1976). Effect of early exposure to patterned sound on unit activity in rat inferior colliculus. *Journal of Neurophysiology, 39,* 1081–1089.

Eggermont, J. J., & Bock, G. R. (Eds.) (1986). Critical periods in auditory development. *Acta Otolaryngologica, Suppl. 429,* 5–64.

Geers, A. E., & Schick, B. (1988) Acquisition of spoken and signed English by hearing-impaired children of hearing-impaired or hearing parents. *Journal of Speech and Hearing Disorders, 53,* 136–143.

Greater Los Angeles Council on Deafness, Ad Hoc Committee on Ear Surgery. (1985, April). *Position paper: Cochlear implant surgery.* Los Angeles, CA: Author.

Groce, N. E. (1985). *Everyone here spoke sign language: Heriditary deafness on Martha's Vineyard.* Cambridge: Harvard University Press.

House, W. F. (1986). Opposition to the cochlear implant in deaf children [Editoral]. *American Journal of Otology, 7.*

Jerger, J., Oliver, T. A., & Chmiel, R. A. (1988). Prediction of dynamic range from stapedius reflex in cochlear implant patients. *Ear and Hearing, 9,* 4–8.

Lane, H. (1984). *When the mind hears: A history of the deaf.* New York: Random House.

National Deaf Children's Society. (1984, October). *Cochlear implants* (NDCS Information Sheet). London: Author.

Norris, C. (Ed.). (1975). *Letters from deaf students.* Eureka, CA: Alinda Press.

Rapin, I. (1979). Effects of early blindness and deafness on cognition. In R. Katzman (Ed.), Congenital and acquired cognitive disorders. *Research Publications: Association for Research in Nervous and Mental Disease, 57,* 189–245.

Rapin, I. (1986). Helping deaf children acquire language: Lessons from the past. *International Journal of Pediatric Otorhinolaryngology, 11,* 213–223.

Ruben, R. J. (1986). Unsolved issues around critical periods with emphasis on clinical application. *Acta Otolaryngologica, Suppl. 429,* 61–64.

Ruben, R. J., & Rapin, I. (1980). Plasticity of the developing auditory system. *Annals of Otology, Rhinology and Laryngology, 89,* 303–311.

Sacks, O. (1986, March 27). Mysteries of the deaf. *The New York Review of Books, 33,* 23–27, 30–33.

Simmons, F. B. (1985). Cochlear implants in young children: Some dilemmas. *Ear and Hearing, 6,* 61–63.

Sloan, C. (1986). *Treating auditory processing difficulties in children.* San Diego, CA: College-Hill Press.

Stark, R. E., Bowman, C. A., Busse, L., Hasenstab, S., House, J. L., & Oller, D. K. (1986). Developmental aspects influencing implantation and rehabilitation of children. *Seminars in Hearing, 7,* 371–382.

Tyler, R. S. (in press). Word recognition with some of the better 3M/Vienna cochlear-implant patients. *Archives of Otolaryngology.*

I N D E X

AUTHOR

Abberton, E., 31, 141
Agelfors, E., 28
Aird, D., 142, 170
Albrektsson, T., 5
Alencewicz, C. M., 193, 233
Alford, B. R., 160
Allsman, C. S., 194, 195
Alpiner, J. C., 43
Andersen, R. A., 287
Andersson, H., 158
Ardell, L. A., 113, 115
Ardito, J. M., 169
Ashbrook, E., 294
Aslin, R., 139

Baccaro, P., 56
Balkany, T. J., 7, 168, 318
Ball, J. B., 172
Ball, V., 11
Banfai, P., 5, 36, 174, 183
Banfai, S., 36
Barker, M. J., 33
Basseres, F., 162

Bates, G. J., 171
Becker, T. S., 169, 191
Beighton, P., 154, 155, 163, 164
Beiter, A. L., 33, 46, 48, 210–214
Belal, A., 160
Bell, B. A., 204, 205
Bell, D. W., 40
Bender, L., 201
Benton, A. L., 287
Berg, K. M., 61
Bergstrom, L., 157, 159
Berkowitz, R., 142, 170
Berliner, K. I., 8, 26, 81, 90, 92, 142,
        183, 186–192, 194–197, 203–205,
        217, 246, 254, 300, 311
Bess, F., 84, 95
Bever, T., 300
Bierman, J. M., 312
Bilger, R. C., 90, 300
Binnie, C. A., 257, 259, 260, 264
Binzer, S. M., 8
Birch, J., 295
Black, F., 300
Black, F. O., 9, 209

I N D E X

SUBJECT

Key: (*A*) indicates Appendix, (*f*) indicated figure, (*t*) indicates table.

Notes

Notes

Notes

Notes

Notes

Notes